Standards and Guidelines for the Psychotherapies

At a time when the psychotherapies were being challenged on many fronts, the Ontario Psychiatric Association in conjunction with the Ontario Medical Association, Section on Psychiatry, commissioned the task force led by Dr Paul Cameron and Dr John Deadman to prepare a definitive statement about the practice of psychotherapies. The outcome of the task force's work has been truly remarkable and has received international attention. The Ontario Psychiatric Association was committed to the dissemination of the definition, guidelines, and standards of the psychotherapies so as to reaffirm the central role of psychotherapies in the care of people with mental health problems. Our association is pleased to endorse and celebrate the completion of this book based on the work of Dr Cameron and colleagues.

DR PAUL LINKS
President, Ontario Psychiatric Assoc'-''

Standards and Guidelines for the Psychotherapies

Edited by

PAUL CAMERON

JON ENNIS

JOHN DEADMAN

UNIVERSITY OF TORONTO PRESS
Toronto Buffalo London

© University of Toronto Press Incorporated 1998
Toronto Buffalo London
Printed in Canada

ISBN 0-8020-0804-6 (cloth)
ISBN 0-8020-7166-X (paper)

Printed on acid-free paper

Canadian Cataloguing in Publication Data

Main entry under title:

Standards and guidelines for the psychotherapies

Includes bibliographical references and index.
ISBN 0-8020-0804-6 (bound)   ISBN 0-8020-7166-X (pbk.)

1. Psychotherapy – Standards – Ontario.   2. Psychotherapy – Practice –
Ontario.   I. Cameron, Paul (Paul M.).   II. Ennis, Jon.   III. Deadman, John.

RC480.5.S72 1998   616.89'14   C98-930585-6

Standards and guidelines described in this book are not intended to serve
as rigid prescriptions for the treatment of all patients. The final decision
concerning the treatment plan for an individual case depends upon the
collaboration between the patient and the treating professional. The treatment
plan for a patient must be arrived at after assessing all the clinical data
available, considering options in view of the psychiatric literature, and the
availability of such options in particular clinical settings.

University of Toronto Press acknowledges the support of the Canada Council
and the Ontario Arts Council for our publishing program.

The editors dedicate this book to their families:

To Barbara, Alison, Jonathan, and Robert,
and to my parents, Robert and Phyllis Cameron

To Janice, Joshua, Miriam, and Naomi,
and to my parents, Julius and Lillian Ennis

To Fran

Contents

Acknowledgments

This book evolved from the work of a task force formed in 1992 to delineate current standards for the practice of psychotherapy, including definitions, knowledge base, training, and other critical issues. The task force was formed by the Council of the Ontario Psychiatric Association (OPA) with the endorsement of the Section on Psychiatry of the Ontario Medical Association (OMA).

This book has been produced primarily through the volunteer work of the task force members and its consultants. The original impetus for the creation of the task force came from John Deadman, who served as chair from 1992 until 1994, when Paul Cameron assumed the duties of chair. Members of the task force were Leopoldo Chagoya, Patrick Conlon, Norman Doidge, Jon Ennis, Ray Freebury, Judith Hamilton, Paul Hoaken, Molyn Leszcz, Rebeka Moscarello, Carolyn Rideout, Richard Swinson, and Martha Wright.

We are indebted to a number of psychiatrists and other consultants with special knowledge in various aspects of psychotherapy who provided peer review and consultation throughout the development of the original task force report and this volume. These were Federico Allodi, Harry Anderson, Jacques Barber, Joan Bishop, Linda Bohnen, Howard Book, Susan Bradley, Jack Brandes, Robert Cardish, Charlotte Chagoya, Ron Charach, Paul Dagg, Arthur Fish, Doug Frayn, Judith Gold, Harvey Golombek, Howard Gorman, Paul Harris, Samuel Izenberg, Ruth Kajander, Art Lesser, Fred Lowy, Roy MacKenzie, Donna Malcolm, Roy Muir, Michael Myers, Clare Pain, Emmanuel Persad, Naomi Rae-Grant, Morton Rapp, Gail Robinson, Gary Rodin, Joel Sadavoy, Mary Seeman,

Paul Steinhauer, Donna Stewart, Ted Waring, Daniel Traub-Werner, and Greg Truant.

The editors would like to acknowledge the support of successive presidents of the Ontario Psychiatric Association (OPA): Dr Pierre Beauséjour, Dr John Deadman, Dr Sam Malcolmson, Dr Joan Bishop, Dr Edward Rzadki, Dr Lucien Faucher, and Dr Paul Links. We also received the support of the chairs of the Section of Psychotherapy of the OPA: Dr Richard Gorman, Dr Martha Wright, Dr Carolyn Rideout, and Dr Sherry Zener; and the chairs of the Section on Psychiatry of the Ontario Medical Association (OMA): Dr Ruth Kajander, Dr Patrick Conlon, and Dr Ray Freebury. We appreciate the financial support of the Section of Psychotherapy of the OPA through the chair, Dr Sherry Zener, and from the Council of the OPA through the president, Dr Joan Bishop. We would also like to acknowledge the administrative and secretarial assistance throughout the project from Helen Killingbeck, the previous executive director of the OPA.

Lynn Marie Flynn, secretary to Dr Cameron, provided excellent coordination and administrative assistance throughout the project. Janice Karlinsky thoughtfully read most of the chapters. Madeline Koch of Wordcraft Services provided valuable support in the production both of the original report and of this volume. The contribution of June Engel, who edited the original report, has been invaluable for the completion of the project. Finally we would like to thank our editors at the University of Toronto Press, Margaret Williams, Anne Forte, and Virgil Duff, who have supported this book from the beginning.

List of Contributors

Martin M. Antony, PhD, CPsych
Associate Professor of Psychiatry
McMaster University

Chief Psychologist and Director,
Centre for the Study of Anxiety
St Joseph's Hospital
Hamilton, Ontario

Morton Beiser, MD, FRCP(C)
David Crombie Professor of Cultural
  Pluralism and Health
Program Head, Culture, Community
  and Health Studies
Clarke Institute of Psychiatry, and
  Department of Psychiatry, Univer-
  sity of Toronto

Director, Centre of Excellence for
  Research on Immigration and
  Settlement
Health Canada National Health
  Scientist
Toronto, Ontario

Howard Book, MD, FRCP(C)
Associate Professor of Psychiatry

Associate Professor of Health Administration
University of Toronto

Coordinator, Brief Psychotherapy
  Resident Training
Director, Post Graduate Brief Psycho-
  therapy Training Program
Clarke Institute of Psychiatry
Toronto, Ontario

Paul M. Cameron, MD, MSc,
  FRCP(C), Co-editor
Professor of Psychiatry
Director of Psychotherapy Training
Department of Psychiatry
University of Ottawa

Director of Psychotherapy Research
  and Teaching Clinic
Ottawa General Hospital
Ottawa, Ontario

Leopoldo Chagoya, MD, FRCP(C)
Associate Professor of Psychiatry
University of Toronto

Head, Couple/Family Therapy
  Clinic
Mount Sinai Hospital
Toronto, Ontario

Patrick Conlon, MD, FRCP(C)
Associate Professor of Psychiatry and
  Family Practice
University of Western Ontario

Consultant Psychiatrist
Alexandra Marine and General
  Hospital

Private Practice
Goderich, Ontario

Simon Davidson, MB, BCh, FRCP(C)
Associate Professor of Psychiatry and
  Paediatrics
University of Ottawa

Chief of Staff and Chief of Psychiatry
Children's Hospital of Eastern
  Ontario
Ottawa, Ontario

John C. Deadman, MD, FRCP(C),
  Co-editor
Associate Professor of Psychiatry
McMaster University

Community Schizophrenia Service
First Place
Hamilton, Ontario

Norman Doidge, MD, FRCP(C)
Assistant Professor of Psychiatry
University of Toronto

Head, Psychotherapy Centre
Clarke Institute of Psychiatry
Toronto, Ontario

Faculty, Center for Psychoanalytic
  Training and Research
Columbia University
New York, New York

Jon Ennis, MD, FRCP(C), Co-editor
Assistant Professor of Psychiatry
University of Toronto

Associate Staff Psychiatrist
The Toronto Hospital
Toronto, Ontario

Arthur Fish, Barrister and Solicitor,
  LLB, BCL, SJD
Chair, Ontario Mental Health
  Foundation
Adjunct Faculty, Department of
  Psychiatry, University of Toronto
Adjunct Faculty, Faculty of Law,
  University of Toronto
Toronto, Ontario

D. Ray Freebury, MBBCh, D(Obst)
  RCOG, FRCP(C)
Associate Professor of Psychiatry
University of Toronto

Staff Psychiatrist, Psychotherapy
  Centre
Clarke Institute of Psychiatry
Director, Toronto Institute of Psycho-
  analysis
Toronto, Ontario

Hazen M. Gandy, MD, FRCP(C)
Assistant Professor of Psychiatry
University of Ottawa

Medical Director, Mental Health
  Patient Service Unit

Children's Hospital of Eastern
Ontario
Ottawa, Ontario

Barry L. Gilbert, MD, FRCP(C)
Staff Psychiatrist, Mood and Anxiety
Division
Clarke Institute of Psychiatry

Psychotherapy Supervisor
The Toronto Hospital
Lecturer in Psychiatry
University of Toronto

Private Practice
Toronto, Ontario

Harvey Golombek, MD, FRCP(C)
Professor of Psychiatry
University of Toronto
Director of Psychotherapy Training,
St. Michael's and Wellesley
Hospitals
Toronto, Ontario

Judith Hamilton, MD, FRCP(C)
Lecturer in Psychiatry
University of Toronto
Chair, Section on Psychiatry
Ontario Medical Association
Toronto, Ontario

Paul C.S. Hoaken, BA, MD, FRCP(C),
DABPN
Professor Emeritus
Department of Psychiatry
Queen's University

Attending Staff
Kingston General Hospital, Hôtel-
Dieu Hospital, and Kingston
Psychiatric Hospital
Kingston, Ontario

Mary Johnston, MD, FRCP(C)
Assistant Professor of Psychiatry
University of Ottawa
Director, Partial Hospitalization
Program
Program Director, Postgraduate
Education
Department of Psychiatry
Ottawa General Hospital
Ottawa, Ontario

Sidney H. Kennedy, MD, FRCP(C)
Professor of Psychiatry
Head, Mood Disorders Program
University of Toronto

Head, Mood and Anxiety Division
Clarke Institute of Psychiatry
Toronto, Ontario

Marshall Korenblum, MD, FRCP(C),
Dip. Child Psych.
Associate Professor of Psychiatry
Director of Postgraduate Education,
Division of Child Psychiatry
University of Toronto

Director, Adolescent Clinical
Investigation Unit
The Hincks Centre for Children's
Mental Health

Consultant, Division of Youth
Psychiatry,
Sunnybrook Health Science Centre
Toronto, Ontario

Molyn Leszcz, MD, FRCP(C)
Associate Professor of Psychiatry
Head, Psychotherapy Program
Department of Psychiatry
University of Toronto

Deputy Psychiatrist-in-Chief
Mount Sinai Hospital
Toronto, Ontario

David M. Magder, MD, CM,
  FRCP(C)
Assistant Professor of Psychiatry
University of Toronto

Staff Psychiatrist, Mood and Anxiety
  Division
Clarke Institute of Psychiatry

Private Practice
Toronto, Ontario

Rebeka Moscarello, MD, FRCP(C)
Assistant Professor of Psychiatry
University of Toronto

Medical Director, Psychiatric/Mental
  Health Out-Patient Clinics
Department of Psychiatry
Women's College Hospital
Toronto, Ontario

Michael F. Myers, MD, FRCP(C)
Clinical Professor of Psychiatry
University of British Columbia

Director of the Marital Discord Clinic
Department of Psychiatry
St Paul's Hospital
Vancouver, B.C.

Carolyn Rideout, MD, FRCP(C)
Consultant Psychiatrist
Mississauga General Hospital

Private Practice
Mississauga, Ontario

Ronald Ruskin, MD, FRCP(C), Dip.
  Psych.
Assistant Professor of Psychiatry
University of Toronto

Staff Psychiatrist
Department of Psychiatry
Mount Sinai Hospital

Senior Research Associate
Trinity College
University of Toronto
Toronto, Ontario

Zindel V. Segal, PhD, CPsych
Associate Professor of Psychiatry and
  Psychology
Head, Psychotherapy Research
Department of Psychiatry
University of Toronto

Head, Cognitive Behaviour Therapy
  Unit
Clarke Institute of Psychiatry
Toronto, Ontario

Michel Silberfeld, MD, MSc,
  FRCP(C)
Assistant Professor of Psychiatry
Member, Joint Centre for Bioethics
University of Toronto

Coordinator, Competency Clinic
Department of Psychiatry
Baycrest Centre for Geriatric Care
Toronto, Ontario

Richard P. Swinson, MD, FRCP(C)
Professor and Chair
Department of Psychiatry
Faculty of Health Sciences

McMaster University
Hamilton, Ontario

Martha Wright, MD, FRCP(C)
Lecturer in Psychiatry
University of Toronto
Private Practice (Psychotherapy and
  Psychoanalysis)
Toronto, Ontario

Ari Zaretsky, MD, Dip. Psych.,
  FRCP(C)
Assistant Professor of Psychiatry
University of Toronto

Head, Cognitive Behaviour Therapy
  Clinic
Mount Sinai Hospital
Toronto, Ontario

Introduction:
Development of the Guidelines

Paul Cameron, Jon Ennis, and John Deadman

The need for a document which outlines how psychotherapy is and should be practised in the 1990s and into the next century emerged in response to four major phenomena – namely:

1 the realization that there were no written guidelines or standards for the practice of medical psychotherapy;
2 the changing forces that now influence health policy and funding, both in the United States and in Canada;
3 the potential for arbitrary de-insurance of some psychiatric procedures in the absence of agreed-upon standards, and without regard for the evidence showing the effectiveness of those procedures;
4 growing concern regarding the problem of sexual abuse of patients by physicians.

Medical psychotherapy, like psychiatry, has origins that date back to the beginnings of human society. However, its modern scientific forms evolved largely within the last hundred years. Hypnotherapy was first practised early in the nineteenth century, but cognitive and behavioural therapies, as well as contemporary forms of psychodynamic psychotherapy, are products of this century.

Medical psychotherapy has undergone intense scrutiny in the past twenty years. More recently, boundary violations within psychotherapy have increasingly become a concern (Epstein, 1994; Gabbard & Lester, 1995). In Ontario this issue led the College of Physicians and Surgeons of Ontario (CPSO), the provincial licensing and regulating body, to establish the Task Force on Sexual Abuse of Patients (McPhedran, 1991). Its report took the position that psychotherapy posed 'special problems [in terms of] the exploitation and abuse of patients.' It emphasized that psychotherapy requires a high level of skill and training, and made several recommendations to redress deficiencies in this area.

The lack of professionally developed and sanctioned guidelines and standards of practice for psychotherapy has hampered the work of professional disciplinary bodies. In Ontario, effective peer review by the CPSO was limited, leading to anomalous situations in complaint and discipline processes. It was at this juncture that the Ontario Psychiatric Association (OPA) undertook the task of developing standards for psychotherapy and, in 1992, established the Joint Task Force on Standards for Medical (Psychiatric) Psychotherapy.

Mandate of the Task Force

The original mandate of the Joint Task Force on Standards for Medical (Psychiatric) Psychotherapy was to develop a document outlining the current acceptable standards of practice for psychotherapy to be used as a reference in the complaints and disciplinary processes of the CPSO. As the task force developed, the need to provide practising physicians, especially psychiatrists, with a comprehensive overview of the art and science of psychotherapy, and with a set of practice guidelines, became apparent.

In its report (Joint Task Force, 1995), the task force attempted to develop practice guidelines rather than standards of medical care. 'Standards of care' are defined by Battista (1993) as 'authoritative statements of: (a) minimum levels of acceptable performance or results, (b) excellent levels of performance or results, or (c) the range of acceptable performance or results' (p. 385). The American Psychiatric Association (APA) (1994b) states: 'Standards of medical care are determined on the basis of all clinical data available for an individual case and are subject to change as scientific knowledge and technology advance and patterns evolve' (p. iv).

The task force interpreted its mandate as restricted to developing and refining definitions, standards, and guidelines for the practice of psychotherapy, the training of medical psychotherapists, the suitability of candidates for practice, and the maintaining of competence. The report included suggestions for sensitizing practitioners to gender and cultural issues that affect psychotherapy outcomes.

It is necessary to distinguish the guidelines set out in the report from regulations made by state-sanctioned regulatory bodies. In Ontario, the CPSO, under the Medicine Act, is the key body responsible for implementing the Regulated Health Professions Act. At times the report considered practices that are clearly proscribed, such as sexual involvement with patients. More often it examined the processes involved in determining the optimal use of the full range of psychotherapeutic actions. The CPSO has established an Education Committee that is using this report, among other documents, in the process of developing more specific standards for the practice of psychotherapy in the province.

Development of the Guidelines

This volume is a revised and expanded version of the 1995 report of the Joint Task Force. Each of the original chapters has been updated, and new chapters have been added that discuss: brief psychotherapy; supportive psychotherapy; psychotherapy with children and adolescents; combining psychotherapy with pharmacotherapy; psychotherapy with patients suffering from severe and persistent mental illness; psychotherapy supervision; cultural issues; and consent issues.

In establishing these guidelines, the contributors recognize that psychotherapy, which has an extensive empirical and research basis, is not only a science, but also an art. Further, while the contributors acknowledge that multiple approaches to similar problems are often valid, they do not endorse a *'laissez-faire'* approach. Where possible, general principles have been developed, from which actions in specific circumstances can be determined.

Defining and establishing guidelines for the psychotherapies has proved to be a complex and daunting task. The majority of attempts at guideline development have focused on defined clinical conditions. For instance, the American Psychiatric Association is currently developing a series of practice guidelines for *DSM-IV* (APA, 1994a) disorders such as eating disorders (APA, 1993a), major depressive disorder in adults (APA, 1993b), bipolar disorder (APA, 1994b), and substance abuse disorders (APA, 1995). Also, the Quality Assurance Project of the Royal Australian and New Zealand College of Psychiatrists has developed treatment outlines for a variety of Axis I and Axis II disorders (The Quality Assurance Project, 1982, 1983, 1991a, 1991b; Andrews, Hadzi-Pavlovic, Christensen, & Mattick, 1987).

Rather than focusing on any particular diagnostic or clinical group or condition, members of the Joint Task Force and the other contributors to this volume have been concerned with defining and maintaining standards for a group of therapeutic modalities, the psychotherapies. Thus it was essential to first arrive at a definition of psychotherapy that is compatible with current standards of medical practice (chapter 1). General guidelines were developed that were common to all forms of psychotherapy across a broad range of patient groups (chapter 2). Specific guidelines for the various modalities of psychotherapy were prepared, including individual psychodynamic psychotherapy (chapters 3 and 4), cognitive/behavioural psychotherapies (chapter 5), brief psychotherapy (chapter 6), couple and family psychotherapy (chapter 7), group psychotherapy (chapter 8), and supportive psychotherapy (chapter 9). Separate chapters were provided on: guidelines for psychotherapy with children and adolescents (chapter 10), guidelines for combining psychotherapy with pharmacotherapy (chapter 11), and guidelines for psychotherapy with patients suffering from severe and persistent mental illness (chapter 12). In developing standards and guidelines for psychotherapy, it is essential that consideration also be given to training (chapter 13) and supervision (chapters 14 and 15). The four final chapters relate to issues considered crucial to the practice of psychotherapy: gender (chapter 16), culture (chapter 17, consent (chapter 18), and record keeping (chapter 19).

The editors and contributors are in agreement with Gray (1996), who argued that practice guidelines for psychotherapy cannot be established solely through outcome-based parameters:

> Although outcome-based parameters have the advantage of their research foundation, they also have its disadvantages. One is a reliance on statistical studies with problematic methodology. Another is that the present funding environment may have influenced researchers to neglect inquiry into the effect of definitive care over the lifetime of an individual. A third is that because few specific interventions have been studied, practice parameters based on outcome studies are incomplete, and psychiatrists therefore encounter obstacles when they try to implement them in daily practice. (p. 226)

The Quality Assurance Project (1982, 1983, 1991a, 1991b, Andrews et al, 1987) combined literature review, the opinions of practising psychiatrists, and the experience of nominated experts to develop treatment outlines for a variety of psychiatric conditions. Andrews et al (1987) emphasized the importance of having consensus procedures for developing guidelines for treatment until the research literature provides more adequate guidance.

We have tried to review and incorporate the outcome-based evidence as much as possible in the development of these guidelines. But we have also used a consensus-based approach. Thus the development of the chapters in this volume has combined literature review with consultation and peer review involving a wide variety of clinicians with expertise in the various modalities.

Unlike the American Psychiatric Association practice guidelines (APA, 1993a, 1993b, 1994b, 1995) and the Australian and New Zealand Quality Assurance Project treatment outlines (1982, 1983, 1991a, 1991b; Andrews et al, 1987), which are organized by psychiatric disorder, the guidelines in this volume are organized by psychotherapeutic modality. This focus reflects the reality that clinicians tend to specialize in the practice of one or two modalities since each modality requires extensive training and experience, but that clinicians should have sufficient knowledge of and experience in all modalities in order to refer patients for appropriate therapies. All psychiatrists should know how to assess a couple or a family and should be proficient in the concurrent use of pharmacotherapy with psychotherapy (see chapter 13, 'Standards and Guidelines for Psychotherapy Training'). Further, many disorders or problems may be responsive to a variety of therapeutic approaches. Therefore, these guidelines focus on applying each therapy appropriately, effectively, and ethically.

The board of directors of the Canadian Medical Association (CMA) has approved and published *Guidelines for Canadian Clinical Practice Guidelines* (1994). These fourteen guidelines fall into three categories: philosophy and ethics, methods, and implementation and evaluation. Although the Joint Task Force adhered to these guidelines in principle, they did not include the final stage in the process recommended for the creation of guidelines. Specifically, there has been no consultation with non-psychiatric physician groups, patients, and other health care providers. With the publication and distribution of this volume, the task force hopes to elicit a response from these stakeholders. Future editions of this work will be enriched by their contribution. Additionally, field trials of these guidelines could lead to further refinements.

Quality Assurance and Peer Review

This volume is intended to be of value in the process of quality assurance, that is, the determination of whether services adhere to minimal standards of appropriate care. Although professional associations agree that standards of professional care should not ignore the economic realities (Cahn & Rickman, 1985; El-Guebaly, 1988), third-party payers have become increasingly concerned with cost containment. In the United States, this has resulted in a shift from retrospective peer review to managed care (Mattson 1984; Beatson & Lancaster, 1993). Beatson, Rushford, Halasz, Lancaster, and Prager (1996) point out that, when the review process was taken away from the medical profession in the United States, the result was breaches of patient confidentiality and loss of professional autonomy. Drawing on the work of El-Guebaly (1988), Beatson and Lancaster (1993) advocate that peer review include the following components: 'an educational focus; review by or including true peers; attention to customary practice rather than normative standards; and the profession having full input into the planning of the peer review and receiving regular feedback concerning the results of review procedures ... *[and]* ... preservation of confidentiality' (p. 317). They emphasize that, in psychotherapy, supervision has been the traditional method of peer review. In a subsequent publication, Beatson et al (1996) report the positive results of a survey of participants in a voluntary program of group peer review.

The Role of Psychiatry

Psychiatry is a medical specialty that is grounded in biological knowledge about human nature. North American psychiatrists generally endorse a 'biopsychosocial model' that recognizes the interplay of biological, psychological, and social factors in the development of psychiatric disorders and in their treatment.

The Joint Task Force strongly endorsed the need to continue to support medical (psychiatric) psychotherapy within the health care system. Psychiatrists have a broad knowledge base and a systematic approach to diagnosis, prognosis, and treatment planning. Psychiatrists receive detailed education in the complex interaction among mind, brain, and body, and therefore are aware of the way that medical disorders, developmental and physical changes, and bodily states influence the mind, and how the mind influences the body. Throughout their training, psychiatrists learn to carry the ultimate clinical responsibility for the management of very ill patients. Psychiatrists have experience with a wide range of mental illnesses, from the minor to the most severe. Psychiatrists can use biological treatments, such as electroconvulsive therapy and pharmacological agents. The literature demonstrates that combined use of medications and psychotherapy is frequently the most appropriate and effective treatment for a number of disorders in many individual patients.

Psychiatrists have a special role within the field of medicine as the interpreters of social and psychological phenomena for their colleagues and their patients. Psychiatry is the only specialty that can act as a specific reference point for the practice of medical psychotherapy.

Although these guidelines have been developed specifically for the practice of psychiatry, the authors do not endorse the position that psychotherapy falls exclusively within the domain of psychiatry. Other medical and non-medical practitioners continue to play important roles in both the practice and the development of psychotherapy.

Licensing bodies, discipline bodies, and other health care providers may find these guidelines and standards helpful in developing their own protocols. The authors definitely expect that, in the future, more accountability and standards will be involved in the practice of the psychotherapies. Informed consent will be a more detailed procedure than has been the common practice up to this time. Also, continuing education and demonstration of competence will likely become mandatory. Ongoing clinical supervision with experts or through peer groups is to be recommended and will likely become the standard of practice.

We anticipate that future editions of this volume will reflect trends in the field of psychotherapy research. Treatment selection will become more refined. The study of cost-effectiveness of the therapies is still rather rudimentary but will become increasingly important. Psychotherapy with three special populations is relatively neglected in this volume: the elderly, the developmentally delayed, and the economically disadvantaged. We hope that the issues related to psychotherapy with these particular populations can be addressed in future editions.

References

American Psychiatric Association (APA). (1993a). Practice guidelines for eating disorders. *American Journal of Psychiatry, 150,* 207–228.

American Psychiatric Association (APA). (1993b). Practice guideline for major depressive disorder in adults. *American Journal of Psychiatry, 150* (Suppl., 4), 1–26.

American Psychiatric Association (APA). (1994a). *Diagnostic and statistical manual of mental disorders* (4th ed.). Washington, DC: Author.

American Psychiatric Association (APA). (1994b). Practice guideline for the treatment of patients with bipolar disorder. *American Journal of Psychiatry, 151* (Suppl., 12), 1–36.

American Psychiatric Association (APA). (1995). Practice guideline for the treatment of patients with substance use disorders: Alcohol, cocaine, opioids. *American Journal of Psychiatry, 152* (Suppl., 11), 1–59.

Andrews, G., Hadzi-Pavlovic, D., Christensen, H., & Mattick, R. (1987). Views of practicing psychiatrists on the treatment of anxiety and somatoform disorders. *American Journal of Psychiatry, 144*, 1331–1334.

Battista, R.N., & Hodge, M.J. (1993). Clinical practice guidelines between science and art. *Canadian Medical Association Journal, 148*, 385–398.

Beatson, J.A., & Lancaster, J.E. (1993). Peer review of psychotherapeutic treatments in psychiatry: A review of the literature. *Australian and New Zealand Journal of Psychiatry, 27*, 311–318.

Beatson, J., Rushford, N., Halasz, G., Lancaster, J., & Prager, S. (1996). Group peer review: A questionnaire-based survey. *Australian and New Zealand Journal of Psychiatry, 30*, 643–652.

Cahn, C., & Richman, A. (1985). Quality assurance in psychiatry: Position of the Canadian Psychiatric Association. *Canadian Journal of Psychiatry, 30*, 148–152.

Canadian Medical Association (CMA). (1994). *Guidelines for Canadian clinical practice guidelines*. Ottawa: Author.

El-Guebaly, N. (1988). Peer review: Empirical data base and practical implications. *Canadian Journal of Psychiatry, 33*, 645–649.

Epstein, R.S. (1994). *Keeping boundaries: Maintaining safety and integrity in the psychotherapeutic process*. Washington, DC: American Psychiatric Press.

Gabbard, G.O., & Lester, E.P. (1995). *Boundaries and boundary violations in psychoanalysis*. New York: Basic.

Gray, S.H. (1996). Developing practice guidelines for psychoanalysis. *Journal of Psychotherapy Practice and Research, 5*, 213–227.

Joint Task Force on Standards for Medical (Psychiatric) Psychotherapy. (1995). *A report to Council of the Ontario Psychiatric Association and to Executive of the Section on Psychiatry, Ontario Medical Association, on the definition, guidelines and standards for medical (psychiatric) psychotherapy*. Toronto: Author.

Mattson, M.R. (1984). Quality assurance: A literature review of a changing field. *Hospital and Community Psychiatry, 35*, 605–616.

McPhedran, M. (Chairperson). (1991, 25 November). *The final report: Task Force on Sexual Abuse of Patients*. An independent task force commissioned by the College of Physicians and Surgeons of Ontario.

The Quality Assurance Project. (1982). A method for preparing 'ideal' treatment outlines in psychiatry. *Australian and New Zealand Journal of Psychiatry, 16,* 153–158.

The Quality Assurance Project. (1983). A treatment outline for depressive disorders. *Australian and New Zealand Journal of Psychiatry, 17,* 129–146.

The Quality Assurance Project. (1991a). Treatment outlines for avoidant, dependent and passive–aggressive personality disorders. *Australian and New Zealand Journal of Psychiatry, 25,* 404–411.

Standards and Guidelines for the Psychotherapies

1. The Definition of Psychotherapy

Jon Ennis

In order to establish standards for the practice of psychotherapy, it is essential first to define 'psychotherapy.' Several issues must be addressed in formulating the definition. Should there be one definition that encompasses all psychotherapies practised by physicians, or should each specific form of psychotherapy be defined separately? Is there a distinction between medical psychotherapy and psychotherapy practised by non-medical therapists? How can the numerous forms of psychotherapy be classified? Can a definition be employed to differentiate psychotherapy from other forms of medical interventions that may not involve the same ethical constraints?

One Definition or Many

Only one of the current editions of the three major American textbooks of psychiatry offers a general definition of psychotherapy. That definition, in the *American Psychiatric Press Textbook of Psychiatry,* is rather vague: 'Psychotherapy, "The Talking Cure," is the generic term for a large number of treatment techniques whose primary means of affecting change is through verbal interchange. Psychotherapy is directed toward changing behavior through the reorganization of mental structures. In the process of this reorganization, both perception and behavior will change' (Ursano & Silberman, 1988, p. 855).

The *Comprehensive Textbook of Psychiatry* (Kaplan & Sadock, 1995) and *Psychiatry* (Michels, 1995) define psychotherapies individually, according to the various major schools. While it is advantageous to arrive at a definition of psychotherapy that encompasses all legitimate forms currently practised, such a definition has certain drawbacks. It may be too vague to establish overall standards. For instance, a technique or practice that might be acceptable for one form of therapy may not be appropriate for another form of therapy. Furthermore, as new forms of therapy are developed, it would be necessary for therapists to justify their procedures, just as manufacturers of new drugs must test them before they are approved. In this instance, the disadvantage of a comprehensive definition is that it may prove too restrictive and inhibit developments in the field. As well, if there is just one definition and set of standards, then only new therapies with techniques that fall outside the limits of these guidelines would require some form of approval.

Medical Psychotherapy

Is there anything that distinguishes medical psychotherapy from non-medical psychotherapy?

In his classic comparative study of psychotherapy, Frank (1974) defines psychotherapy as characterized by three common features:

1. a trained, socially sanctioned healer, whose healing powers are accepted by the sufferer and by his social group or an important segment of it
2. a sufferer who seeks relief from the healer
3. a circumscribed, more or less structured series of contacts between the healer and the sufferer, through which the healer, often with the aid of a group, tries to produce certain changes in the sufferer's emotional state, attitudes, and behavior. All concerned believe these changes will help him. Although physical and chemical adjuncts may be used, the healing influence is primarily exercised by words, acts, and rituals in which sufferer, healer, and – if there is one – group, participate jointly. (pp. 32–3)

Frank states that these features are common not only to all forms of psychotherapy, but also to methods of primitive healing, religious conversion, and brainwashing.

Although psychotherapy may be practised by a variety of 'healers' and shares common features with primitive and religious practices, it is specifically a medical term. The *Oxford English Dictionary* defines psychotherapy as 'the treatment of disease by "psychic" methods.' It notes that the term was first used in the late nineteenth century to denote medical treatment, initially hypnosis. Walter Cooper Dendy first introduced the term 'psychotherapeia' in 1853. He defined it as prevention and remedy (of disease) by psychical influence and predicted that it would become valuable in psychiatry (Colpe, 1995).

Medical psychotherapy has two distinguishing features. The 'healer' is a physician, and the 'sufferer' is seeking relief from a recognized medical disorder. In other words, the therapist assesses the patient according to a standard medical diagnostic system.

Is psychotherapy practised by a physician necessarily different from that practised by a non-physician? In other fields, many recognized medical procedures are performed by non-medical personnel, for example, optometrists, midwives, and nurse practitioners.

A recent report by the Group for the Advancement of Psychiatry (1992) describes the current de-medicalization of psychotherapy in the United States and predicts that, in the future, psychotherapy will be practised largely by non-medical therapists. Our challenge is not to prove that non-physicians are unqualified to practise psychotherapy, but to prove that there is a unique place for physicians in the practice of psychotherapy.

However, two recent trends – the re-medicalization of psychiatry and the growth of biological psychiatry – raise questions about the validity of psychotherapy as a medical procedure. Although the 'medical model' (Ludwig & Othmer, 1977) is far narrower and more restrictive than psychiatry's prevailing biopsychosocial model, its adoption can, in part, be understood as a reaction to trends in the 1960s and 1970s that tried to separate psychiatry from medicine. Writing in 1980, Marmor described the newer psychotherapies as a 'third revolution' in psychotherapy. These newer therapies, such as gestalt therapy, primal therapy, bioenergetics, and transcendental meditation, depart from the classic psychoanalytic therapies and behaviour therapies in two ways. They do not depend on a 'disease' model and they are not based on scientific theories. Although Marmor sees little evidence that these therapies produce lasting positive results and warns that they can pose several dangers for patients, he believes that the development of these techniques has enriched the practice of more conventional therapies.

Nevertheless, one can differentiate forms of therapy and therapeutic techniques that fall within a scientific framework from those that do not. Furthermore, the American Psychiatric Association's development of *DSM-III* (APA, 1980), *DSM-III-R* (APA, 1987), and *DSM-IV* (APA, 1994), which replace the term 'disease' with 'disorder,' facilitates the practice of psychotherapy within a medical context. The concept of 'disorder' is especially relevant in maintaining a medical approach to the assessment and treatment of patients whose distress is best understood within a social or family context. For instance, recent work on post-traumatic stress disorder (Herman, 1992) examines the phenomenology and treatment of victims of family violence and other traumatic events.

The recent growth of biological psychiatry may ultimately both enrich our understanding of the psychotherapeutic process and facilitate our therapeutic techniques (Gottschalk, 1990; Mohl, 1987). As Mohl states, 'psychotherapy *is* a biological treatment that acts through biological mechanisms (interneuronal synaptic facilitation, provision of external physiological regulation, exploration of hippocampal memory processing) on biological problems (deficits in gene–environment interactions, erroneous synaptic facilitation, inappropriate locus ceruleus gate activity). Medication, dream interpretation and empathy simply become various ways to alter different neurotransmitters, presumably in different parts of the brain' (p. 325).

It is not advantageous to create a rigid differentiation between psychotherapy as a medical act and psychotherapy as carried out by non-medical therapists. For many patients with medical disorders or Axis I disorders requiring medical intervention, psychotherapy may be carried out by a non-medical therapist working collaboratively with a physician. Although some individuals without *DSM-IV* diagnoses who seek therapy for personal growth or understanding may prefer non-medical therapists, studies of practice patterns reveal that psychiatrists tend to treat patients with diagnosable *DSM-IV* conditions (Doidge, Simon, Gillies, & Ruskin, 1994).

There are compelling reasons to continue using the services of medical (and especially psychiatric) therapists within our health care system. Medical psychotherapists have had a long and intensive immersion in modern medicine, including the benefits of a systematic approach to diagnosis, prognosis, and treatment planning. Psychiatrists receive a detailed education in the complex, ongoing interaction among mind, brain, and body, so that they are aware of the way that medical disorders, developmental and physical changes, and bodily states influence the mind, and how the mind influences the body. They have experience in diagnosing and treating psychosomatic conditions. As part of their training, they are also taught to carry a high level of clinical responsibility in managing many very ill patients. They have experience with a wide range of mental illnesses, from minor forms to the most severe. By virtue of their training, they have been exposed to the painful realities of human frailty, sickness, death, and dying, enabling them to help patients deal with these matters as they occur in the course of life and therapy. They have experience working in hospitals and in the community, and they are acquainted with the full range of health services. Psychiatrists are trained to use biological treatments such as electroconvulsive therapy (ECT) and medication. Through the experience of working in hospital emergency departments, they develop the ability and expertise to remain 'cool under fire.' They are experts in the differential diagnosis of psychiatric disorders.

In order to be regarded as medical psychotherapy, any form of psychotherapy must meet three sets of standards: technical standards, ethical standards, and scientific standards.

1 *Technical standards:* All forms of psychotherapy consist of a theoretical framework and a (not necessarily finite) number of techniques. The techniques must correlate with the theory. A therapist must be knowledgeable in and competent to practise the basic techniques of any form of therapy undertaken.
2 *Ethical standards:* Medical psychotherapy must conform to the ethical standards of the medical profession.
3 *Scientific standards:* To qualify as medical psychotherapy, a form of psychotherapy must be scientifically valid with regard to both theory and technique. Theory should be constructed of potentially testable hypotheses and should not depend on previously falsified or discredited hypotheses. In addition, the efficacy of the therapy should be scientifically testable.

Current Definitions

In his book on psychotherapy, Wolberg (1977) reviewed thirty-seven definitions of psychotherapy and arrived at the following composite definition:

> Psychotherapy is the treatment, by psychological means, of problems of an emotional nature in which a trained person deliberately establishes a professional relationship with the patient with the object of (1) removing, modifying, or retarding existing symptoms, (2) mediating disturbed patterns of behavior, and (3) promoting positive personality growth and development. (p. 3)

A more recent variation of this definition appears in the *International Dictionary of Medicine and Biology*:

Any form of treatment for mental disorders or emotional disturbances in which a suitably trained person establishes a professional relationship with an identified patient for the purpose of removing or modifying symptoms of the disorder, or of promoting character growth and development so as to strengthen the patient's ability to cope with the problems of living. The relationship established between patient and therapist is used to influence the patient to unlearn old, maladaptive patterns and to learn and test new approaches. Psychotherapy includes guidance, counselling, psychoanalysis, behavior therapy, conditioning, hypnotherapy, and all other forms of treatment in which the major technique employed is communication, rather than drugs or other somatic agents. (Landau, 1986, p. 2348)

The current definition of psychotherapy used by the Ontario Hospital Insurance Plan (OHIP), Canada's largest provincial health insurance plan, resembles the above definitions:

Psychotherapy is any form of treatment for mental illness, behavioural maladaptions, and/or other problems that are assumed to be of an emotional nature, in which a physician deliberately establishes a professional relationship with a patient for the purpose of removing, modifying, or retarding existing symptoms, or attenuating or reversing disturbed patterns of behaviour and of promoting positive personality growth and development. (Ontario, Ministry of Health, 1991, p. xv)

Further, OHIP distinguishes between counselling and psychotherapy:

Counselling is distinct from psychotherapy and is that form of activity in which the physician engages in an educational dialogue with the patient(s) on an individual or group basis wherein the goal of the physician and patient(s) is to become aware of the patient's problems or situation and of modalities for prevention and/or treatment. Counselling is not to be claimed for the advice that is a normal part of any consultation or other assessment, nor as ongoing treatment. (Ontario, Ministry of Health, 1991, General Preamble, p. xv)

The Canadian Psychiatric Association approved the following definition in 1985:

Medical Psychotherapy: A series of medical procedures carried out by a physician trained to treat mental, emotional, and psychosomatic illness through a relationship with the patient in an individual, group, or family setting, utilizing verbal or non-verbal communication with the patient. Medical psychotherapy always entails continuing medical diagnostic evaluations and responsibility and may be carried out in conjunction with drug and other physical treatments.

Medical psychotherapy recognizes that the psychological and physical components of an illness are intertwined and that at any point in the disease process, psychological symptoms may give rise to, substitute for, or run concurrently with physical symptoms and vice versa. (Katz, 1986, p. 458)

Proposed Definition

The following definition was proposed by the Joint Task Force on Standards for Medical (Psychiatric) Psychotherapy of the Ontario Psychiatric Association and the Section on Psychiatry, Ontario Medical Association (Joint Task Force, 1995):

Psychotherapy is any form of psychological treatment for psychiatric disorders, behavioural maladaptions and/or other problems that are assumed to be of a psychological nature, in which a physician deliberately establishes a professional relationship with a patient for the purpose of removing, modifying or retarding existing symptoms, or attenuating or reversing disturbed patterns of behaviour, and of promoting positive personality growth and development.

Treatment or therapy is initiated after a thorough assessment of the patient's presenting complaints, including exploration of biological, psychological, social and cultural factors contributing to the patient's disorder. The relationship established between patient and physician is used to facilitate changes in maladaptive patterns and to encourage the patient to learn and test new approaches.

The treatment should be based on general standards of practice developed from: (a) professional standards and practice guidelines generally endorsed by peer-reviewed professional literature and/or taught in university departments of psychiatry, and (b) ethical standards of practice as adapted by professional licensing bodies.

Psychotherapy includes psychoanalysis, psychodynamic psychotherapy, cognitive therapy, behaviour therapy, conditioning, hypnotherapy, couple therapy, group therapy and all other forms of treatment in which the major technique employed is communication, although drugs or other somatic agents may be used concurrently. (p. 15)

Forms of Psychotherapy

Although there are numerous forms of psychotherapy, they can be abstracted into four overlapping, heterogeneous 'orientations': psycho-dynamic, cognitive/behavioural, strategic/systems, and experiential. Within each orientation, therapies can be provided in one of three for-mats: individual, group, and family (Clarkin, Frances, & Perry, 1991). Interactions between orientations and formats are summarized in table 1. The list of psychotherapies in the table is not meant to be exhaustive, but to offer examples. Psychotherapists increasingly are integrating aspects of different forms of therapy in the treatment of individual patients.

Not all psychotherapies listed in table 1.1 could be regarded as 'medi-cal psychotherapy.' Therapies based on a non-medical model, such as self-help groups, would by definition be non-medical therapies. Further, therapies that do not conform to the ethical or scientific standards of medical psychotherapy would also be excluded. For instance, therapies based on 'pelvic bonding' or regression to past lives, or those that attempt to discover the cause of symptoms in supposed 'abduction by aliens,' would certainly not conform to the accepted scientific standards of medical psychotherapy.

New therapeutic approaches can generally be incorporated into the grid. For instance, the treatment of male batterers would appear as cog-nitive/behavioural orientation, group format. Some psychotherapeutic treatment strategies involve multiple forms of psychotherapy. For instance, in outlining the treatment of post-traumatic stress disorder, Herman (1992) advocates the use of combined treatments involving several orientations and formats. Just as physicians who prescribe phar-macotherapy must bear in mind the potential for drug interactions, psy-chotherapists must understand the optimal approaches and drawbacks of combining psychotherapies.

Transference and the Definition of Psychotherapy

There is a common misconception that psychotherapy can be differenti-ated from other clinical interactions, such as counselling, by the pres-ence of transference. Problems arising from such a misunderstanding are illustrated by the following example.

The primary goal of the Joint Task Force in establishing standards for the practise of psychotherapy was to ensure that medical psychothera-

Table 1.1: Forms of Psychotherapy

Orientation	Format		
	Individual	Group	Family
Psychodynamic	Psychoanalysis Focal therapy Psychodynamic psychotherapy	Insight-oriented heterogeneous group therapy (Wolf)	Insight-oriented marital/family therapy (Ackerman, Framo)
Cognitive Behavioural	Cognitive treatment of depression (Beck) Rational-emotive therapy (Ellis)	Group treatment of agoraphobia Assertiveness training groups	Behavioural marital/family treatment (Falloon, Jacobson, Patterson)
Strategic/ Systems	'Uncommon therapy' (Erikson)	Most heterogeneous group therapies	Structural family therapy (Minuchin) Strategic family therapy (Haley) Paradoxical family therapy (Palazolli)
Experiential	Client-centred therapy (Rogers) Existential therapy (May)	Gestalt (Peris) Psychodrama (Moreno) Most homogeneous group therapies	Experiential family therapy (Whitaker)

Source: Clarkin, Frances, & Perry, 1991, p. 2

pists practice within the ethical, scientific, and technical standards relevant to the practice of psychotherapy as a medical procedure. The proposed definition was constructed to include all legitimate forms of psychotherapy. Any physician–patient interaction that does not conform to the definition would not be considered psychotherapy.

At the request of the College of Physicians and Surgeons of Ontario (CPSO), the task force was asked to define psychotherapy for a different purpose. In order to implement recommendations from the *Final Report* of the CPSO Task Force on Sexual Abuse of Patients (McPhedran, 1991), the CPSO requires a definition of psychotherapy that will differentiate it from other forms of physician–patient interaction, specifically 'supportive counselling.' This is based on the assumption that there are ethical constraints on the practice of psychotherapy that do not apply to other forms of medical care.

In a letter to members of the CPSO, the president stated:

Specifically, the Council has adopted the principle that physicians should have no sexual contact with a former patient for a period of one year following the date of the last professional contact, even if the professional contact has terminated. In looking at professional relationships involving psychotherapy or psychoanalysis, the Council has agreed in principle that no sexual contact should ever be permitted between physicians and former patients because the power of transference lasts long after the professional relationship has formally ended and possibly forever. (Edney, 1992)

The recommendations approved by CPSO Council state further:

There is overwhelming evidence to support the fact that special safeguards are needed to govern sexual contact between doctors and patients after the termination of a professional relationship that involved psychoanalysis or psychotherapy. The phenomenon of transference, the necessary creation of dependency and the inequality in the power balance between doctor and patient puts these relationships in a special category. Moreover, transference does not end when the professional relationship ends, as many studies have documented. Rather, a successful therapist has an importance and presence in the patient's life which is deeply felt long after treatment has ended. (CPSO, 1992)

The use of the definition of psychotherapy proposed in this volume to differentiate psychotherapy from other forms of physician–patient contact would be problematic. Although many forms of contact such as 'counselling' are distinct from psychotherapy, all doctor–patient relationships encompass many aspects of psychotherapeutic relationships. Under ideal circumstances, all medical acts would be performed by psychotherapeutically informed physicians.

There is ample evidence that transference, dependency, and power imbalance are not confined to psychotherapy. In fact, the phenomenon of transference is considered to be ubiquitous in human relations (Orr, 1954; McLaughlin, 1981). Orr states that 'transference in its widest sense is regarded as a universal phenomenon in interpersonal relationships' (p. 621).

According to Greenberg and Mitchell (1983), 'the concept of transference suggests that the "object" of the patient's experience (be it analyst, friend, lover, even parent) is at best an amended version of the actual other person involved. People react to and interact not only with an actual other but also with an internal other, a psychic representation of a person which in itself has the power to influence both the individual's affective states and his overt behavioral reactions' (p. 10) Greenson (1967) defined transference as 'the experiencing of feelings, drives, attitudes, fantasies, and defenses toward a person in the present which do not befit that person but are a repetition of reactions originating in regard to significant persons of early childhood, unconsciously displaced onto figures in the present. The two outstanding characteristics of a transference reaction are: it is a repetition and it is inappropriate' (p. 155).

In developing his ideas about transference, Freud (1912/1958) explicitly stated that transference develops not only in psychoanalysis, but also in other forms of treatment. These manifestations may be just as intense, but are not necessarily recognized for what they are. He understood transference as a manifestation of the patient's neurosis rather than as a product of the treatment.

There are several ways in which the manifestation of transference in psychotherapy differs from that in other relationships. The most vital difference is that, in psychodynamic forms of psychotherapy, the therapist uses the transference to understand the patient. According to Gabbard (1990), 'the dynamic psychiatrist recognizes the pervasiveness of transference phenomena and realizes that the relationship problems of which the patient complains will eventually manifest themselves in the patient's relationship with the treater. What is unique then about the doctor–patient relationship in dynamic psychiatry is not the presence of transference, but the fact that it is therapeutic material to be understood' (p. 10). Even in this quoted material, Gabbard is not specifically addressing psychotherapy. It is a central thesis of his textbook that dynamic psychiatrists will enrich their treatment of patients by an understanding of transference, even when they are using forms of treatment other than psychotherapy.

However, only in psychodynamic forms of psychotherapy is transference formally addressed. In the contemporary interpretations of dynamic psychotherapy, supportive psychotherapy and insight-oriented psychotherapy are no longer regarded as distinct. Rather, the interventions that therapists employ fall on a continuum from supportive to expressive (Gabbard, 1990; Luborsky, 1984). Although a therapist may tend to use predominantly expressive or predominantly supportive interventions, depending on the characteristics of the particular patient, 'the effective dynamic therapist will shift flexibly back and forth along the expressive–

supportive continuum, depending on the needs of the patient at a given moment in the psychotherapy process' (Gabbard, 1990, p. 72).

The specific manner in which the transference is addressed varies considerably along the expressive–supportive continuum. In formal psychoanalysis, at the most expressive end of the continuum, a certain amount of regression is fostered in order to facilitate the development of the transference neurosis. According to Freud (1920/1955), the psycho-analytic patient is 'obliged to *repeat* the repressed material as a contem-porary experience instead of *remembering* it as something belonging to the past. These reproductions are invariably acted out in the sphere of the transference, of the patient's relation to the physician. When things have reached this stage, it may be said that the earlier neurosis has now been replaced by a fresh "transference neurosis"' (p. 18). With certain vulnerable patients, the therapist will operate at the most supportive end of the continuum and will attempt to minimize regression as well as avoiding interpretation of the transference.

In summary, psychodynamic psychotherapy cannot be differentiated from other forms of medical intervention by the presence of transference alone. Further, as is evident in the *Final Report* of the CPSO Task Force on Sexual Abuse of Patients (McPhedran, 1991), dependency and inequal-ity of power balance between doctor and patient are not exclusive to psychotherapeutic relationships. The report documents many cases of sexual abuse of patients by physicians that did not occur in the context of psychotherapy.

References

American Psychiatric Association (APA). (1980). *Diagnostic and statistical manual of mental disorders* (3d ed.). Washington, DC: Author.

American Psychiatric Association (APA). (1987), *Diagnostic and statistical manual of mental disorders* (3d ed., revised). Washington, DC: Author.

American Psychiatric Association (APA). (1994). *Diagnostic and statistical manual of mental disorders* (4th ed.). Washington, DC: Author.

Clarkin, J.F., Frances, A.J., & Perry, S.W. (1995). The psychosocial treatments. In R. Michels (Chairman, Editorial Board), *Psychiatry.* Philadelphia: Lippincott.

College of Physicians and Surgeons of Ontario (CPSO). (1992, 26 May). *Recom-mendations approved by Council: Guidelines for personal relationships between physicians and former patients.* Toronto: Author.

Colpe, R. (1995). Psychiatry: past and future. In M.I. Kaplan and B. Sadock

(Eds.), *Comprehensive textbook of psychiatry* (6th ed.). Baltimore: Williams & Williams.

Doidge, N., Simon, B., Gillies, L.A., & Ruskin, R. (1994). Characteristics of psychoanalytic patients under a nationalized health plan: DSM-III-R diagnoses, previous treatment and childhood traumata. *American Journal of Psychiatry, 151,* 586–590.

Edney, R. (1992, June). Letter to members of the College of Physicians and Surgeons of Ontario.

Frank, J.D. (1974). *Persuasion and healing: a comparative study of psychotherapy* (Rev. ed.). New York: Schocken.

Freud, S. (1958). The dynamics of transference. In J. Strachey (Ed. and Trans., *The standard edition of the complete psychological works of Sigmund Freud* (Vol. 12). London: Hogarth Press. (Original work published 1912)

Freud, S. (1955). Beyond the pleasure principle. In J. Strachey (Ed. and Trans., *The standard edition of the complete psychological works of Sigmund Freud* (Vol. 18). London: Hogarth Press. (Original work published 1920)

Gabbard, G.O. (1990). *Psychodynamic psychiatry in clinical practice.* Washington, DC: American Psychiatric Press.

Gottschalk, L.A. (1990). The psychotherapies in the context of new developments in the neurosciences and biological psychiatry. *American Journal of Psychotherapy, 44,* 321–339.

Greenberg, J.R., & Mitchell, S.A. (1983). *Object relations in psychoanalytic theory.* Cambridge, MA: Harvard University Press.

Greenson, R.R. (1967). *The technique and practice of psychoanalysis* (Vol. 1). New York: International Universities Press.

Group for the Advancement of Psychotherapy (GAP). Committee on Therapy. (1992). *Psychotherapy in the future.* Washington, DC: Author/American Psychiatric Press.

Herman J.L. (1992). *Trauma and recovery.* New York: Basic.

Joint Task Force on Standards for Medical (Psychiatric) Psychotherapy. (1995). *A report to Council of the Ontario Psychiatric Association and to Executive of the Section on Psychiatry, Ontario Medical Association, on the definition, guidelines and standards for medical (psychiatric) psychotherapy.* Toronto: Author.

Kaplan, H.I., & Sadock, B.J. (Eds.). (1995). *Comprehensive textbook of psychiatry* (6th ed.). Baltimore: Williams & Wilkins.

Katz, P. (1986). The role of the psychotherapies in the practice of psychiatry: The position of the Canadian Psychiatric Association. *Canadian Journal of Psychiatry, 31,* 458–465.

Landau, S.I. (Editor-in-Chief). (1986). *International dictionary of medicine and biology.* New York: Wiley.

Luborsky, L. (1984). *Principles of psychoanalytic psychotherapy: A manual for supportive–expressive treatment*. New York: Basic.

Ludwig, A.M., & Othmer, E. (1977). The medical basis of psychiatry. *American Journal of Psychiatry, 134*, 1087–1092.

Marmor, J. (1980). Recent rends in psychotherapy. *American Journal of Psychiatry, 137*, 409–416.

McLaughlin, J.T. (1981). Transference, psychic reality, and countertransference. *Psychoanalytic Quarterly, 50*, 639–664.

McPhedran, M. (Chairperson). (1991, 25 November) *The final report: Task Force on Sexual Abuse of Patients*. An independent task force commissioned by the College of Physicians and Surgeons of Ontario.

Michels, R. (Chairman, Editorial Board). (1995). *Psychiatry*. Philadelphia: Lippincott.

Mohl, P.C. (1987). Should psychotherapy be considered a biological treatment? *Psychosomatics, 28*, 320–326.

Ontario. Ministry of Health. (1991, 1 April). *Schedule of benefits, physicians' services under the Health Insurance Act*. Toronto: Author.

Orr, D.W. (1954). Transference and countertransference: A historical survey. *Journal of the American Psychoanalytic Association, 2*, 621–670.

Ursano, R.J., & Silberman, E.K. (1988). Individual psychotherapies. In J.A. Talbott, R.E. Hales & S.C. Yudofsky (Eds.), *American Psychiatric Press textbook of psychiatry*. Washington, DC: American Psychiatric Press.

Wolberg, L.R. (1977). *The technique of psychotherapy* (3d ed.). New York: Grune & Stratton.

2. General Guidelines for the Practice of Psychotherapy

Ray Freebury, Jon Ennis, Carolyn Rideout, and Martha Wright

Development of the Guidelines

In general, standards of psychotherapeutic practice are based on two related components: the ethical aspects and the technical aspects of professional practice.

Ethical standards of practice are regulated by professional licensing bodies, such as the College of Physicians and Surgeons of Ontario (CPSO). Professional bodies, such as provincial and national medical and psychiatric associations, have also been instrumental in developing ethical standards. The Canadian Medical Association (CMA) maintains a Code of Ethics and issues periodic policy summaries on ethical issues. For example, the CMA has recently published a policy summary titled 'The Patient–Physician Relationship and the Sexual Abuse of Patients' (Canadian Medical Association [CMA], 1994a).

Technical standards of practice for psychotherapy are derived from the peer-reviewed professional literature and taught in university departments of psychiatry. Professional bodies, such as the Canadian and American psychiatric and psychoanalytic associations, also help to formulate these standards.

The development of practice guidelines by professional organizations is a recent advance (CMA, 1994b). The American Psychiatric Association (APA) is currently developing a series of practice guidelines for *DSM-IV* (APA, 1994a) disorders such as eating disorders (APA, 1993a), major depressive disorder in adults (APA, 1993b), bipolar disorder (APA, 1994b), and substance abuse disorders (APA, 1995b). As those guidelines focus on the treatment of specific disorders, their development process could reflect the evidence-based literature.

In this chapter we delineate guidelines applicable across the range of psychotherapeutic modalities, and not specific to the treatment of any psychiatric disorder. In discussing the development of practice guidelines for psychoanalysis in the treatment of depression, Gray (1996) argues that achievement of a broad consensus among practitioners is more relevant than outcome-based parameters to developing guidelines for the psychotherapies. The development process employed by the APA (1995a) in producing practice guidelines for psychiatric evaluation of adults can serve as a model for these types of clinical guidelines. The process involved in developing the material in this chapter was not nearly as exhaustive. The task force that produced these guidelines did not have the resources of the APA. Further, the focus was much broader. Essentially this material was developed through a series of drafts based on literature review, consultation with a wide variety of psychiatrists external to the task force, and consensus among a group of psychiatrists with expertise in a variety of psychotherapeutic modalities. The material was included in a report (Joint Task Force, 1995) which was approved by the Council of the Ontario Psychiatric Association and the Executive of the Ontario Medical Association, Section on Psychiatry. The report was then widely circulated in Canada among provincial and national psychiatric associations and academic psychiatrists. Comments and suggestions, as well as a review of recent literature, have been incorporated in this chapter.

The ethical practice of psychotherapy involves a number of related aspects. First and foremost, the therapist must respect the privileged patient–physician relationship. Therapy is initiated following a thorough assessment of the patient's presenting complaints, including an exploration of the biological, psychological, social, and cultural factors that contribute to the disorder. A specific therapeutic modality is chosen only if the patient meets the appropriate selection criteria for that modality. The therapist must be adequately trained in the specific therapeutic modality chosen, and must have kept up his or her competence in that therapy through continuing-education activities.

The Foundation of Psychotherapy: Respecting the Patient–Physician Relationship

In a recent policy summary, the CMA defines physician abuse of patients as 'any behaviour that transgresses the patient–physician relationship in an exploitive manner by a physician's words or actions. Exploitation implies that physicians are acting for their own advantage against their patients' interests' (CMA, 1994a, p. 1884A). In recent years, sexual abuse of patients by physicians has come under increasingly intense scrutiny. Additional types of abuses of the patient–physician relationship include breaches of confidentiality, unethical financial practices, abusive speech or behaviour, and neglectful behaviour.

BOUNDARIES IN PSYCHOTHERAPY

In the maintenance of respectful therapist–patient relationships, the concept of boundaries is crucial. Gutheil and Gabbard (1993) extensively reviewed the concept of boundaries in clinical practice. They emphasized the role of the 'therapeutic frame,': 'The analyst or therapist constructs the elements of the frame partly consciously and partly unconsciously. These elements include regular scheduling of appointments, the duration of the appointments, arrangements for payment of the fee, and the office setting itself.' They defined a boundary violation as a 'harmful crossing, a transgression, of a boundary' (p. 190).

Deviations from the standard therapeutic frame can be problematic because they may involve a blurring or crossing of a boundary without necessarily being harmful. Deviations from the standard therapeutic frame may be made on technical grounds. In this event they should fulfil certain criteria. Such deviations may be undertaken in order to sustain the treatment – for example, intervening on the patient's behalf with an employer to provide time for treatment – or to alleviate unnecessary suffering or resolve an impasse in treatment – for instance, when a therapist accompanies a phobic patient into situations that cause anxiety and avoidance. Each time such a deviation is undertaken, the therapist should have a therapeutic rationale for his or her action. Any major changes in the frame, or deviations from technical neutrality, should be documented. Subsequent treatment should aim to remove the need for deviation and explain the circumstances that necessitated it, elucidating the meaning that the process has had for the patient. Such safeguards are essential to maintain a trusting doctor–patient relationship and to achieve the success of psychotherapy. Although sexual misconduct usually begins with relatively minor boundary violations, such violations do not in themselves constitute misconduct.

Examples of problematic boundary violations include patients or therapists entering each other's homes, therapists presenting patients with gifts, and therapists disclosing personal details of their lives to patients. It is difficult to establish precise principles for the conditions under which such deviations from the standard therapeutic frame might be appropriate. It is essential, however, that therapists be aware that these *are* deviations, and that they understand the rationale for their use and recognize the potential meanings that they could have for patients. Therapists who depart from the standard therapeutic frame must be prepared to accept responsibility for the risks to their patients of such actions. Consultation with colleagues can be helpful when using unconventional techniques.

Psychotherapy occurs within the context of a human relationship. Involvement in such relationships is genuinely stimulating and rewarding for therapists. However, there is a risk that therapists can purposefully or inadvertently exploit the relationship for their own gratification without benefiting the patient. Patients will often view their therapists as powerful or idealized figures. It can be very gratifying for therapists to have an admiring patient take their advice in business or personal affairs, or laugh at their jokes. However, it is crucial that therapists understand these reactions in the context of the therapeutic relationship.

Although inviting patients to enter the therapist's home generally constitutes a boundary violation, an exception occurs where the therapist maintains a home office. Having an office at home is a time-honoured medical practice for psychotherapists. Physicians who adopt this practice generally ensure that the office is well separated from the rest of the home, the files remain confidential, and noise leakage is avoided. The home office may not be an optimal arrangement for certain types of patients with poor reality testing or highly demanding transferences.

It is inappropriate for a psychotherapist to treat his or her family members, or those with whom he or she has a current social or business relationship. However, it is appropriate for the therapist to refer such patients to a colleague.

It is generally problematic for a psychotherapist to treat concurrently a patient and that patient's close relatives, friends, or lovers. However, it may be appropriate to provide to a relative or a lover of a patient a consultation and referral for further treatment. In certain situations, such as in underserviced areas, a therapist may provide continued treatment to these intimates because no other competent clinician is available. The clinician should then document the reasons for that decision and recognize how this unusual situation influences the treatment. Examples of the complications arising from concurrent treatment of relatives or lovers with psychodynamic psychotherapy are elaborated in chapter 3, 'Guidelines for the Practice of Individual Psychodynamic Psychotherapy.'

RULES OF CONDUCT

The rules of conduct for psychotherapy are part of the overall frame of psychotherapy, but are most elaborate in psychodynamic psychotherapy (outlined in chapter 3). On the expressive–supportive continuum, to which psychodynamic psychotherapy and psychoanalysis belong, even clinical physical examination may be experienced as a boundary violation if undertaken during the course of therapy. If there is a concern about physical illness, the clinician has a responsibility to ensure that the patient is referred to a general physician. It goes without saying that the physician-psychotherapist is not precluded from responding appropriately when some unexpected, life-threatening emergency occurs.

In psychotherapies, there is no rationale for technical procedures that involve real or simulated corporal punishment, physical sexual contact, or disrobing as part of the therapeutic process. It should be noted that cognitive/behavioural therapies do have some well-documented procedures such as aversive conditioning or masturbation training. These procedures, however, do not normally take place in unchaperoned private-office settings, as is the case with psychodynamic psychotherapy and psychoanalysis (see chapter 5, 'Guidelines for the Practice of Cognitive/Behavioural Psychotherapy').

ERADICATING SEXUAL ABUSE

In its recent policy summary, 'The Patient–Physician Relationship and the Sexual Abuse of Patients' (CMA, 1994a), the Canadian Medical Association defines abuse of patients by physicians and describes policies developed to prevent such abuse. We fully endorse this position. In addition, we endorse the principle of 'zero tolerance of sexual abuse,' recommended by the College of Physicians and Surgeons of Ontario (CPSO) Task Force on Sexual Abuse of Patients (McPhedran, 1991). Standards of practice regarding the sexual abuse of patients are essentially the same for the practice of psychotherapy as for any other physician–patient relationship. But, because of the central role of this relationship in psychotherapy, and because psychotherapy is often intense and prolonged, patients in psychotherapy are especially vulnerable to sexual abuse by unethical practitioners.

The CMA defines sexual abuse of patients as 'any behaviour that transgresses the patient–physician relationship in a sexually exploitive manner by a physician's words or actions' (CMA, 1994a, p. 1884B). Any form of sexual activity between a therapist and a patient constitutes abuse, regardless of who initiated it. Although the patient's perception of the boundaries of acceptable behaviour may differ from the physician's, it is the responsibility of the physician to establish and maintain the boundaries or limits of behaviour for him- or herself and the patient.

In its most blatant forms, sexual behaviour is easily defined. It includes sexual intercourse, touching, kissing, embracing, and disrobing by either party. Except under certain specific circumstances, there is generally no clinical justification for any physical contact between therapist and patient beyond a handshake as part of the psychotherapeutic procedure.

However, under exceptional circumstances it is appropriate to touch a patient. For instance, in the psychotherapeutic treatment of patients with debilitating or stigmatizing physical illnesses, it is often necessary for the therapist to physically touch the patient. This touch is meant to facilitate the experience of human contact and acceptance. It would generally consist of a handshake or a touch on the arm or shoulder. There are also occasions when it is appropriate for therapists to return a spontaneous physical display of affection initiated by a patient. For instance, it is not unusual for a patient to give a hug as an expression of warm farewell when treatment is terminated. In such circumstances, it is the responsibility of the therapist to ensure that these gestures will be unambiguously perceived by the patient as non-sexual. The underlying assumption is that the therapist's response will be appropriately determined by knowledge of the patient's psychopathology.

The psychotherapist's use of language can be problematic. In some instances, in its most blatant form the therapist's use of language can constitute sexual impropriety. Examples include sexually demeaning comments, frank sexual suggestions or invitations to a patient, gratuitous sexual comments, and inappropriate or demeaning sexual humour. Similarly, revelations of the therapist's private sexual life, behaviour, or fantasies can also constitute sexual impropriety.

Determining what constitutes sexual abuse is far more difficult in the area of verbal communication than in that of physical contact. After all, whereas physical contact plays a minimal role within psychotherapy, psychotherapies are essentially 'talking therapies.' Specifically, talking with patients about sexual issues is appropriate within psychotherapy and is not considered sexually abusive. Inquiring about sexual behaviour, concerns, and history is, in fact, an essential aspect of clinical interviewing and decision making. Because colloquial language often relies on current sexual metaphors to express strong feelings, therapists may use sexual language to help patients express their emotions. Verbal communications are thought to constitute sexual abuse only when they exploit or abuse the patient. Ethical practice requires that therapists be sensitive to the impact of language on their patients. Therapists must also recognize that some particularly sensitive patients require an explanation of why it is often necessary to use sexually explicit language within the clinical situation. Psychiatrists practising psychotherapy and psychoanalysis treat individuals with serious character pathology such as severe narcissistic disorders, borderline character pathology, and paranoid character structures. Patients in these categories may have distortions of reality perception that render them highly sensitive to slights and to minor empathic failures by the therapist. Neutral comments may be interpreted by such patients as demeaning or as having a sinister connotation. As Gedo (1993) notes, 'in circumstances of that kind, the lexical meaning of words gets lost; communication takes place primarily in terms of the affects, especially as they are conveyed by the paraverbal aspects of speech. Hence it may become necessary to speak with strong emphasis or even in an angry manner' (p. 286). In determining whether verbal communication constitutes sexual or some other form of impropriety, it is essential to consider the therapist's intention.

The definition of sexual abuse extends to the relationship between the therapist and the patient's family or others whose involvement in the treatment and welfare of a patient requires direct interaction with the physician. A therapist's sexual involvement with the spouse, parent, child, or sibling of a patient clearly transgresses and abuses the relationship between therapist and patient.

Only in exceptional circumstances are planned contacts with patients outside the therapeutic setting justifiable. For example, a behavioural approach to phobic disorders often requires the therapist to accompany a patient in confronting a feared situation. This type of contact would not be considered social.

The issue of romantic and sexual involvement between therapists and former patients is a controversial one among psychotherapists. For instance, in the province of Ontario, the College of Physicians and Surgeons (CPSO), the provincial licensing and regulatory body, passed the following guidelines in 1992: 'Where the doctor–patient relationship has, at any time, involved psychotherapy of such duration that it may be seen to have been a *significant component* of treatment, sexual contact with the patient is also prohibited at any time after termination of treatment. "Significant component" is defined as distinct from superficial, supportive psychotherapy administered infrequently or on isolated occasions and as incidental to the overall doctor–patient relationship' (Dempsey & Eccles, 1994, p. 11). This position was supported by the Council of the Ontario Psychiatric Association in 1995. The Canadian Psychiatric Association (CPA) adopted an even stronger position in a position statement approved by the CPA board of directors in September 1995: 'The Canadian Psychiatric Association deems sexual relationships with former patients to be unethical' (CPA, no date).

An intimate personal relationship with a current patient, or the termination of treatment for the purpose of pursuing such a relationship, is antithetical to all forms of psychotherapy, without exception. Although it is generally agreed that such a relationship is inadvisable after treatment has ended, some psychiatrists oppose a lifetime ban on intimate personal relationships between patients and former therapists. They believe that such a ban not only infringes on the patient's rights to freedom of association, but also prejudicially implies that patients who have undergone psychotherapy or psychoanalysis will never be able to make healthy judgments about such relationships (OMA, 1992). However, as Gabbard and Lester (1995) state, 'ethical standards do not require a demonstration that a particular behaviour always results in harm ... Ethics codes are generally based on the *potential* to harm' (p. 156).

RESPECTING PATIENT CONFIDENTIALITY

The privileged nature of the physician–patient relationship is an essential feature of psychotherapy. For therapy to be effective, therapists must be unwavering in their protection of their patients' confidentiality.

Breaches of confidentiality may take a variety of forms and can result from different motives. It is unethical for a therapist to use information obtained as a result of the patient's expectation of confidentiality for the therapist's personal gain. Examples include insider trading on the stock market or other investment decisions based on privileged communication, seeking endorsement from an influential patient, encouraging a patient to bequeath money to the therapist (or some personal contact of the therapist's), and taking advantage based on knowledge of a patient's alienation from a spouse or other close acquaintance for any form of personal gain or social acquaintance with that other person.

Therapists may also breach confidentiality by revealing the identity of their patients. At times, this may result from carelessness or from a desire to impress friends or colleagues. Whenever discussing patients with colleagues, be it informal consultation or formal presentation at rounds or conferences, it is imperative that therapists strive to protect patient confidentiality and not reveal the patient's identity. It is often advisable to obtain informed consent from patients before publishing clinical material in technical and scientific papers.

There are some circumstances when therapists are required by law to disclose information obtained in confidence. This includes the reasonable suspicion of child abuse and, in some jurisdictions, the suspicion of sexual abuse of a patient by a regulated health care provider. It may also include the reasonable suspicion that a patient will or may harm another person. In such circumstances, disclosing information without the patient's permission should be done only after encouraging the patient to report him- or herself; seeking permission from the patient to make a report; and, finally, informing the patient that the physician will make a report.

MAINTAINING ETHICAL FINANCIAL PRACTICES

Charging fees for psychotherapy or related services when such charges are not legal or exceed the legal fee constitutes a breach of the physician–patient relationship. At times, a therapist may believe that a fee prohibited by law is justified by the therapist's level of training or expertise or by particular circumstances. Nevertheless, charging the fee or encouraging the patient to pay it voluntarily is an example of unethical exploitation of the physician–patient relationship for the therapist's financial gain.

Psychiatrists practising psychotherapy, whether they receive payment directly from a third-party payer, such as a government health insurance plan, or bill the patient directly and submit claims to a third-party payer on the patient's behalf, should clearly spell out the terms of the therapeutic contract. In establishing this contract, psychiatrists are bound by the regulations of the provincial or state licensing bodies. For instance, in the province of Ontario, the fee must not exceed that paid by the Ontario Health Insurance Plan (OHIP). The Ontario Medical Association (OMA, 1994) has published the *Physicians' Guide to Third-Party and Other Uninsured Services*. Under OHIP regulations, physicians may charge patients for missed appointments only if the patient has given less than twenty-four hours' notice of cancellation. An exception is psychotherapy practices in which a reasonable written agreement exists between the patient and the physician. In this circumstance, billing for missed appointments is at the discretion of the therapist. The contract may also itemize those uninsured services listed by the College of Physicians and Surgeons of Ontario for which payment may be the patient's responsibility in the event that they are required.

It is unethical for a therapist to enter into a business arrangement with a patient outside the therapeutic relationship. This includes investing in a patient's business or encouraging a patient to invest in a business venture initiated by the therapist. It is also unethical for a therapist to lend money to or borrow money from a patient.

Guidelines for Treatment Selection

Psychiatric psychotherapy is a highly specialized form of psychotherapy whose practice requires a medical degree and a specialty qualification in psychiatry. The medical base is a prerequisite for the full understanding of the complex interaction of body and mind. Medical knowledge is also vital for appreciating the psychiatric sequelae of physical illnesses, and the potential consequences of medical and surgical treatments.

A thorough grounding in basic neuroscience and a knowledge of the various models of psychotherapy are essential prerequisites for the selection of treatment modalities appropriate to the patient's psychiatric diagnosis, constitution, psychological make-up, and sociocultural circumstances. These requirements are intended to ensure an accurate diagnosis and selection of appropriate treatment. Models of psychotherapy fall into four broad categories – namely, psychodynamic, cognitive/ behavioural, strategic/systems, and experiential (described later in this section). Psychiatrists should be knowledgeable about the appropriate application of all effective modalities. However, individuals usually develop expertise in one or two models and refer patients to an appropriate colleague if they believe that another modality would better suit the patient's needs.

REFERRAL PROCESSES

- Referral for psychotherapy may come from other physicians, community agencies, or other health care professionals, or can be initiated by patients themselves.

- The psychiatrist must ensure that an appropriate medical work-up has been completed, where indicated.
- The referral source may be an important factor in assessing the patient's motivation for treatment and change. For example, patients seeking treatment in compliance with demands from third parties, such as courts, insurance companies, or family members, may have little motivation for change.

PSYCHIATRIC EVALUATION

Psychotherapy can begin only after a thorough psychiatric evaluation. The American Psychiatric Association has recently published its 'Practice Guideline for Psychiatric Evaluation of Adults' (APA, 1995a). The guideline outlines the following domains of the clinical evaluation:

A. *Reason for the evaluation*
B. *History of the present illness*
C. *Past psychiatric history*
D. *General medical history*
E. *History of substance abuse*
F. *Psychosocial/developmental history (personal history)*
G. *Social history*
H. *Occupational history*
I. *Family history*
J. *Review of systems*
K. *Physical examination* – where psychotherapy is to be a major component of treatment, the physical examination is generally performed by another physician. In circumstances where the psychiatrist elects to conduct a physical exam, it is essential to be aware of the patient's concerns about boundaries and potential meanings to the patient of physical touch by the therapist. Where psychotherapy is not to be a major component of the treatment, a nurse should be present whenever the psychiatrist performs a physical examination of a patient. Even when psychotherapy is a major component of the treatment, it is generally appropriate for the psychiatrist to perform certain aspects of the physical exam, such as neurological examinations and blood pressure. Therapists will consider the potential meanings of these actions for the patient. Regardless of who conducts the physical exam, it is an essential component of any psychiatric evaluation.
L. *Mental-status examination:*
   1. Appearance and general behaviour

    2. Expressions of mood and affect
    3. Speech and language
    4. Movement and posture
    5. Current thoughts and perceptions:
       a. spontaneous worries, concerns, impulses, and perceptual expe-
          riences
       b. cognitive and perceptual symptoms of specific mental disorder,
          usually elicited by specific questioning
       c. suicidal, homicidal, violent, or self-injurious thoughts, feelings,
          or impulses
    6. Features of the patient's associations
    7. Patient's understanding of his or her current situation
    8. Cognitive status:
       a. level of consciousness
       b. orientation
       c. attention and concentration
       d. language functions
       e. memory
       f. fund of knowledge
       g. calculation
       h. drawing
       i. abstract reasoning
       j. executive functions
       k. quality of judgment
M. *Functional assessment* – when appropriate
N. *Diagnostic tests* – includes psychological tests, structured interviews,
    questionnaires when appropriate
O. *Information derived from the interview process* – includes patient's
    response to the interviewer, ability to communicate about emotional
    issues, defence mechanisms displayed

Using the information obtained in the evaluation, the clinician develops a differential diagnosis, case formulation, and initial treatment plan.

Diagnosis: This includes a differential and provisional diagnosis based
on a recognized diagnostic system such as *DSM-IV* using Axes 1–5 and
V codes. If psychotherapy is to be undertaken, the psychiatrist will take
into account the patient's personality, and interpersonal and intrapsychic functioning, according to the particular theoretical model on which
the treatment plan is based.

Formulation: This is a hypothesis that tries to explain the clinical picture presented by the patient. It includes biological, psychological, and socio-cultural factors, and is crucial in planning treatment.

Initial Treatment Plan: See 'Selection of Psychotherapeutic Approach' (below).

FACTORS INFLUENCING OUTCOME

There are many factors that influence psychotherapy outcomes. These include variables within the patient, therapist, and environment (Hadley & Strupp, 1976; Crown, 1983).

a. *Therapist factors:* The therapist's training, experience, self-awareness, relational skills, personality, warmth, and ability to form collabora-tive working relationships determine his or her ability to arrive at an accurate diagnosis and select an appropriate treatment modality, also influencing the outcome of the therapeutic process. Additionally, research has shown that other factors such as the patient–therapist fit are crucial in determining outcome.
b. *Patient factors:* These include diagnosis, past treatment response, bio-logical factors such as intelligence and memory, genetic factors, psy-chological factors such as the capacity for trust and commitment, and motivation for change.
c. *Environmental factors:* These include sociocultural influences such as family, social conditions, cultural attitudes, as well as travel distance and workplace flexibility. Language in common may also influence outcome.

SELECTION OF PSYCHOTHERAPEUTIC APPROACH

Choosing the Treatment Format

There are many factors involved in the choice of treatment format. A person with a particular diagnosis may benefit from a variety of treat-ment modalities. Therapeutic alliance is enhanced if the person is given a choice and takes part in selecting the treatment modality.

a. *Individual:* This is indicated when the locus of the problem is thought to be within the patient, for example, relational difficulties, internal conflict, or problematic behaviours.

b. *Family or couple:* This is indicated in the case of marital or family conflict, in situations where there are poor communication skills and unhealthy alliances within the family, and where a family has fixed, severe functional deficits.

c. *Group:* This is often preferred for those with interpersonal, interactional problems. Group therapy is contraindicated in certain diagnostic categories such as manic, acutely psychotic, or suicidal patients. Some patients with paranoid or schizoid personalities may also do poorly in group therapy. Specialized groups may be very helpful as part of a comprehensive treatment strategy for conditions such as anorexia nervosa, bulimia nervosa, and drug abuse. Self-help groups such as those provided by Alcoholics Anonymous can be a useful part of treatment programs for alcoholism.

Choosing a Treatment Orientation

a. *Psychodynamic psychotherapy (psychoanalytic):* The primary aim is for the patient to increase his or her understanding of internal conflict, deficits, and defensive compromises, and to develop increased awareness of affects, leading to symptom relief and personality change.
   – The data sources include developmental history, unconscious derivatives in dreams, fantasies, free association, transference, and countertransference.
   – The therapist's stance is one of a neutral, empathic, and abstinent (relatively inactive) listener, thus allowing the therapist to serve as a transference object.
   – The strategies include observation, empathic listening, clarification, confrontation, interpretation, and reconstruction.
   – The therapeutic categories include psychoanalysis and long-term or brief dynamic psychotherapy.

b. *Cognitive/behavioural:* The primary aim is to change maladaptive behaviours and to help patients enhance or learn new adaptive behaviours.
   – The data sources include history of symptoms, behavioural sequences, habit patterns, behavioural analysis, and cognitive analysis.
   – The therapist's stance is that of expert, adviser, teacher, and parent surrogate.

- The strategies include functional analysis, self-monitoring, psychoeducation, homework assignments, cognitive restructuring, hypothesis testing, exposure, skills training, relaxation training, biofeedback, and problem-solving training.
- The therapeutic categories include cognitive therapy, behavioural therapy, biofeedback, and reciprocal inhibition.

c. *Strategic/systems:* The primary aim is modification of behaviour within a given system or modification of the entire system. Insight is seen as antithetical to change unless it is imparted according to a strategic plan.
- The strategies include direct advice, paradoxic injunctions, reframing, symptom prescription, boundary marking, and positive connotation.
- The therapeutic categories include structural, strategic, and paradoxical family therapy; 'uncommon therapy'; and heterogeneous group therapy.

d. *Experiential:* The primary aim is the sharing of experience and feelings.
- The data source derives from the 'here and now' experience and the therapist's empathic awareness. The therapy is largely ahistorical.
- The therapist stance is non-authoritarian and empathically reflective.
- The strategies include abreaction, empathy, sharing, identification, imitation, and confrontation.
- The therapeutic categories include Rogerian therapy, gestalt therapy, primal therapy, logotherapy, and existential therapy.

e. *Eclectic:* Psychotherapists may use more than one approach with a patient. One approach may prepare a patient to move to another. For example, a directive–supportive technique may prepare a patient to move into a more intensive exploratory framework (Clarkin, Frances, & Perry, 1994).

Factors Affecting the Duration and Frequency of Psychotherapy

Factors that affect the duration and frequency of psychotherapy include diagnosis and prognosis, duration of illness, social context, therapist and patient treatment goals, patient motivation, secondary gain, therapeutic techniques, therapist's skill, and therapist–patient fit.

a. *Diagnosis and prognosis:* Conditions such as severe personality disorders, chronic dysthymia, or eating disorders, for which psychotherapy remains an important part of a strategic plan, require prolonged treatment. Conditions such as simple phobias, acute grief reactions, or situational maladjustments usually respond to brief therapies.

b. *Onset and duration of illness:* Disorders such as personality disorders, in which there is a history of disturbed behaviour and difficulties in relationships over many years, prolong the duration of treatment. In contrast, when the onset of illness is recent and there are precipitating or traumatic life events, and when symptoms are focal in nature, treatment can be brief.

c. *Social context:* This may play a major role in the duration of treatment. Treatment length may be affected by the patient's employment conditions or by the necessity to move to another city. Treatment may also be prematurely terminated or prolonged in cases where there is spousal opposition, and spousal abuse may be a significant factor in early termination.

d. *Treatment goals:* When treatment goals, jointly agreed-upon by patient and therapist, are ambitious and aim for multiple and major changes, the duration of therapy increases. When the goals are more limited and focal in nature, treatment tends to be shorter.

e. *Treatment models:* The treatment model selected can affect the frequency as well as the duration of treatment.
   – Techniques that increase frequency and duration are insight and uncovering, restructuring the personality, free-ranging exploration, destabilizing the defences, provoking affect, modifying thought, and reorienting attitude and behaviour.
   – Techniques that limit frequency and duration are suppressive or covering, problem solving, focused examination, strengthening defences, affect-reducing, behaviour modification, and stabilization.

f. *Other factors:* These tend to be individual-specific and include the patient's motivation for change; secondary gain in remaining ill, which in turn may be affected by the social context in which the patient lives; the therapist's skill; and the patient–therapist fit. There is a considerable body of knowledge related to the influence of therapist–patient relationships on the outcome of psychotherapy. Therapists' qualities of accurate empathy, non-possessive warmth, and genuineness have been defined as three main factors (Truax et al., 1966). Similar value systems of patient and therapist, embodying factors of 'mutual attraction' and 'influence,' have also been correlated with good outcomes (Kessel & McBrearty, 1967).

Treatment Goals

Treatment goals must be mutually elaborated by therapist and patient and should be reassessed and re-evaluated periodically during the course of treatment. Goals may range from symptom-reduction to improved intrapsychic and interpersonal functioning (improved self-esteem and relationships). Other goals may include improved work performance and satisfaction, and decreased utilization of medical services. Evidence shows that psychotherapy reduces the utilization of general medical services (Mumford, Schlessinger, Glass, Patrick, & Cuerdon, 1984).

Concurrent Use of Medication

(See chapter 11, 'Guidelines for Combining Pharmacotherapy with Psychotherapy')

Psychotherapy is often used in conjunction with medication. Sometimes it is the secondary modality, as is usually the case with schizophrenia or severe depression; at other times it is the primary modality, with medications used to control symptoms. It is necessary to recognize the meanings that patients might attach to such combined treatment.

In some disorders in which pharmacological treatment is clearly indicated, the psychiatrist may be obliged to treat the patient with psychotherapy alone, for example, because the patient's physical state precludes the use of medication, or because the patient refuses to take medication or fails to respond to it. In such circumstances, it is advisable for the physician to document the rationale for this clinical decision.

Although medical psychotherapists are trained in psychopharmacology, the therapist may choose to have a colleague manage the medication. This usually occurs when there is a concern that the act of prescribing may constitute a breach of the therapeutic frame. When psychiatrists work in collaboration with other physicians or with non-medical therapists in prescribing medication, each must recognize the possibility that a patient may play one off against the other, as occurs in splitting.

Psychotherapy with Children and Adolescents

(See chapter 10, 'Guidelines for the Practice of Psychotherapy with Children and Adolescents')

Managing therapeutic relationships in work with children and adolescents demands greater flexibility than that with adults. In particular, the impact of developmental stage and surrounding context (school, family, peer, community) needs to be considered in therapy with this age group.

For instance, the therapist generally tries to help the child/adolescent better understand his or her parents, while at the same time fostering empathy with, and insight into, the child from the parental perspective. In this sense, child therapy is systemic and holistic. It usually requires a greater degree of activity as well. With younger children, this takes the form of play, games, or sports. With adolescents, neutrality can be construed as passivity, which is anathema to most teenagers, and so the therapist may need to incorporate humour, active listening, verbal limit-setting, and creative endeavours (e.g., encouraging poetry, prose, or art), along with clarification and interpretation.

Special considerations such as boundaries to physical contact, confidentiality, self-disclosure, and involvement of child-welfare agencies are covered more fully in Chapter 10, 'Guidelines for the Practice of Psychotherapy with Children and Adolescents.'

Recommendations for Special Situations

Stalemated Treatments: Many treatments reach a point at which improvement is limited, stalled, or stalemated in a manner that signals more than temporary resistance. In such cases, it is recommended that the clinician discuss this circumstance with a colleague and seek supervision, or refer the patient for a formal consultation.

Treatment Contracts: Treatment contracts are often valuable with patients who have failed in previous treatments because of behaviour that interfered with the therapy. Examples of such behaviour are stalking the therapist, repeatedly calling about threatened suicide and hanging up, not talking in sessions for prolonged periods, manipulative suicide attempts, threatening the therapist, damaging the therapist's office, and refusing to leave the office at the end of sessions. In such cases, the clinician drafts a contract with the patient, stating that treatment can be conducted only under certain conditions. If the patient contravenes these conditions by engaging in behaviour that makes treatment impossible, the clinician will end treatment. This makes it clear to the patient that the success of treatment depends upon the patient's collaboration, and that treatment is not magic and may not be possible. It also makes it clear that the patient has some responsibility for treatment, and that the therapeutic frame is not to be used simply for acting out, but rather for positive purposes. These contracts also protect clinicians treating patients who may not otherwise receive treatment.

Recovered Memories of Childhood Sexual Abuse: Childhood sexual abuse is a complex and pervasive problem in North America that has historically gone unacknowledged. The large majority of adults who were sexually abused as children do, in fact, remember all or part of what happened to them. It is possible that, in some cases, long-repressed memories of abuse can be recovered years later. However, research indicates that some individuals who 'recover' memories of being abused as children have constructed so-called pseudo-memories. In addition, memories of actual events can be shaped by varying degrees of accuracy as time passes. No symptom pattern has been identified that validates a person's claims of being the victim of childhood sexual abuse. Under questioning, memories can be significantly influenced by a therapist or other trusted person, and repeated questioning can even lead people to report 'memories' of traumatic events that did not take place. In a public statement issued in 1993, the American Psychiatric Association encourages psychiatrists to 'maintain an empathic, nonjudgemental, neutral stance toward reported memories of sexual abuse.' Further, they recommend that 'care must be taken to avoid pre-judging the cause of the patient's difficulties or the veracity of the patient's reports. A strong prior belief by the psychiatrist that sexual abuse or other factors are or are not the cause of the patient's problems is likely to interfere with appropriate assessment and treatment' (APA, 1996).

A position statement titled 'Adult Recovered Memories of Childhood Sexual Abuse' was approved by the board of directors of the Canadian

Psychiatric Association (Blackshaw, Chandarana, Garneau, Merskey, & Moscarello, 1996). The conclusion and recommendations are as follows:

- Sexual abuse at any age is deplorable and unacceptable and should always be given serious attention. All spontaneous reports should be treated with respect and concern and be carefully explored. Psychiatrists must continue to treat patients who report the recollection of childhood sexual abuse, accepting the current limitations of knowledge concerning memory, and maintain an empathic, nonjudgmental, neutral stance.
- Lasting serious effects of trauma at an early age very probably occur, but children who have been sexually abused in early childhood may be too young to accurately identify the event as abusive and to form a permanent explicit memory. Thus, without intervening cognitive rehearsal of memory, such experiences may not be reliably recalled in adult life.
- Reports of recovered memories of sexual abuse may be true, but great caution should be exercised before acceptance in the absence of solid corroboration. Psychiatrists should be aware that excessive emphasis on recovering memories may lead to misdirection of the treatment process and unduly delay appropriate therapeutic measures.
- Routine inquiry into past and present experience of all types of abuse should remain a regular part of psychiatric assessment. Psychiatrists should take particular care, however, to avoid inappropriate use of leading questions, hypnosis, narcoanalysis, or other memory enhancement techniques directed at the production of hypothesized hidden or lost material. This does not preclude traditional supportive psychotherapeutic techniques, based on strengthening coping mechanisms, cognitive psychotherapy, behaviour therapy, or neutrally managed exploratory psychodynamic or psychoanalytic treatment.
- Since there are no well-defined symptoms or groups of symptoms that are specific to any type of abuse, symptoms that are said to be typical should not be used as evidence thereof.
- Reports of recovered memories that incriminate others should be handled with particular care. In clinical practice, an ethical psychiatrist should refrain from taking any side with respect to their use in accusations directed against the family or friends of the patient or against any third party. Confrontation with alleged perpetrators solely for the supposed curative effect of expressing anger should not be encouraged. There is no reliable evidence that such actions are therapeutic. On the contrary, this type of approach may alienate relatives and cause a break-

down of family support. Psychiatrists should continue to protect the best interests of their patients and of their supportive relationships.
- Further education and research in the specific areas of childhood sexual abuse and memory are strongly recommended. (pp. 305–306)

Termination of Treatment

The following quotation is from the position paper of the Canadian Psychiatric Association, 'The Role of Psychotherapies in the Practice of Psychiatry' (Katz, 1986).

> One of the more controversial topics being discussed is termination of treatment. It is very difficult to set guidelines for termination. Achieving the original goals is often an irrelevant guideline because the goals are frequently reset as the patient gains insight into his or her condition. An impasse in treatment may be difficult to assess, as treatment often stalls at a plateau for varying periods of time before proceeding again. The therapist's philosophy of termination will affect the guidelines – some therapists see 'termination' as an ending to the treatment relationship, requiring very careful and thorough preparation. Other therapists see 'termination' as an interruption in what will most likely be an ongoing series of periods of therapy. The latter approach applies particularly to adolescents whose emotional lability affects their motivation for treatment, and to patients with severe psychopathology, who often require a number of periods of psychotherapy, as they face changing life situations over the course of many years. The usual guideline is an agreement between the patient and the therapist that the patient has achieved what can reasonably be expected from psychotherapy. (p. 463)

In a recent position paper, the CPA has outlined guidelines for unilateral termination of treatment (UTT) by a psychiatrist (Tapper, 1994). The following justifications for UTT are described:

1. no treatment is indicated after full consideration of the situation;
2. further treatment would not produce additional benefit;
3. the specified treatment, for which the doctor and patient contracted, has been completed;
4. the psychiatrist does not feel competent to provide the treatment necessary after assessment of the condition;
5. the psychiatrist is ceasing practice or relocating to a distant place;

6. the psychiatrist is markedly altering the nature of his practice, for instance from office based, general adult psychiatry to university based, psychopharmacological research;
7. the patient has initiated legal proceedings against the physician;
8. the patient has assaulted or harassed the psychiatrist, his or her family or friends;
9. boundary violations, for instance of a sexual nature, of the psychiatrist–patient relationship are a significant risk;
10. transference or countertransference is persistently, therapeutically destructive;
11. this has been chosen as a constructive, therapeutic maneuver; and/or
12. the patient is consistently non-compliant with appointment times, medications, explicit conditions of treatment or simple treatment recommendations. (p. 2).

The patient should be informed of the reasons for UTT and, if further treatment is indicated, the psychiatrist should make arrangements for the services of another suitable physician. A psychiatrist may unilaterally terminate treatment with an unstable patient only after rigorous examination of the circumstances. Consultation with another psychiatrist is generally indicated in such circumstances. It is advisable for the initial psychiatrist to continue treatment after UTT for one or two months to facilitate the transfer.

The following information should be fully documented in the patient's chart: 'the reasons for UTT, all relevant correspondence, verbal discussions with the patient, family and colleagues and the arrangements made for the provision of the patient's future care' (p. 3).

Maintaining Competence

Medical psychotherapists maintain their competence through a variety of activities, including reading articles and texts; undertaking projects in continuing medical education; traineeships; self-assessment programs; teaching, research, publication, or presentations; using audiotapes, videotapes, or computer learning programs; and attending courses, rounds, conferences, journal clubs, and workshops. In order to maintain competence in psychotherapy, it is essential to be knowledgeable about current advances in diagnosis and psychiatric treatments, including pharmacology, as well as advances in psychotherapy. In some jurisdictions, formal continuing-education requirements are necessary to maintain licensure.

In Canada, although there are no such requirements, it is advisable for psychiatrists to participate in the Maintenance of Competence Program (MOCOMP) of the Royal College of Physicians and Surgeons of Canada (Fox, 1993).

Quality Assurance and Assessment of Competence

It is essential, in all instances, that assessors be fully conversant with and trained in the modality of psychotherapy practised by the clinician who is undergoing evaluation.

Therapist Errors

It is important to acknowledge that psychotherapists can make errors that influence outcome of psychotherapy. Luborsky, McLellan, Woody, O'Brian, and Amelbach (1985) have demonstrated that individual therapists' success with a variety of clients is largely dependent on the ability to establish good therapeutic alliances. Therefore, the failure both to recognize the importance of therapeutic alliance and to develop it can lead to major errors for psychotherapists. Safran (1993) demonstrated that repairing a rupture or a disturbance in the therapeutic alliance is extremely effective in obtaining a good outcome, whereas failing to recognize a rupture or to take action is a significant error.

Henry, Schacht and Strupp (1986, 1990) demonstrated that therapist errors occur when therapists become locked into negative cycles with patients. They also point out that errors occur when therapists respond to patient hostility with their own counter-hostility.

According to Hadley and Strupp (1976), therapist errors include therapist's hostility, criticism, blame, exploitativeness, and excessive need to make patients change. They also cite technical problems, including: technical rigidity; unclarified attacks on defences; destructive interpretations; and misplaced focus of treatment. Rakoff, Sigal, and Epstein (1975) have demonstrated that premature interpretations involving transference may result in high drop-out rates. Frayn (1992) confirmed this finding in his research on premature termination of psychotherapy. Furthermore, Frayn suggests that improper assessment, failure to recognize vulnerability of patients, and to evaluate ego strength can be therapist errors that influence drop-out from treatment.

In a review of negative effects of psychotherapy, Crown (1983) suggests that harmful impacts on spouses or children may occur, especially if the psychotherapist excludes involvement of spouses or family. Crown attributes negative effects to the personality of therapist and to technique. Poor insight, emotional insecurity, and psychopathology in therapists may lead to negative results. Excessive rigidity of technique, incomplete assessment, improper selection of treatment, invalidation of the patient, and inadequate training are all examples of error which lead to poor outcome, and occasionally to worsening of symptoms.

Cost-Effectiveness

Cost-effectiveness must be taken into consideration for clinical practice guidelines to be relevant and valid. However, the current status of models of cost-effectiveness that are available to us in medicine are not fully refined. There is no empirically tested consensus about the right way to do cost-effective studies in psychiatry. Frank (1993) states that few existing studies of psychotherapy indicate that treatments are cost-effective. However, as most treatments have not been studied, Frank warns of the risk of falsely rejecting cost-effective treatments that have not been studied. He states that, should clinical-practice guidelines or government positions endorse paying only for cost-effective treatments, certain effective treatments would be unavailable to patients. In reviewing cost-effectiveness studies of psychotherapy, Gabbard, Lazar, Hornberger, and Spiegel (1997) found that, in 80 per cent of clinical studies with random assignment and 100 per cent of studies without random assignment, psychotherapy reduced the total cost of the disorder studied.

References

American Psychiatric Association (APA). (1993a). Practice guidelines for eating disorders. *American Journal of Psychiatry, 150,* 207–228.

American Psychiatric Association (APA). (1993b). Practice guideline for major depressive disorder in adults. *American Journal of Psychiatry, 150* (Suppl., 4), 1–26.

American Psychiatric Association (APA). (1994a). *Diagnostic and statistical manual of mental disorders* (4th ed.). Washington, DC: Author.

American Psychiatric Association (APA). (1994b). Practice guideline for the treatment of patients with bipolar disorder. *American Journal of Psychiatry, 151* (Suppl., 12), 1–36.

American Psychiatric Association (APA). (1995a). Practice guideline for psychiatric evaluation of adults. *American Journal of Psychiatry, 152* (Suppl., 11), 65–80.

American Psychiatric Association (APA). (1995b). Practice guideline for the treatment of patients with substance use disorders: Alcohol, cocaine, opioids. *American Journal of Psychiatry, 152* (Suppl., 11), 1–59.

American Psychiatric Association (APA). (1996). Memories of sexual abuse, [on line] Available: www.psych.org/public_info/MEMOR~1.MTM [1996, Jan. 1]

Blackshaw, S., Chandarana, P., Garneau, Y., Merskey, H., & Moscarello, R. (1996). Position statement: Adult recovered memories of childhood sexual abuse. *Canadian Journal of Psychiatry, 41,* 305–306.

Canadian Medical Association (CMA). (1994a). CMA policy summary: The patient–physician relationship and the sexual abuse of patients. *Canadian Medical Association Journal, 150,* 1884A–1884F.

Canadian Medical Association (CMA). (1994b). *Guidelines for Canadian clinical practice guidelines.* Ottawa: Author.

Canadian Psychiatric Association (CPA). (No date). Position statement on sexual misconduct [on line] Available: cpa.medical.org/cpa/public2/papers/position.papers/estat16.htm [1997, Nov. 18]

Clarkin, J.F., Frances, A.J. & Perry, S.W. (1995). The psychosocial treatments. In R. Michels (Chairman, Editorial Board), *Psychiatry.* Philadelphia: Lippincott.

Crown, S. (1983). Contraindications of psychotherapy. *British Journal of Psychiatry, 143,* 436–441.

Dempsey, L., & Eccles, J. (1994, November). Understanding the dating guidelines. The College of Physicians and Surgeons of Ontario, *Members' Dialogue,* 9–11.

Fox, R.D. (1993). The foundations of the Maintenance of Competence Program. *Royal College of Physicians and Surgeons of Canada Annals, S28.*

Frank, R.G. (1993) Cost–benefit evaluations in mental health: Implications for financing policy. *Advances in Health Economics and Health Services Research, 14,* 1–16.

Frayn, D. (1992) Assessment factors associated with premature psychotherapy terminations. *American Journal of Psychotherapy, 46,* 250–261.

Gabbard, G.O., Lazar, S.G., Hornberger, J. & Spiegel, D. (1997). The economic impact of psychotherapy: A review. *American Journal of Psychiatry, 154,* 147–155.

Gabbard, G.O., & Lester, E.P. (1995). *Boundaries and boundary violations in psychoanalysis.* New York: Basic.

Gedo, J. (1993). In impasse and innovation. In J.E. Gedo & M.J. Gehrie (Eds.), *Psychoanalysis: Clinical case seminars* (p. 286). Hillsdale, NJ: The Analytic Press.

Gray, S.H. (1996). Developing practice guidelines for psychoanalysis. *Journal of Psychotherapy Practice and Research, 5,* 213–227.

Gutheil, T.G., & Gabbard, G.O. (1993). The concept of boundaries in clinical practice: Theoretical and risk-management dimensions. *American Journal of Psychiatry, 150,* 188–196.

Hadley, S.W., & Strupp, H.H. (1976). Contemporary views of negative effects in psychotherapy. *Archives of General Psychiatry, 33,* 1291–1303.

Henry, W.P., Schacht, T.E., & Strupp H.H. (1986) Structural analysis of social behavior: Application to a study of interpersonal process in differential psychotherapeutic outcome. *Journal of Consulting and Clinical Psychology, 54,* 27–31.

Henry, W.P., Schacht, T.E., & Strupp, H.H. (1990) Patient and therapist introject, interpersonal process, and differential psychotherapy outcome. *Journal of Consulting and Clinical Psychology, 58,* 768–774.

Joint Task Force on Standards for Medical (Psychiatric) Psychotherapy. (1995). *A report to Council of the Ontario Psychiatric Association and to Executive of the Section on Psychiatry, Ontario Medical Association, on the definition, guidelines and standards for medical (psychiatric) psychotherapy.* Toronto: Author.

Katz, P. (1986). The role of the psychotherapies in the practice of psychiatry: The position of the Canadian Psychiatric Association. *Canadian Journal of Psychiatry, 31,* 458–465.

Kessel, P., & McBrearty, J.F. (1967). Values and psychotherapy: A review of the literature. *Perceptual Motor Skills, 25,* 669–690.

Luborsky, L., McLellan, A.T., Woody, G.E., O'Brien, C.P., & Amelbach, A. (1985). Therapist success and its determinants. *Archives of General Psychiatry, 42,* 602–611.

McPhedran, M. (Chairperson). (1991, 25 November). *The final report: Task Force on Sexual Abuse of Patients.* An independent task force commissioned by the College of Physicians and Surgeons of Ontario.

Mumford, E., Schlesinger, H.J., Glass, G.V., Patrick, C., & Cuerdon, T. (1984). A new look at evidence about reduced cost of medical utilization following mental health treatment. *American Journal of Psychiatry, 141,* 1145–1158.

Ontario Medical Association (OMA). (1992, September). Section on Psychiatry position statement. *Ontario Medical Review,* 17–24.

Ontario Medical Association (OMA). (1994, November). *Physicians' guide to third-party and other uninsured services.* Toronto: Author.

Rakoff, V., Sigal, J., & Epstein, N. (1975). Predictions of therapeutic process and progress in conjoint family therapy. *Archives of General Psychiatry, 32,* 1013.

Safran, J.D. (1993). Breaches in the therapeutic alliance: An arena for negotiating authentic relatedness. *Psychotherapy, 30,* 11–24.

Tapper, C.M. (1994). Position paper: Unilateral termination of treatment by a psychiatrist. *Canadian Journal of Psychiatry, 39,* 2–3.

Truax, C.B., Wargo, D.G., Frank, J.D. Imber, S.D., Battle, G.C., Hoehm-Sanic, R., Nash, E.H., & Stone, A.R. (1966). The therapist's contribution to accurate empathy, non-possessive warmth, and genuineness in psychotherapy. *Journal of Clinical Psychology, 22,* 331–334.

3. Guidelines for the Practice of Individual Psychodynamic Psychotherapy

Norman Doidge and Ray Freebury

Individual psychodynamic psychotherapy is based on principles derived from psychoanalytic theory and practice. Other terms for this form of treatment include 'psychoanalytic psychotherapy,' 'insight-oriented psychotherapy,' 'uncovering psychotherapy,' and 'expressive–supportive psychotherapy.' Individual psychodynamic psychotherapy is the form most frequently practised by psychiatrists in North America (Luborsky, Docherty, Barber, & Miller, 1993). This form of treatment can be used alone or together with other treatments, including medication and conjoint psychotherapies (Gabbard, 1994). The guidelines described here frequently make reference, for empirical support, to chapter 4, 'Empirical Evidence for the Core Clinical Concepts and Efficacy of the Psychoanalytic Psychotherapies: An Overview.'

Rationale for Prescribing Individual Forms of Psychodynamic Psychotherapy

Psychoanalytic psychotherapy is a broad-spectrum treatment for a number of disorders. Originally developed by Freud as a treatment for individuals, it gave rise to techniques that can be used with groups, couples, and families. It is prescribed as treatment for an *individual* when the clinician has reason to believe that:

1 the origins of the difficulties that bring a patient to treatment are sufficiently specific to warrant detailed exploration and tailor-made interventions that cannot occur in group settings;
2 the nature of the patient's difficulties are based, in significant part,

upon psychic conflicts that ward off unconscious affects, memories, fantasies, wishes, and thoughts that result in intense shame, guilt, or anxiety. A patient often feels able to discuss such distressing material only with a single clinician who has earned his or her trust, in an atmosphere of privacy and confidentiality;

3 the dyadic, or interpersonal, component of individual treatment is needed to promote the therapeutic process and provide opportunities to relearn and change relationships, and cognitive, affective, and defensive patterns, and undo developmental inhibitions – a process called 'working through.'

Tailoring Treatment to Individual Patients

Individual psychotherapy is tailored to the individual at several levels:

1 At a micro level, within treatment sessions, the content, timing, and form of the clinician's interventions are geared to the patient's individual psychodynamic formulation and current state of mind, which includes current activated affects, defences, and transferences. This level of tailoring is too specific to be dealt with in general guidelines.
2 For each level of psychiatric disorder or disability, clinicians tailor the dose and frequency of sessions and the frame of treatment, usually at the outset of treatment, modifying them as clinical conditions change.
3 At the level of the patient's ego functions (Gabbard, 1994), the clinician may tailor treatment by titrating the balance of insight-oriented interventions that aim to facilitate the patient's self-reflective capacities and supportive measures that can ready the patient for insight-oriented interventions. This level of tailoring is often decided on at the start of treatment and modified within sessions.

General Theoretical Concepts

Common to all psychoanalytic theory is the assumption that we, as psychological beings, have specific genetic constitutions, developmental histories, and unique internal or imaginative responses to external events. Many of these internal responses become part of unconscious thought patterns, which, along with conscious thought, influence the person and his or her symptoms.

In cases of psychopathology, a patient's developmental history may be inhibited, fixated, or arrested. Since Freud's (1905/1953) early work on development suggested that children's passionate attachments unfold in a developmental sequence, psychoanalytic theories have explored various aspects of childhood development, including the formation of mental representations of the external world, and cognitive and affective development. Pine (1988) has reviewed four broad categories in which current developmental theories can be classified. These points of view are artificially separated for heuristic reasons. In practice they are interwoven and interdependent.

a. *Drive theory:* This considers the individual in terms of innate instinctual drives that are our evolutionary endowment and are represented in conscious and unconscious fantasies. These drives include sexual reproductive, affiliative, self-preservative, and aggressive instincts. Drives can be deferred, channelled, blocked, or opposed by other drives, and these modified expressions are necessary from time to time as individuals interact with others or try to control themselves. The process produces ongoing intrapsychic conflicts between instinctual desires and reality, or between instinctual desires and conscience. Freud's studies of infantile drives have been corroborated and expanded by Roiphe and Galenson (1981), and Weil (1989a, 1989b). Bowlby (1980) has studied the ethological and instinctual components of human attachment. Freud argued that instinctual drives are experienced by the subject somatically in terms of pleasure and pain, and mentally as having a specific aim, which is to interact in a particular way with a human object.

b. *Ego-psychology theory:* This sees the individual in terms of the slow acquisition of the capacity for adaptation, reality testing, and defence (Blanck & Blanck, 1974, 1979). This aspect of psychoanalytic theory has incorporated developments in cognitive psychology to understand how the ego forms its particular psychological outlook (Wolff, 1960; Greenspan, 1979, 1981). An extremely important part of the ego is the unconscious superego, or unconscious conscience, which frequently contributes to symptoms and character formation (Freud, 1923/1961);

c. *Object-relations theory:* This group of theories views the individual as the carrier of an internal drama derived from childhood, in which he or she repeatedly lives out one or more childhood roles. Relationship patterns, which include self, object, and affect representations, are unconsciously encoded but can be altered in long-term therapy. These representations are a combination of the infant's subjective experience of external events, coloured by: his or her level of development at the time; defences, fantasies, memories; and biological constitution (Kernberg, 1988). When affective thresholds are altered by psychiatric illnesses of biological origin, these representations will be fundamentally altered.

d. *Self-development theory:* Empirical work by Mahler, Pine, and Bergmann (1975), Stern (1985), Greenspan (1979, 1981), Grunberger (1989), and others has shown that the sense of self develops largely in the context of interpersonal relationships. Mahler et al (1975) have shown that this is a gradual process, leading to the formation of boundaries of the self and achievement of self-constancy. The work of Kohut (1971) on narcissistic personality disorders, which led to the development of self-psychology, traces how certain deficiencies in early caretaking can influence the development of the self and self-esteem. The priority of the theory is the experience of the self by the patient in terms of cohesiveness, solidness, and needs for certain functions from others, including the analyst. These functions are described as self–object functions. The major self–object needs of patients are classified as follows: idealizing, mirroring, adversarial, and efficacy.

These four theories attempt to relate how external events, including traumatic ones, are given meaning by the subject. Freud, with Breuer, first coined the term 'psychic trauma' (Freud, 1910/1957), attempting to understand the impact of traumatic events on patients, as influenced by the child's mind and particular phase of development. The fact that many patients have experienced childhood trauma does not mean that such trauma is *always* present in people who develop neurotic conditions.

Clinical Concepts and Techniques

While clinicians may differ in the mix of developmental theory they use to gain insight into patients, mainstream psychodynamic psychotherapists employ the following fundamental concepts and techniques:

a. *Free association:* Referred to as the 'fundamental' or the 'basic' rule, it underlies all expressive–supportive therapies. In a non-judgmental, neutral climate (technical neutrality), the patient is encouraged to speak freely of whatever comes to mind, in order to make conscious painful emotions, thoughts, memories, and wishes that have been kept out of awareness, but have contributed to symptoms or character difficulties. There is a movement from highly abstract, planned thought, with logical connections, towards more personal, concrete, emotionally laden language, and, at times, dream-like images. The therapist's non-judgmental listening is a therapeutic manoeuvre to promote free association (Kris, 1991). Asking patients to free-associate to thoughts and feelings before acting on them facilitates self-reflection, but does not mean that the goal of treatment is for people never to act or make judgments. Rather, it means that therapy aims to encourage patients to explore the full range of their thoughts, as a tactic to help undermine pathological adaptations, symptoms, or inhibitions. There is empirical evidence that progress in treatment correlates with the increased use of less-guarded, less-abstract, more emotionally laden language (Fretter, Bucci, Broitman, Silberschatz, & Curtis, 1994).

b. *Transference:* Transference is the universal *unconscious* tendency to transfer scenes from the past onto the present, often in the hope of re-experiencing scenes or people from the past, or in the hope of gaining satisfaction where one had formerly failed (Freud, 1910/1957). Transference occurs to varying degrees in all human relationships and is not confined to therapeutic relationships (Freud, 1912/1958). Transference is a subjective mental experience, coloured by the past, that does not accurately match the current scene, and hence seems distorted or inappropriate in quality or intensity to an objective observer (Greenson, 1967). Patients who are significantly disturbed can transfer aspects of themselves, or their own wishes, onto other people in a situation called part–object transference' (Kernberg, Selzer, Koenigsberg, Carr, & Appelbaum, 1989). The maladaptive consequence of transference is that it can engender a compulsion to repeat. The adaptive consequence lies in the extent to which transference reflects an urge to master the past (Roth, 1987).

In expressive–supportive psychotherapy, with sessions as infrequent as once weekly, after eight or nine months the transference can assume a quality in which the patient may no longer dispute the unreality of the perceptions and affects associated with it. This is the 'transference neurosis,' in which the patient's difficulties take on a new meaning in relation to the therapist (Roth, 1987). The transference now lends itself to more effective interpretation. Transference has been extensively studied empirically and can be reliably rated. In successful therapies, more adaptive responses occur as transferences are made conscious.

c. *Countertransference:* The therapist can, in response to the patient's transference, especially if it is intense, become involved in the transference scene, and have his or her own transferences in response. These responses, called 'countertransference,' if unrecognized, unacknowledged, or unanalysed, may render therapeutic efforts ineffective. For this reason, many psychotherapists undertake personal therapy or personal analysis. Countertransference can, when properly harnessed and analysed, provide invaluable information about the patient's transference.

d. *The unconscious and the defences:* Psychoanalytic theory assumes that behaviour is frequently determined by factors that lie outside conscious awareness and are kept out of awareness because they are disturbing or conflict with other wishes. The unconscious consists of the preconscious, to which attention can be drawn by a simple change of focus, and the unconscious proper, which consists of mental contents that are censored because they are unacceptable and resist efforts at being made conscious. The contents of the unconscious appear in dreams or may find expression through parapraxes (forgetting important events, slips of the tongue, etc.). Empirical evidence for the unconscious mind is currently illustrated by subliminal experiments and studies of defences that ward off painful thoughts. Shevrin and Bond (1993) describe the current empirical approach to this area, and Perry (1993) has reviewed the empirical data on defences. Mature defences correlate longitudinally with mental health, immature ones with mental illness.

e. *Resistance:* Resistance can be defined as a defence against insight, either cognitive or emotional, or defensive activity that interferes with the therapeutic process. It is an effort by the patient to preserve the status quo, to resist giving up defensive compromises that represent attempts to deal with the painful affects associated with previous experiences. The therapist aims to understand and interpret resistance rather than proscribe it at the expressive end of the continuum. At the supportive end of the therapeutic continuum, defences associated with resistance can sometimes be reinforced. Graff and Luborsky (1977) found that, in successful psychoanalyses, levels of both transference and resistance were high in the early phases. In mid-phase, transference stabilized and resistance ratings fell. In unsuccessful analyses, resistance ratings did not fall. Resistance may show itself as subtle cognitive disturbances or forgetfulness during sessions (Luborsky, 1993a). These studies show a statistically significant activation of transference and conflict themes in forgetting versus control segments. Resistance can also decrease following interventions that do not confirm unconscious fears (Fretter et al, 1994).

f. *The therapeutic alliance and transference interpretation:* The concept of therapeutic alliance derives from Freud's notion that rapport is required to conduct psychoanalysis and psychodynamic psychotherapy. The specific techniques for developing it are outlined by Greenson (1967). A meta-analysis by Luborsky, Crits-Christoph, Mintz, and Auerbach (1988) shows that the greater the alliance, as measured by operationalized measures, the better the outcome. Alliance measures include items that ask whether the patient believes the therapist is helping, understanding, and dependable; wants the patient to achieve goals; and collaborates. When maladaptive transference patterns are clarified, the therapeutic alliance frequently improves (Luborsky, 1993b).

(See chapter 4, 'Empirical Evidence for the Core Clinical Concepts and Efficacy of the Psychoanalytic Psychotherapies: An Overview,' for an overview of the empirical studies of free association, transference, the unconscious, defences, resistance, and the therapeutic alliance.)

Clinical Interventions

Clinical interventions come under a number of categories along an expressive–supportive continuum (see Gabbard, 1994; Kris, 1991; Greenson, 1967):

a. *Interpretation:* An explanatory statement that links a feeling, thought, symptom, or behaviour to its unconscious meaning. Analysis of transference and defence or conflict occurs through interpretation. There is empirical evidence (Crits-Christoph, Barber, Baranackie, & Cooper, 1993) that accurate interpretation of transference conflicts correlates with improved outcomes (see chapter 4).
b. *Confrontation:* This involves bringing together two different aspects of the patient's mental experience or behaviour that seem to be connected but have not yet been consciously linked by the patient (Greenson, 1967). The confrontation is not between the patient and the clinician, but, rather, is a case of the clinician addressing things that the patient does not want to accept or would rather avoid confronting in him- or herself. The therapist clearly identifies the issues being avoided, without being too blunt or aggressive. This step often precedes interpretation.
c. *Clarification:* This means rephrasing the patient's words in order to convey a more coherent view of the material being communicated, or asking questions to get more clinical information (Greenson, 1967).

d. *Encouragement to elaborate:* By showing interest or by direct questions, the therapist may invite more information about a patient's thoughts, feelings, wishes, and memories.

e. *Empathic validation:* This is a therapist's empathic attunement with the patient's internal state, demonstrated by understanding or elaborating on the patient's communications through clarification and interpretation, or by non-verbal means. Empathy in psychodynamic psychotherapy requires that the therapist attempt to empathize with the patient's conscious *and* unconscious thoughts, affects, and wishes to help patients integrate warded-off material.

Interventions at the supportive end of the continuum (described in detail by Rockland [1989] include:

f. *Advice and praise:* This refers to direct suggestions about ways to behave, or the reinforcement of adaptive behaviours by direct approval. As this intervention may undermine the atmosphere of technical neutrality, it must be used with care in a manner consistent with expressive techniques. Patients must feel free to reveal to the clinician a variety of behaviours, not only praiseworthy ones. Since clinicians are trained to be experts in the treatment of psychopathology, any advice or praise they offer should generally be confined to that area of expertise. Thus, it may be appropriate to give praise to someone who does not realize that he or she has broken through an important threshold or inhibition. But it is inappropriate to laud patients' tastes just because they parallel the clinician's views on art, politics, sociology, economics, music, or other matters. The same restriction applies to advice, which should always be confined to areas relevant to the patient's psychopathology. Thus, it might be appropriate to tell a patient to visit a doctor he or she was avoiding because of denial, despite symptoms that signalled an emerging, treatable condition. But it would be outside the therapeutic mandate to give a patient advice on non-therapeutic areas, such as the stock market, religious matters, politics, or business.

g. *Affirmation:* This entails simple supportive comments that encourage patients to continue.

h. *Limit-setting:* Here a potentially life-threatening or treatment-threatening behaviour (e.g., destroying the therapist's office, refusing to speak for many sessions, multiple missed sessions) is forbidden by the therapist, and the patient is asked to discuss the urges rather than act on them (Rockland, 1989; Kernberg et al, 1989). The goal of these limits is to preserve life and to facilitate therapeutic resolution of difficulties.

This list does not exhaust all the psychoanalytic interventions, some of which have been classified in other ways (Wallerstein, 1986). Many common techniques, such as providing an opportunity for catharsis, can be both supportive and expressive.   ·

All psychodynamic psychotherapies belong to what has been called the *expressive–supportive continuum* (Gabbard, 1994). Individual psychotherapy invariably contains both expressive (insight-oriented) and supportive elements, with one or the other predominating, depending on the clinical picture at any given stage of treatment. Clinical interventions at both ends of the continuum contribute to good outcomes (Wallerstein, 1986; Luborsky, 1993b). When working at the expressive end of the continuum, therapists seek to maximize the patients' ability to self-reflect and, ultimately, achieve mature autonomy by helping patients to understand behaviours, thoughts, and feelings, and to decide for themselves how to direct them. When working at the supportive end, the therapist seeks to support the patient in some way compatible with mature dependence. However, all major textbooks (e.g., Greenson, 1967; Gabbard, 1994) point out the distinguishing aspect of psychodynamic treatment as an accurate interpretation of unconscious phenomena. When clinicians choose to move to a supportive treatment and deviate from technical neutrality, they must be mindful of both the gains and the potential losses of the ability to analyse (Warme, 1994). Thus, in general, if a patient with intact reality testing were working at the expressive (insight-oriented) end of the continuum and asked for advice (which might be given in supportive psychodynamic psychotherapy) on a matter that he or she was capable of dealing with independently, it would be clinically sound to help the patient analyse the doubts and understand the longing for advice. Ultimately, it would be more beneficial for that patient to have learned to make such decisions. For patients with severe mental disorders, however, therapists might appropriately give advice on occasion. When working with severely disturbed patients with borderline personalities, it is often helpful to order hierarchically the issues to be dealt with, distinguishing those that threaten life from those that threaten treatment, or are less threatening (Kernberg et al, 1989).

It is critical to distinguish 'support in psychotherapy' from supportive psychotherapy (Rockland, 1989). In the former, the principle of choice between supportive and expressive interventions is often summarized as: 'Be as expressive as you can be, and as supportive as you have to be' (Wallerstein, 1986, p. 688). In this case, even supportive interventions are used in a way that takes into account the need to facilitate, preserve, or improve the therapeutic frame (see below) and not permanently undermine future free association or technical neutrality. In the case of pure supportive psychotherapy, the principal goal may be to support a patient's ego functions, and the psychodynamic formulation will help the clinician to understand what to support and when. It is helpful to distinguish between the clinician's intention and the outcome of an intervention. For instance, advice that is ill-founded may turn out to be especially non-supportive. Some of the expressive measures, such as accurate interpretations, may be experienced as quite supportive. In expressive–supportive psychotherapy, many supportive manoeuvres can be analysed or interpreted after the fact so that the patient understands their impact.

How Does Change or Benefit Occur?

Change in psychodynamic psychotherapy occurs in many ways. Luborsky's recent review of the empirical literature concludes that 'the main curative factors in dynamic psychotherapy come about through working toward three changes: achieving a helping relationship, achieving understanding and incorporating the gains of treatment. Each is fostered by the technical ability of the therapist' (Luborsky, 1993b, p. 519). The importance of the therapeutic alliance was underscored. Empirical studies of changes in the Core Conflictual Relationships Theme (CCRT) treatment, brought about by accurate interpretation, show that, as the unconscious is made conscious, aspects of the CCRT are altered. Luborsky and Crits-Christoph (1990), studying medium-length treatments, have shown that, while the wishes do not alter, how the patient reacts to them alters significantly. Weiss, Sampson, and the Mount Zion Psychotherapy Research Group (1986) have developed a measure of transference that accurately measures not just particular transference images, but also how the patient seeks to put the entire transference plan into effect, in an attempt to repeat and possibly disconfirm the pathogenic beliefs behind it.

While the therapist's understanding of patients correlates with patient progress, it is by no means the only factor, and patient insight has no simple one-to-one correlation with outcomes. Luborsky (1993b) found that early insight correlates with good outcomes. But the psychoanalytic notion of insight contains both cognitive and affective components.

Indeed, it has been argued that many curative factors operate at an unconscious level (Strachey, 1934). Loewald (1960) showed that positive identification with the therapist is formed slowly. Instruments to measure how patients identify with therapists have been reviewed by Orlinsky and Geller (1993). Another aspect of psychoanalytic treatment is the interpretation of maladaptive defences. Preliminary evidence suggests that, as therapy progresses, patients start to use more mature defences. Follow-up studies show that patients develop an analysing ability and can reflect upon themselves with critical distance (Schlesinger & Robbins, 1975, 1983).

The therapeutic alliance (which some see as an effect of positive transference, and others see as separate from it) permits the transference relationship and eventually, in most cases, a transference neurosis. The therapist's understanding of the emerging transference is conveyed to the patient at the most propitious time. This interpretation enables the patient to appreciate repeated patterns of maladaptive behaviour and the basis on which they occur. It is only through repeated experience – through continual discovery, rediscovery, and working through – that permanent change is likely to occur.

Indications for Psychodynamic Psychotherapy

This form of treatment can be beneficial only if the caregiver understands how the patient's personality affects his or her participation in the treatment process, an understanding fundamental for collaborative treatment relationships (Kahana & Bibring, 1964). This is equally essential for mental illnesses generally considered to have an underlying biological component. For example, in schizophrenics, grandiose delusions or hallucinations frequently follow an insult to the patient's self-esteem (Garfield, 1985).

The prescription of psychotherapy is determined by several factors, including perceived etiology, diagnosis, personality, onset and duration of symptoms, and aberrant behaviour, as well as the strengths and weaknesses of the patient (Wallace, 1983; Ursano, Sonnenberg, & Lazar, 1991). Thus far, the best guideline is that shorter treatments are best for focal conflicts that may involve working with one transference paradigm. Longer-term, higher-frequency modalities of up to several times a week or psychoanalysis is indicated as the need to analyse diffuse disorders, multiple transference paradigms, or pathology of early onset increases.

Consensus-based guidelines as described by Gray (1996) are based on the prevailing practices of experienced clinicians, and acknowledge the complexity of the individual patient. While there are a number of outcome studies of psychoanalytic psychotherapy (see chapter 4), outcome-based research does not provide sufficient detail to replace practice guidelines. Some of the limits on using outcome-based research for guidelines for individual psychotherapy include: (1) important subject-matter, which will relate to the patient's outcome, cannot be articulated by the patient at the onset of treatment because it is warded off, and it may be left out of the baseline history; (2) outcomes are unique and specific to each individual case in individual psychodynamic psychotherapies, but the research is less specific; (3) the funding environment for research has tended to neglect inquiry into the very long-term effects of therapies.

At this time, we recommend the general guidelines for psychoanalysis and psychoanalytic therapy endorsed by both the American Psychiatric Association and the American Psychoanalytic Association.

The American Psychiatric Association's (APA) *Peer Review Guidelines for Psychoanalysis* (1985) has provided a sophisticated decision tree not only for psychoanalysis, but also for the psychodynamic psychotherapies. These complex but clinically sensitive guidelines take into account etiology, type of disorder, and patient's ability to use treatment according to ego function. Table 3.1 summarizes the criteria that must be satisfied before psychoanalysis can be indicated. Table 3.2 also contains information for determining the choice of long-term or briefer forms of psychodynamic psychotherapy.

The APA's *Peer Review Guidelines for Psychoanalysis* and a number of key texts (e.g., Gabbard, 1994; Blanck & Blanck, 1974; Bachrach & Leaff, 1978) provide guidelines for determining the choice of psychodynamic psychotherapies and psychoanalysis. These criteria enable us to make appropriate differential treatment choices. These choices will be further refined by other factors. The following are a few examples of how these criteria are useful in choosing various forms of individual psychodynamic psychotherapy or psychoanalysis.

- Patients who qualify for criterion A (i.e., that the symptoms are based on chronic intrapsychic conflict) but not criterion B (i.e., the patient has no inhibitions, fixation, or deviations of development). If there is reason to believe that the intrapsychic conflicts are focal, a trial of psychodynamic psychotherapy might be indicated and the therapist may reasonably believe that high-dose psychoanalysis is not necessary. These conflicts must be fairly close to consciousness, as in patients

Table 3.1: American Psychiatric Association Peer Review Indications for Psychoanalysis

---

Psychoanalysis is the treatment of choice for repetitive, long-standing, maladaptive problems involving personality or character, and chronic, repetitive behavioural, affective or mental disturbances or symptoms that do not respond to cheaper, or quicker, forms of treatment. Generally, it is used for all the character disorders or personality disorders except the antisocial and schizotypal disorders, as well as numerous symptom disorders, discussed below. Terms not familiar to the reader are defined in the *American Psychiatric Association Peer Review Manual*, 3d ed. (1985), published by the American Psychiatric Association, Washington, DC.

Primary Indicators for Psychoanalysis

Psychoanalysis is indicated
  I. For each *DSM* category for whom A and B [below] are true:
      A. Chronic symptoms, predominantly reflecting intrapsychic conflict, are present.
      B. Chronic symptoms reflecting partial or complete inhibition of development, developmental fixation, or arrest.
AND
  II. For whom a qualifying indicator for psychoanalysis C or D or E [below] is true:
      C. Chronic symptoms will not respond, or will worsen, or development will not proceed with other treatment methods, e.g., chronic symptoms either embedded in rigid character structure or occurring in the presence of fragile or brittle defences whose failure would be threatening to the patient; or
      D. Relief of chronic symptoms is achievable with other treatment only at excessive personal or social cost (e.g., risk of chronic dependency upon anti-anxiety medication, when prescribed in proper dosage; or retreat to a self-depreciating job to avoid mastering anxiety through understanding); or
      E. Temporary relief, particularly of acute symptoms related to current stress, may be obtained with other treatment methods; however, the presenting chronic symptom (or other equivalent disability) is likely to recur.
AND
  III. For those patients who fulfil Criteria for Analysability, which include the capacity to form, maintain, and eventually to relinquish a therapeutic relationship with particular reference to the following that have not be explicitly covered in I and II above. The psychological strengths and weaknesses of the patient must be taken into consideration in the final choice of treatment.
      The following list of factors correlates with increased analysability, and better prognosis. Not all of the factors need be present or weighted equally. When prescribing psychoanalysis, for instance, since the treatment goes on without non-verbal feedback from the analyst, the ego strength of reality testing must be present. Other factors, such as the presence of early trauma, are not contraindications, and indeed a large number of analytic patients have experienced trauma. Such factors are on this list because, as the level of early trauma rises in intensity and quality, the likelihood of being analysable tends to decrease:

• Stable current and prospective life situations providing possibilities for change. (This is necessary because this is a long-term treatment, and requires that the patient be in a position to maintain the treatment.)

Table 3.1: (*Concluded*)

- Evidence of successful social functioning and the ability to use intellect, e.g., in school, on job.
- An adequate ability to communicate verbally.
- Adequate capacity for introspection and with the possibility of access to fantasy life.
- Adequate tolerance for anxiety, frustration, depression, and adequate impulse control.
- Adequate potential for sublimation.
- Capacity to tolerate and to utilize therapeutic regression – ability to alternately experience and observe self.
- Internal object constancy (i.e., some sense of self and others as stable over time).
- Adequate capacity for self–object differentiation and high level of reality testing.
- Ability to form reciprocal as well as nurturant object relationships.
- Relative absence of significant early trauma.

AND

IV. Patients for whom a dynamic formulation is presented that makes use of data from the analyst's history, interview, assessment of current psychological function, and the analyst's empathetic response to these. The formulation should reflect the documentation of I, II, and III, using the following categories: (1) History; (2) Assessment of Current Psychological Functioning (Including Mental Status); and (3) Quality of Interaction.

Source: Adapted from APA, 1985

with a fairly good level of premorbid functioning who have experienced recent stressors or changes that expose underlying conflicts or exacerbate symptoms. These treatments tend to be short (including those with patients receiving psychoanalytically oriented crisis intervention) or medium length.

- Patients who meet criteria A (chronic intrapsychic conflict) and B (chronic symptoms reflecting inhibited, arrested, fixated, or deviant development) and C or D or E, but who do not meet the criteria of analysability. An assessment of ego strengths (table 3.1, section III) is required to help determine which patients have insufficient ability to tolerate regression, to observe themselves, or to test reality. Such patients may reach a point at which it is advisable to convert their therapy to analysis. In practice, this group represents a large number of patients, and treatment is often long-term.
- Patients who meet the criteria for psychoanalysis but for whom psychodynamic psychotherapy is indicated include those who do not have stable-enough living arrangements to make it possible or who lack the motivation for psychoanalysis.
- Psychodynamic psychotherapy with supportive elements may be indicated for patients who have had good premorbid functioning and in whom a recent trauma has exposed chronic symptoms reflect-

Table 3.2: Some Examples of the Border between Psychoanalysis and Psychodynamic Psychotherapy

Conflict	Inhibited Development	C or D or E*	Analysable	Psychosis	Treatment	Selected Examples of Some Disorders Typical for this Category
Chronic	True	True	++	No	Psychoanalysis, good prognosis	Obsessive–compulsive personality disorder and dysthymia; Mixed personality disorder, anxiety NOS, sexual dysfunction; Avoidant personality disorder with intimate relational difficulties, special conditions for loving, based on unresolved childhood conflict
Chronic	True	True	+–	No	Psychoanalysis, less favourable prognosis	Narcissistic personality disorder; Borderline personality disorder with some impulse control
Chronic	True	True	–	No	Psychoanalysis with guarded prognosis	Borderline personality disorder, can tolerate non-verbal environment
Chronic	False	N/A	N/A	No	Psychodynamic psychotherapy, predominantly expressive, but with support	Recent-onset sexual dysfunction, dysthymia, post-traumatic anxiety following interpersonal trauma; Recent loss, with unresolved past losses

Table 3.2: (*Concluded*)

Conflict	Inhibited Development	C or D or E*	Analysable	Psychosis	Treatment	Selected Examples of Some Disorders Typical for this Category
Acute	False	N/A	N/A	Yes	Supportive psychodynamic psychotherapy	Bipolar patient, getting over mood episode, while on medication
				No		Anxiety NOS in a man whose daughter was recently in a disabling car accident
				No		Burn victim with Major Depression
None	True	N/A	–	No	Psychodynamic psychotherapy +/– CBT interventions	Certain paraphilias
Acute	N/A	N/A	N/A	No	Psychodynamic psychotherapy	Patient with good premorbid functioning with unresolved grief

*C, D, or E are explained in table 3.1. In brief:

C = chronic symptoms that will not respond, or will worsen, or development will not proceed with other treatment methods.
D = Relief of chronic symptoms is achievable with other treatment, only at excessive personal or social cost (e.g., risk of chronic dependency upon anti-anxiety medication, retreat into self-deprecating job to avoid mastering anxiety related to conflicts).
E = Temporary relief, particularly of acute symptoms related to current stress, may be obtained with other treatment methods; however, the presenting chronic symptom (or equivalent disability) is likely to recur.

Please note that the type of therapy may change as the patient's condition changes. For instance, a patient who was raised by a bipolar parent, and who had a traumatic childhood on account of the parent's illness, and then himself develops bipolar disease, may benefit from supportive psychodynamic psychotherapy during episodes, along with medication, and some more expressive work when well stabilized on medication. *The criterion of analysability (column 4) is more crucial in determining the treatment of choice than is the patient's diagnosis or disorder, or level of disability.* Thus, for example, some narcissistic patients may be analysable, and others not at all. At times, analysability has to be determined by a trial of psychoanalysis or psychoanalytic psychotherapy. The scientific literature describes numerous cases of seriously ill patients, who, because they are quite analysable, end up with a good outcome. Similarly, many patients who are less seriously ill may prove to be less analysable, owing to the configuration of their resistances to insight.

ing intrapsychic conflict or given rise to new symptoms, but not developmental inhibitions (i.e., don't meet criterion B). The length of these treatments varies according to the post-traumatic reaction and whether it is acute or has evolved into a chronic form.

- Patients who meet criteria A or B, and either C or D or E, but because of a co-morbid Axis I disorder (e.g., a psychotic disorder) may require a largely supportive treatment.

As can be seen from the guidelines included in table 3.1, the choice of the most appropriate psychoanalytic therapy requires a complex assessment of the patient's psychiatric or emotional disorder, the etiology of the disorder, the patient's ego strengths and weaknesses, and whether other treatments would likely give as good a result with less effort, and without causing harm or undue risk. Such an evaluation does not mean that less-intensive forms of therapy must always be attempted first, before undertaking analysis or another more intensive psychoanalytic psychotherapy, if it is likely that the less-intensive form would be insufficient, as this would drag out the patient's illness and suffering, and clearly waste resources. There are many cases in medicine where the first-line treatment is intensive.

Summary of Factors that Determine the Choice of Treatment

1 *Duration of symptoms or maladaptive behaviour:* If the psychopathology is chronic and there are signs of intrapsychic conflict or long-standing evidence of arrested development, deviant development, or maladaptive coping mechanisms, long-term psychodynamic psychotherapy or psychoanalysis is indicated. When the symptoms or atypical behaviour are recent and of brief duration, and if they were likely provoked by stressful psychological or environmental events, briefer forms of psychotherapy might be indicated. An example might be someone who previously functioned at a high level but suddenly became incapacitated after a stressful event.

2 *Severity of the illness:* Taken in conjunction with the nature of onset and the severity of the illness, the presence or absence of the aforementioned strengths (table 3.1, section III) can guide the psychotherapist in designing appropriate treatment for the patient (Freebury, 1986).

If the person has psychological strengths, and if the onset of severe symptoms is accompanied by precipitating stressors, brief expressive therapies are probably the best choice. In patients with severe, acute illnesses who reveal few strengths, the treatment of choice will be closer to the supportive end of the psychotherapeutic continuum and may require brief active intervention and pharmacotherapy. If the illness is severe and chronic, as in the case of repeated failures in work or intimate relationships, but the patient reveals several psychological strengths, a more expressive approach may be attempted, with increased frequency and longer sessions. Intensive long-term psychodynamic psychotherapy or psychoanalysis might be the best treatment.

Severe and chronic illnesses, in which failures in work or relationships have long since given way to withdrawal from relationships or any effort to work, and in which the patient has few psychological strengths, may call for supportive, possibly long-term psychotherapy. With mild illnesses, the treatment will most frequently be brief. It should be designed to complement the person's strengths and might focus on particular areas of difficulty, such as performance anxiety, or shore up weaknesses, as in the reinforcement of existing defences (Lowy, 1981).

3 *Multiple transference paradigms:* When there are multiple transference paradigms to be analysed, longer-term psychotherapies or psychoanalysis will be required.

Recommendations by Psychiatric Disorder

While the recommendation for psychodynamic psychotherapy is not based solely upon diagnosis or the disorder, certain disorders tend to do well in this form of treatment, and others poorly.

These guidelines are in agreement with *DSM-IV* (APA, 1994), acknowledging that the *DSM-IV* system is not the only diagnostic system in use, and that at times psychiatrists will treat conditions that are not well described in the manual or that are described well in other systems. As is stated in the *Diagnostic and Statistical Manual of Mental Disorders* (4th ed.) (APA, 1994), 'the specified diagnostic criteria for each mental disorder are offered as guidelines for making diagnoses, because it has been demonstrated that the use of such criteria enhances agreement among clinicians and investigators ... These diagnostic criteria ... reflect a consensus of current formulations of evolving knowledge in our field. They do not encompass, however, all the conditions for which people may be treated or that may be appropriate topics for research' (p. xxvii).

There are some disorders, such as bereavement (APA, 1994, V 62.82), in which psychiatric attention may be humane and helpful, although the patient may not meet other criteria. In keeping with the complexity of human psychopathology, the authors have introduced 'not otherwise specified (NOS)' categories in each area of diagnosis for patients suffering from a mental disorder who may not meet formal diagnostic criteria but do meet some of the criteria. Although the *DSM-IV* criteria list is not exhaustive, the majority of patients for whom this form of treatment is indicated qualify for *DSM-IV* disorders.

The empirical data on which the following guidelines are based are outlined in chapter 4, 'Empirical Evidence for the Core Clinical Concepts and Efficacy of the Psychoanalytic Psychotherapies: An Overview.' These guidelines are based upon a review of extensive published case histories and expert literature reviews (such as *Treatment of Psychiatric Disorders: The DSM-IV Edition* [Gabbard, 1995]), outcome studies, empirical studies of the types of patients psychodynamic clinicians treat, and a review of major psychodynamic psychotherapy texts. The disorders are listed according to the *DSM* categories, usually *DSM-IV*, but at times according to earlier *DSM* categories if the relevant studies were conducted when an earlier edition of *DSM* was in place.

AXIS I DISORDERS

1 *Psychoactive substance abuse:* In these conditions, psychotherapy is frequently a significant part of treatment.

2 *Psychotic disorders:* Supportive psychodynamic psychotherapy can be used, in conjunction with medication and family therapy. However, some will not, or for medical reasons cannot, take medication, and supportive psychodynamic psychotherapy can be used alone. Stanton, et al (1984) assigned non-chronic schizophrenics to either a more supportive or a more expressive psychodynamic psychotherapy, and found the supportive group did better in terms of recidivism and role performance, and the expressive group did better in terms of ego functioning and cognitive improvement. In general, these guidelines recommend a mixed approach that favours the supportive end of the continuum, but ventures into expressive measures at times if the patient's condition is stabilized.

3 *Mood disorders:* Most outcome studies of psychoanalysis or psychodynamic psychotherapy have included patients from this category, usu-

ally with dysthymia, but at times with other depressive disorders (see chapter 4). Interpersonal therapy, a modified form of psychodynamic psychotherapy, has been shown effective in relieving depression and in reducing recurrent episodes (Frank, Kupfer, & Perel, 1989). Psychotherapy is used in conjunction with antidepressant medication during acute phases of depression, but may be used alone for prophylactic reasons during remission. Patients with manic episodes often have difficulty using the treatment, but may benefit once settled.

4 *Anxiety disorders:* In a number of studies, including the Menninger (Wallerstein, 1986) and the Penn (Luborsky et al, 1988) studies, some patients with anxiety disorders improved in psychodynamic psychotherapy or psychoanalysis.

   a. *Post-traumatic stress disorders or related anxiety Not Otherwise Specified (NOS):* Patients with anxiety NOS may include those who do not quite meet the criteria for post-traumatic stress disorder. Psychodynamic psychotherapy, often with some support, is frequently used for these conditions.
   b. *Panic attacks:* These respond to pharmacotherapy in the short term. Cooper (1985) noted that some panic attacks are clearly triggered by psychophysiological or environmental events, and such patients may use characteristic defences. In such cases, psychotherapy can help to reduce or eliminate panic episodes (Milrod, Busch, Cooper, & Shapiro, 1997).
   c. *Phobias:* Zitrin, Klein, and Woener (1978) showed that, in combination with imipramine, both supportive psychotherapy and behaviour therapy were effective in 70–86 per cent of cases. There were no relapses in 83 per cent of cases at follow-up one year later. Simple phobias respond to psychodynamic psychotherapy, but in most instances may be more effectively treated with behavioural approaches.
   d. *Generalized anxiety disorder:* Medication is, at best, a short-term adjunct to psychotherapy. In the course of psychotherapy, patients must learn to tolerate anxiety as a meaningful signal of the need for adaptive responses to known stressors (Gabbard, 1994). Patients with this disorder improved in the Penn study of psychodynamic psychotherapy (Luborsky et al, 1988).

5 *Somatoform disorders:* Conversion disorders were among the first treated by psychoanalysis. This category also includes hypochondri-

asis. One of the expressive–supportive psychotherapies will be the treatment of choice in most cases.

6 *Dissociative disorders:* This includes patients who are diagnosed with multiple personality disorder (now called 'dissociative identity disorder'). Modified psychodynamic psychotherapy is used in these treatments, and many patients previously sexually abused or beaten as children are treated with this type of psychotherapy.

7 *Sexual and gender identity disorders:* This group includes:

a. *Sexual-dysfunction disorders.* Sexual-dysfunction disorders have a good prognosis and are quite prevalent in patients in psychoanalysis and psychotherapy (Wallerstein, 1986; Doidge, Simon, Gillies, & Ruskin, 1994). Underlying personality and psychological issues often become the focus of treatment.

b. *Paraphilias.* The paraphilias are generally difficult to treat, and most patients come to therapy as a result of coercion. Prospects for successful psychotherapy are best in those patients who continue to come for therapy after external pressures have been relaxed. As with sexual dysfunction, underlying personality disorders often become the focus of treatment and may bring some improvement. The prognosis is better for those with higher levels of personality organization who can tolerate some anxiety and frustration.

c. *Gender-identity disorders.* As with the paraphilias, underlying personality disorders often become the focus of treatment. Prognosis is best for those with higher levels of personality organization who can tolerate some anxiety and frustration.

8 *Eating disorders:* Psychotherapy is frequently a significant part of treatment, especially if personality factors are involved.

9 *Sleep disorders:* Insomnia is common in patients undergoing psychodynamic treatment and is usually related to psychic conflict. Psychoanalysis or psychodynamic psychotherapy is the treatment of choice for those sleep disorders that result from unresolved psychic conflict. Where abnormal sleep patterns appear to be learned, cognitive/behavioural approaches are helpful.

10 *Impulse disorders:* There are many case histories about treatments of gambling and kleptomania. Psychodynamic psychotherapy can be used if these problems exist together with other personality problems.

11 *Adjustment disorders:* Generally, briefer forms of psychodynamic psychotherapy are indicated.

AXIS II DISORDERS

Cluster-A Personality Disorders

1 *Paranoid personality disorder:* Although this disorder is difficult to treat, psychodynamic psychotherapy offers hope for change in selected cases.
2 *Schizoid and schizotypal personality disorder:* Individual psychodynamic psychotherapy, often in conjunction with group psychotherapy, offers the best hope of change. Patients with schizoid personality disorder may benefit from psychoanalysis (Guntrip, 1969).

Cluster-B Personality Disorders

1 *Borderline personality disorder:* Psychodynamic psychotherapy and modified psychoanalysis may be used in conjunction with other treatment modalities, including hospitalization, and family and group therapy (Kernberg, 1984).
2 *Narcissistic personality disorder:* Psychodynamic psychotherapy or psychoanalysis is the treatment of choice (Kohut, 1984; Kernberg, 1984).
3 *Histrionic personality disorder:* Psychodynamic psychotherapy or analysis is classically the treatment of choice for this disorder, formerly called 'hysterical personality disorder' (Gabbard, 1994; Gunderson, 1988).

Cluster C Personality Disorders

1 *Obsessive–compulsive personality disorder:* 'The preferred treatment of obsessive-compulsive personality disorder is usually a form of dynamic psychotherapy ... Psychoanalysis may be effective in bringing about a profound change in the defensive structure of some individuals' (Gunderson, 1988, p. 353; see also Salzman, 1985).
2 *Avoidant personality disorder:* Individual psychodynamic psychotherapy or psychoanalysis alone, or in combination with group psychotherapy, is the preferred treatment for this condition. Many of these patients are classified as schizoid in the psychoanalytic literature (Gabbard, 1994).
3 *Dependent personality disorder:* As with avoidant personality disorder, this is seldom used as a single diagnosis as the problem frequently occurs in conjunction with dysthymia, depression, or anxiety. Individ-

ual psychotherapy or psychoanalysis is the treatment of choice, depending upon the accompanying problem.

4 *Passive–aggressive personality disorder:* According to Gunderson (1988, p. 354), 'individual psychotherapy is generally considered the treatment of choice. Therapists must be ready to confront and interpret the patient's inevitable (conscious and unconscious) efforts to frustrate agreed-upon goals ... Short-term psychotherapy and group therapy are often sufficient for identifying, interpreting, and clarifying the reasons for the maladaptive aspects of passive aggressive behaviors. If the trait is broadly displayed, more extensive dynamically oriented therapies, including psychoanalysis, may be indicated. Behavioral therapy techniques directed at assertiveness training can be useful.'

Personality Disorders Not Otherwise Specified (NOS)

This category is for specific personality features that are of sufficient magnitude to lead to clinical impairment (e.g., personality disorder NOS with narcissistic and obsessional features). The treatment of this category depends on the predominant feature of the disorder. Psychoanalysts frequently treat a condition known as 'masochistic or depressive personality disorder' (or 'self-defeating personality') that, while not a *DSM-IV* disorder, includes people who are 'habitually bored by nice people' and attracted to 'abusive' people, and are rigid enough to have personality difficulties. (Or, they may fall under the depressive personality disorder in the *DSM-IV* appendix.) The masochistic personality or self-defeating traits have been extensively documented in psychoanalytic literature, and are frequently diagnosed in these patients (Doidge et al, 1994). For the treatment of masochistic or self-defeating disorders, 'dynamic therapies are often useful in helping to unravel the aggressive inhibitions, problems of self-esteem, and interpersonal needs of masochistic persons. Long-term exploratory therapies, including psychoanalysis, may be needed to uncover and provide perspective on the core issues' (Gunderson, 1988, p. 355).

Intensive forms of psychodynamic psychotherapy and psychoanalysis, which require a patient to be truthful, may also be contraindicated for certain Axis II disorders, for example, as an outpatient treatment for people with antisocial personality disorder and a history of lying. Some Axis I disorders such as bipolar disorders or schizophrenia do not respond to expressive supportive forms of psychotherapy alone. However, as noted, well-designed psychotherapy can be a useful adjunct to comprehensive treatment programs.

OTHER CONDITIONS THAT MAY BE A FOCUS OF
CLINICAL ATTENTION

Other disorders that qualify for psychodynamic psychotherapy or psychoanalysis include those that involve:

1 *Psychological factors affecting medical conditions:* Some personality traits or defensive styles affect medical conditions. These conditions may benefit from brief psychodynamic interventions, with consultation to help patients adapt to illness, understand stressors, or deal with psychological resistance to compliance with recommended treatments.

The *DSM-IV* V codes include an array of important conditions that may be the focus of clinical attention, including:

2 *Relational problems:* This new category involves interpersonal relationship problems that influence general medical conditions; parent–child relations; or work, partner, and sibling relations. Individual psychodynamic interventions can help patients discover how their defences, conflicts, and transferences cause distress to themselves and others.
3 *Problems related to abuse or neglect:* In this category, patients neglect or abuse another person sexually or physically. Often these people have themselves been abused or neglected as children and repeat the pattern in adulthood. Psychodynamic psychotherapy can help them work through the childhood trauma.
4 *Additional conditions that may be a focus of clinical attention:* Several other conditions may benefit from short-term intervention if they are not co-morbid, for instance, bereavement, and occupational, academic, identity, religious or spiritual, acculturation, and phase-of-life problems.

The Frame of Expressive–Supportive Psychoanalytic Therapies

The frame refers to the practical arrangements and technical aspects of psychotherapy, including (Kernberg, 1988):

1 *The duration, regularity, and frequency of sessions:* The most intensive

form of treatment, in terms of dose, is usually psychoanalysis, with frequent meetings in which the patient lies on a couch with the clinician seated behind and out of sight. In psychodynamic psychotherapies – other than psychoanalysis – sessions are less frequent and can be face-to-face, with both parties seated. Sometimes, a single interview based on psychodynamic principles can be therapeutic.

2 *The contractual arrangements:* This refers to the way financial arrangements are handled.

3 *The setting and the physical arrangements:* This includes the way in which the office and waiting-room are set up, privacy issues, how interruptions are handled, and the use of a couch or face-to-face positions for interviews.

4 *The rules of the therapeutic process:* Described above, these are the rules of free association; how the therapist listens and speaks; and the therapist's relative abstinence, neutrality, and maintenance of confidentiality.

FACTORS AFFECTING THE FRAME

- *Changes in frame:* Any major changes in the frame or deviations from technical neutrality should be documented. Such changes might include alterations in the originally proposed treatment, for example, having a patient on the psychoanalytic couch sit up if a psychotic transference develops; visiting a seriously ill patient in hospital; changing the frequency of visits from three times to once a week (owing to an unworkable transference) or increasing the frequency in order to increase the visibility of transference. It is wise to document how the intervention affected treatment.

- *Policies regarding holidays and missed appointments:* Any regular form of psychodynamic psychotherapy requires commitment by both patient and clinician. Clinicians who practise intensive psychotherapy almost universally hold regular hours free for patients and frequently form an arrangement by which the patient must pay for missed sessions. This practice has been recognized and approved by the College of Physicians and Surgeons of Ontario (CPSO). Policies about long holidays vary. In general, long interruptions are counterproductive to psychodynamic psychotherapy, and clinicians therefore encourage patients, if they can, to take holidays in a way that minimizes interruption of therapy. (Of course, not all patients can choose when to take holidays.) Therapists generally balance the patient's needs, the therapist's needs, and issues of resistance in considering a response to a patient's absence or missed session.

- *Home offices:* Having an office at home is a well-established practice for many physicians as well as psychodynamic psychiatrists. In such cases, physicians must ensure that the office should be in such a location in the home as to ensure reasonable and sufficient privacy for the patient, that the files remain confidential, and that noise leakage is avoided. A home office may not be an optimal arrangement for patients with poor reality testing or highly demanding transferences.
- *Telephone contacts:* At times, phone sessions are needed to speak with patients in crisis. Many patients travel to earn their income, and increasingly therapists conduct sessions by telephone, with good effect.
- *Treatment contracts:* Several investigators (Yeomans, Selzer, & Clarkin, 1992; Kernberg et al, 1989) support the use of treatment contracts with patients who have failed in previous treatments because of behaviours that interfered with therapy. Examples of such behaviour are stalking the therapist, repeatedly calling to threaten suicide and hanging up, refusing to talk in sessions for long periods, manipulative suicide attempts or threats, threatening the therapist, damaging the therapist's office, and refusing to leave the office at the end of sessions. For these patients, treatment is often the only chance of getting better. In such cases, the clinician drafts a contract with the patient, stating that treatment can be conducted only under certain conditions that, if contravened by the patient, will make treatment impossible so that the clinician will have to end treatment, and it will be the patient's responsibility to seek further care. This makes it clear to the patient that the success of treatment depends upon his or her collaboration, that treatment is not magic, and that it may not be possible to continue. It also makes it clear that the patient has some responsibility for treatment, and that the therapeutic frame is not to be used simply for acting out, but, rather, for positive purposes. These contracts also protect clinicians treating patients who may not otherwise receive any treatment.

Contraindications to Psychodynamic Psychotherapy

The fact that psychotherapy can cause negative effects was pointed out by Freud (1923/1961). Over the years, studies have revealed which patients do and which do not benefit from this treatment and, when patients are carefully assessed, the number of patients who actually get worse in psychodynamic psychotherapy is very low. In the Penn study, only 1 per cent of patients got worse (Luborsky et al, 1988). A survey of

150 expert psychotherapists concerning the existence and nature of negative effects produced a list of such effects (Hadley & Strupp, 1976). Negative effects – those generally harmful to the patient or those that impede the goals of therapy – include exacerbation of existing symptoms or the appearance of new symptoms. Of course, some or all of these symptoms could be the products of the natural progress of a difficult-to-treat illness.

Even these negative symptoms must be taken in a clinical context, for all patients are different and what is good for one can be bad for another. For instance, some symptoms such as the ability to feel sadness, grief, depression, or guilt about past deeds in a person whose conscience was warded off or inhibited might signify therapeutic progress. Decreased grandiosity (a pathological form of self-esteem) or the appearance of depression might be a sign of progress in a narcissistic person (Zetzel, 1965). Patients who break off destructive relationships in the course of treatment may feel more lonely, until they form new and better relationships. The ability to experience anxiety in someone previously unable to feel anxiety or who warded it off with denial may be a sign of progress (Zetzel, 1970). But decreased anxiety in a highly anxious person would also be a sign of progress. There is a well-documented phenomenon, called the 'negative therapeutic reaction' (Sandler, Dare, & Holder, 1992), in which patients transiently feel worse off despite progress when:

- progress interferes with a lifelong neurotic equilibrium;
- they feel more connected to the therapist;
- progress elicits envy of the therapist, stirring up guilt and fear of success.

The negative therapeutic reaction is to be expected in many cases. Other reasons for negative effects include inadequate diagnostic assessment, deficiencies in the therapist's training, and misapplications of therapy or technique. Many patients find that symptoms return transiently with the termination of meaningful, long-term treatment because loss of the therapeutic relationship activates grief and old conflicts. The termination phase also provides an opportunity to work through separation conflicts.

Medical treatment at times involves discomfort; psychotherapy is no exception. The potential for negative effects in and of themselves is not a contraindication for treatment, but rather may contraindicate certain therapeutic goals and techniques. For example, using psychodynamic techniques in some patients with poorly defined boundaries may lead to a psychotic transference in which reality testing is lost (Kernberg et al, 1989). Similarly, explorative psychotherapy may be stressful in certain cases of post-traumatic stress disorder (Krystal, 1988).

Training of Psychodynamic Psychotherapists and Psychoanalysts

The Task Force of the Association for Academic Psychiatry and the American Association of Directors of Psychiatric Residency Training identified some major reasons for teaching psychodynamic psychotherapy (Mohl et al, 1990), including the following:

- Psychodynamic psychotherapy is an effective treatment for many mental disorders.
- Psychodynamic concepts are intimately related to the psychological and social concepts of all doctor–patient relationships.
- Psychodynamic psychotherapy allows observation of complex pathological and normal functioning over time.
- Training in psychodynamic psychotherapy enhances a psychiatrist's ability to anticipate, analyse, and avoid ethical dilemmas and transgressions.
- The observations required for such work enhance intellectual rigour and discipline in observing behaviour, developing hypotheses, and analysing theories and data.

The American task force outlined a model curriculum, setting goals for each of four training years, the minimum goals being:

- to provide an adequate basic background so that psychiatrists can achieve competence as psychodynamic psychotherapists with additional training;
- to provide the general psychiatrist with a starting language and basic concepts for understanding dyadic interaction and unconscious forces;
- to make the general psychiatrist aware of the omnipresent role of unconscious forces in every clinical situation;
- to sensitize the general psychiatrist to the complicated process and evolution of clinical relationships in all therapeutic settings.

These requirements recognize the vital role of further training in psychodynamic psychotherapy for psychiatrists who wish to specialize. In the case of psychoanalysis practised by physicians, the standards of training as set by the International Psychoanalytic Association (having a personal analysis with an accredited training analyst, adequate supervision, hours of providing supervised psychoanalyses, and numbers of patients supervised) are the minimum for someone to become a psychoanalyst, or to represent himself or herself to the public as a psychoanalyst. In Ontario, these standards involve a four-year program of didactic lectures and a minimum of 160 hours of supervision spread over three supervised cases with sessions at least four times a week.

Quality Assessment

Assessment of the quality of psychotherapy is based primarily on the standards displayed by the psychotherapist in his or her evaluation of the patient's illness. The psychodynamic formulation, goals of treatment, treatment plans, appropriateness of the therapy plan to the diagnosis, and the patient's psychological capacities must be demonstrated by the therapist.

We recommend careful documentation of a psychodynamic formulation, outlining core conflicts and inhibitions of development. Since every patient is different, it can be expected that each psychodynamic formulation will display a patient's unique difficulties, narratives, defences, and so on. An example of a full psychodynamic formulation and an explanation of the necessary data base for this formulation are provided by MacKinnon and Yudofsky (1986). This ideal psychodynamic formulation extends beyond the minimum standards described in this volume in chapter 19, 'Standards and Guidelines for Psychotherapy Record Keeping.'

Quality assurance cannot be based on short-term changes in a patient, because significant progress cannot be made in psychodynamic psychotherapy without temporary regressions, nor can progress occur without periods of painful affects when past losses are re-experienced. In fact, as already mentioned, the ability to experience sad or depressive affects can signal progress towards the capacity for concern and improved relationships, or changes in a maladaptive intrapsychic equilibrium (Joseph, 1989). Temporary regressions or apparent worsening of symptoms may make inexperienced observers think that the therapist is incompetent or has made an inappropriate choice of treatment. However, these changes often signify the patient's trust in the therapist as forgotten or repressed traumatic life experiences are recovered.

Those assessing quality assurance for psychodynamic psychotherapies should be fully accredited practitioners of the type of psychodynamic psychotherapy being assessed, be well respected in their field, and spend a large part of their day practising that form of treatment. The same courtesy applies to other modalities, and licensing bodies such as the College of Physicians and Surgeons of Ontario (CPSO) usually honour this request.

Recommendations for Special Situations

- *Building therapeutic alliances with explanations:* We recommend informing patients about those aspects of the therapeutic encounter that seem unfamiliar or beyond their normal experience, to decrease misunderstanding and improve the therapeutic alliance (Greenson, 1967). This is most necessary at the expressive end of the continuum, where some attempt should be made to explain the purpose of techniques such as free association, technical neutrality, relative abstinence, and relative anonymity – concepts probably unfamiliar to patients.
- *Concurrently treating a patient's relatives and intimates:* While it is usual in some forms of treatment (such as family and couple therapy) to treat family members conjointly, in individual psychodynamic psychotherapy it is not generally recommended that the physician undertake concurrent treatment of a patient's family members, cohabitants, very close intimates, or lovers, as the physician may become an important transference figure in the family, leading to an unanalysed group process and various enmeshments. To illustrate, if a physician treated both a husband and a wife who themselves were in conflict about triangular Oedipal issues, a triangular transference would be enacted that might be difficult for the patients to work through. One party may use free association to tell secrets, enacting a triangular situation. The physician, obligated to honour confidentiality, would then hold information that creates opportunities for inadvertent breach of confidence. In these cases, the physician could stumble into conflicts of interest that emerge when treating both patients. In general, it is preferable to refer close relatives, lovers, or intimates to someone else. This recommendation does not mean that it would necessarily be inappropriate to perform a consultation for the relative or lover of a patient, and then refer him or her on. Patients often request this once trust is established. Clinicians may at times treat a patient's more distant relatives concurrently. When assessing whether to treat a patient's friend concurrently, the clinician should view the following factors as complicating treatment: the relationship includes a history

of destructive enactments; the relationship is volatile; the two are very close, see each other very frequently, are rivals, have been lovers together; at least one expresses a wish to become a lover; at least one has poor reality testing. When any of these is likely to create major difficulties for the therapeutic process, the clinician is advised to refer the patient on. Sometimes two of a clinician's patients will turn out to know each other, or meet by chance and become very close. Obviously it would be problematic to automatically break off treatment for one of them. As in all cases, the clinician should continue to analyse the feelings and fantasies that each patient has about the situation, the clinician, and the clinician's relationship with the other person, should it come up, and interpret resistances to free association as they arise, treating the situation as grist for the therapeutic mill.

Psychodynamic clinicians are no different from other medical practitioners in that they vary in skill, training, approach, experience, and expertise; people seeking treatment know this, and it is natural and often sensible for them to seek to be treated by a clinician who comes recommended by someone they know well and trust, such as a friend. The psychodynamic clinician, aware that transference and unconscious fantasy, and, at times, unrealistic idealization, play a role in referrals, should try to anticipate how such factors may play out. Since treatments of people who are friendly can work out well, there is no absolute contraindication for psychodynamic psychotherapy in such situations. When in doubt, a clinician would do well to consult with a colleague outside the transference–countertransference field before going beyond consultation with such a patient. If significant doubt persists, we recommend the clinician be inclined to err on the side of referring such patients on if possible. In some situations, as in underserviced areas, the above recommendation may be overlooked if no other clinician with comparable expertise is available. Even so, the clinician should document the reasons for this unusual situation and how it influences treatment.

- *Recommendations for dealing with psychotic or delusional, paranoid, and erotized transferences:* At times, patients with certain disorders (for example, borderline, paranoid, narcissistic, and antisocial disorders) may develop a psychotic, paranoid, or erotized transference. Patients may begin to act on these ideas, in or out of therapy. According to Kernberg et al (1989), the therapeutic task is to help convert these actions into self-reflection about intrapsychic motives by acknowledging the difference in perspective, clarifying the extent to which the patient can make use of reality testing, and, if possible, discussing the meaning of these transferences. If these measures do not succeed in converting the actions into self-reflections, and if they extend beyond the transference despite accurate interpretation, the therapist may, depending upon their severity, seek consultation, change the treatment frame, and try medication or hospitalization.

- *Hospitalization:* When outpatients are hospitalized, their care is often taken over by staff psychiatrists. In some cases, ongoing therapy with the outpatient therapist may be helpful for continuity, if approved by the inpatient staff.

References

American Psychiatric Association (APA). Committee on Peer Review. (1985). *Manual of psychiatric peer review, Peer review guidelines for psychoanalysis,* (3d ed.). Washington, DC: Author.

American Psychiatric Association (APA). (1994). *Diagnostic and statistical manual of mental disorders* (4th ed.). Washington, DC: Author.

Bachrach, H.M., & Leaff, L.A. (1978). Analyzability: A systematic review of the clinical and quantitative literature. *Journal of the American Psychoanalytic Association, 20,* 881–920.

Blanck, G., & Blanck, R. (1974). *Ego psychology: Theory and practice.* New York: Columbia University Press.

Blanck, G., & Blanck, R. (1979). *Ego psychology II: Psychoanalytic developmental psychology.* New York: Columbia University Press.

Bowlby, J. (1980). *Attachment and loss. Vol. 3. Loss, sadness, and depression.* New York: Basic.

Cooper, A.M. (1985). Will neurobiology influence psychoanalysis? *American Journal of Psychiatry, 142,* 1395–1402.

Crits-Christoph, P., Barber, J., Baranackie, K., & Cooper, A. (1993). Assessing the therapist's interpretations. In N.E. Miller, L. Luborsky, J.P. Barber, & J.P. Docherty (Eds.), *Psychodynamic treatment research: A handbook for clinical practice.* New York: Basic.

Doidge, N., Simon, B., Gillies, L.A., & Ruskin, R. (1994). Characteristics of psychoanalytic patients under a nationalized health plan: DSM-III-R diagnoses, previous treatment and childhood traumata. *American Journal of Psychiatry, 151,* 586–590.

Frank, E., Kupfer, D.J., & Perel, J.M. (1989). Early recurrence in unipolar depression. *Archives of General Psychiatry, 46,* 397–400.

Freebury, D.R. (1986). The prescription of psychotherapy. *Canadian Journal of Psychiatry, 29,* 449–503.

Fretter, P.B., Bucci, W., Broitman, J., Silberschatz, G., & Curtis, J.T. (1994). How the patient's plan relates to the concept of transference. *Psychotherapy Research,* 4, 58–72.

Freud, S. (1953). Three essays on sexuality. In J. Strachey (Ed. and Trans.), *The standard edition of the complete psychological works of Sigmund Freud* (Vol. 7). London: Hogarth Press. (Original work published 1905)

Freud, S. (1957). Five lectures on psycho-analysis. In J. Strachey (Ed. and Trans.), *The standard edition of the complete psychological works of Sigmund Freud* (Vol. 11). London: Hogarth Press. (Original work published 1910)

Freud, S. (1958) The dynamics of transference. In J. Strachey (Ed. and Trans.), *The standard edition of the complete psychological works of Sigmund Freud* (Vol. 12). London: Hogarth Press. (Original work published 1912)

Freud, S. (1961). The ego and the id. In J. Strachey (Ed. and Trans.), *The standard edition of the complete psychological works of Sigmund Freud* (Vol. 19). London: Hogarth Press. (Original work published 1923)

Gabbard, G. (1994). *Psychodynamic psychiatry in clinical practice: The DSM-IV edition.* Washington, DC: American Psychiatric Association.

Gabbard, G. (Ed.). (1995). *Treatments of psychiatric disorders: The DSM-IV edition.* Washington, DC: American Psychiatric Press.

Garfield, D. (1985). Self-criticism in psychosis: Enabling statements in psycho-therapy. *Dynamic Psychotherapy,* 3, 129–137.

Graff, H., & Luborsky, L. (1977). Long-term trends in transference and resistance: A quantitative analytic method applied to four psychoanalyses. *Journal of the American Psychoanalytic Association,* 25, 471–490.

Gray, S.H. (1996) Developing practice guidelines for psychoanalysis. *Journal of Psychotherapy Practice and Research,* 5, 213–227.

Greenson, R.R. (1967). *The technique and practice of psychoanalysis* (Vol. 1). New York: International Universities Press.

Greenspan, S.I. (1979). *Intelligence and adaptation: An integration of psychoanalytic and Piagetian developmental psychology.* New York: International Universities Press.

Greenspan, S.I. (1981). Psychopathology and adaptation in infancy and early childhood: Principles of clinical diagnosis and preventive interven-tion. *Clinical infant reports* (No. 1). New York: International Universities Press.

Grunberger, B. (1989). *New essays on narcissism* (David Macey, Ed. and Trans.). London: Free Associations.

Gunderson, J.G. (1988). Personality disorders. In A.M. Nicholi, Jr (Ed.), *The new Harvard guide to psychiatry* (pp. 337–359). Cambridge, MA: Belknap Press of Harvard University Press.

Guntrip, M. (1969). *Schizoid phenomena, object relations and the self.* New York: International Universities Press.

Hadley, S.W., & Strupp, H.H. (1976). Contemporary views of negative effects in psychotherapy. *Archives of General Psychiatry, 33,* 1291–1303.

Horvath, A., Gaston, L., & Luborsky, L. (1993). The therapeutic alliance and its measures. In N.E. Miller, L. Luborsky, J.P. Barber, & J.P. Docherty (Eds.), *Psychodynamic treatment research: A handbook for clinical practice.* New York: Basic.

Joseph, B. (1989). Towards the experiencing of psychic pain. In *Psychic equilibrium and psychic change: Selected papers of Betty Joseph.* London: Tavistock/ Routledge.

Kahana, R., & Bibring, G. (1964). Personality types in medical management. In N.E. Zinberg (Ed.), *Psychiatry and medical practice in a general hospital.* New York: International Universities Press.

Kernberg, O.F. (1984). *Severe personality disorders: Psychotherapeutic strategies.* New Haven, CT: Yale University Press.

Kernberg. O.F. (1988). Object relations theory in clinical practice. *Psychoanalytic Quarterly, 57,* 481–504.

Kernberg. O.F., Selzer, M.A., Koenigsberg, H.W., Carr, A.C., & Appelbaum, A.H. (1989). *Psychodynamic psychotherapy of borderline patients.* New York: Basic.

Kohut, H. (1971). *The analysis of the self.* New York: International Universities Press.

Kohut, H. (1984). *How does analysis cure?* Chicago: University of Chicago Press.

Kris, A.O. (1991) Psychoanalysis and psychoanalytic psychotherapy. In R. Michels (Ed.), *Psychiatry* (Vol. 1). Philadelphia: Lippincott.

Krystal, H. (1988). *Integration and self healing: Affect, trauma, alexithymia.* Hillsdale, NJ: Analytic Press.

Loewald, H. (1960). On the therapeutic action of psychoanalysis. *International Journal of Psycho-Analysis, 41,* 16–33.

Lowy, F. (1981). The role of psychoanalysis in contemporary psychiatry. Panel Presentation, 31st Annual Meeting, Canadian Psychiatric Association.

Luborsky, L. (1993a). Documenting symptom formation during psychotherapy. In N.E. Miller, L. Luborsky, J.P. Barber, & J.P. Docherty (Eds.), *Psychodynamic treatment research: A handbook for clinical practice.* New York: Basic.

Luborsky, L. (1993b). How to maximize the curative factors in dynamic psychotherapy. In N.E. Miller, L. Luborsky, J.P. Barber, & J.P. Docherty (Eds.), *Psychodynamic treatment research: A handbook for clinical practice.* New York: Basic.

Luborsky, L.M., & Crits-Christoph, P. (1990). *Understanding transference: The CCRT method.* New York: Basic.

Luborsky, L., Crits-Christoph, P., Mintz, J., & Auerbach, A. (1988). *Who will benefit from psychotherapy? Predicting therapeutic outcomes.* New York: Basic.

Luborsky, L., Docherty, J.P., Barber, J.P., & Miller, N.E. (1993). How this basic handbook helps the partnership of clinicians and clinical researchers: Preface. In N.E. Miller, L. Luborsky, J.P. Barber, & John P. Docherty (Eds.), *Psychodynamic treatment research: A handbook for clinical practice*. New York: Basic.

MacKinnon, R.A., & Yudofsky, S.C. (1986). *The psychiatric evaluation in clinical practice*. Philadelphia: Lippincott.

Mahler, M.S., Pine, F., & Bergmann, A. (1975). *The psychological birth of the human infant*. New York: Basic.

Milrod, B.L., Busch, F.N., Cooper, A.M., & Shapiro, T. (1997). *Manual of panic-focused psychodynamic psychotherapy*. Washington, DC: American Psychiatric Press.

Mohl, P.C., Lomax, J., Tasman, A., Chan, C., Sledge, W., Summergrad, P., & Notman, A. (1990). Psychotherapy training for the psychiatrist of the future. *American Journal of Psychiatry, 147*, 7–13.

Orlinsky, D.E., & Geller, J.D. (1993). Patient's representations of their therapists and therapy: New measures. In N.E. Miller, L. Luborsky, J.P. Barber, & J.P. Docherty (Eds.), *Psychodynamic treatment research: A handbook for clinical practice*. New York: Basic.

Perry, J.C. (1993). Defenses and their effects. In N.E. Miller, L. Luborsky, J.P. Barber, & J.P. Docherty (Eds.), *Psychodynamic treatment research: A handbook for clinical practice*. New York: Basic.

Pine, F. (1988). On the four psychologies of psychoanalysis and the nature of the therapeutic impact. In A. Rothstein (Ed.), *How does treatment help?* Madison, CT: International Universities Press.

Rockland, L.H. (1989). *Supportive therapy: A psychodynamic approach*. New York: Basic.

Roiphe, H., & Galenson, E. (1981). *Infantile origins of sexual identity*. New York: International Universities Press.

Roth, S. (1987). *Psychotherapy: The art of wooing nature*. New York: Jason Aronson.

Salzman, Leon. (1985) *Treatment of the obsessive personality*. New York: Jason Aronson.

Sandler, J., Dare, C., & Holder, A. (1992). The negative therapeutic reaction. In *The patient and the analyst* (2d ed., rev. and expanded by Joseph Sandler and Ursula Dreher). Madison, CT: International Universities Press.

Schlessinger, N., & Robbins, F. (1975). The psychoanalytic process: Recurrent patterns of conflict and change in ego functions. *Journal of the American Psychoanalytic Association, 23*, 761–782.

Schlessinger, N., & Robbins, F. (1983). *A developmental view of the psychoanalytic process*. New York: International Universities Press.

Shevrin, H., & Bond, J.A. (1993). Repression and the unconscious. In N.E. Miller, L. Luborsky, J.P. Barber, & J.P. Docherty (Eds.), *Psychodynamic treatment research: A handbook for clinical practice*. New York: Basic.

Stanton, A.H., Gunderson, J.G, Knapp, P.H., Frank, A.F., Vannicelli, M.L. Schnitzer, R., & Rosenthal, R. (1984). Effects of psychotherapy on schizophrenic patients, I: Design and implementation of a controlled study. *Schizophrenia Bulletin, 10,* 520–563.

Stern, D.N. (1985). *The interpersonal world of the infant: A view from psychoanalysis and developmental psychology*. New York: Basic.

Strachey, J. (1934). The nature of the therapeutic action of psycho-analysis. *International Journal of Psycho-Analysis, 38,* 140–157.

Ursano, R., Sonnenberg, S., & Lazar, S. (1991). *Concise guide to psychodynamic psychotherapy*. Washington, DC: American Psychiatric Association.

Wallace, E.R. (1983). *Dynamic psychiatry in theory and practice*. Philadelphia: Lea & Febiger.

Wallerstein, R.S. (1986). *Forty-two lives in treatment. A study of psychoanalysis and psychotherapy*. New York: Guilford.

Warme, G. (1994). *Reluctant treasures: The practice of analytic psychotherapy*. Northvale, NJ: Jason Aronson.

Weil, J.L. (1989a). *Instinctual stimulation of children* (Vol. 1). Madison, CT: International Universities Press.

Weil, J.L. (1989b). *Instinctual stimulation of children* (Vol. 2). Madison, CT: International Universities Press.

Weiss, J., Sampson, H., & the Mount Zion Psychotherapy Research Group. (1986). *The psychoanalytic process: Theory, clinical observations and empirical research*. New York: Guilford.

Wolff, P.H. (1960). The developmental psychologies of Jean Piaget and psycho-analysis. In *Psychological Issues* (Monograph 5). New York: International Universities Press.

Yeomans, F.E., Selzer, M.A., & Clarkin, J.F. (1992). *Treating the borderline patient: A contract-based approach*. New York: Basic.

Zetzel, E. (1965). Depression and the incapacity to bear it. In Max Shur (Ed.), *Drives, affects and behaviour* (Vol. 2). New York: International Universities Press.

Zetzel, E. (1970). Anxiety and the capacity to bear it. In *The capacity for emotional growth: Theoretical and clincial contributions to psychoanalysis, 1943–1969*. New York: International Universities Press.

Zitrin, C., Klein, D., & Woener, M. (1978). Behavior therapy, supportive psychotherapy, imipramine and phobias. *Archives of General Psychiatry, 35,* 307–316.

4. Empirical Evidence for the Core Clinical Concepts and Efficacy of the Psychoanalytic Psychotherapies: An Overview

Norman Doidge

Part I: Introduction to the Empirical Study of the Psychoanalytic Psychotherapies

There is a wealth of empirical evidence supporting the efficacy of the psychoanalytic psychotherapies and the core concepts on which they are based. Though there are more than a hundred different types of psychotherapy, a recent review of the forty major international psychotherapy research programs found that eighteen of these programs are mainly psychoanalytic in orientation (Beutler & Crago, 1991). Thus the psychoanalytic psychotherapies, from the various forms of face-to-face psychoanalytic (sometimes called 'psychodynamic') psychotherapies to psychoanalysis, not only have been, but continue to be, among the most intensively studied treatments (Doidge, 1997; Sledge, 1997).

The psychoanalytic psychotherapies are the most widely practised of the major forms of psychotherapy, valued by psychiatrists and other mental health professionals (Luborsky, Docherty, Barber, & Miller, 1993; Wiener, 1994). This form of individual treatment remains the mainstay of psychotherapy training in a wide variety of psychiatric settings (Tasman, 1993). A national survey of psychotherapists by the American Psychological Association found that a psychodynamic orientation predominates among clinical psychologists (Norcross, Proschaska, & Gallagher, 1989). Even among those who call themselves eclectic, 44 per cent have integrated psychoanalytic principles (Norcross & Prochaska, 1988).

Psychoanalytic psychotherapy is derived from psychoanalysis.

Whereas psychoanalysis involves four to five sessions per week with the patient on the couch, psychoanalytic psychotherapy typically involves one to three sessions per week, conducted with clinician and patient sitting face to face. The major underlying principles of psychoanalysis and psychoanalytic psychotherapy techniques have been formulated and written about in well-known texts (Fenichel, 1941; Glover, 1955; Greenson, 1967; Giovacchini, 1972; Bergmann & Hartman, 1976; Thomä & Kächele, 1987; Etchegoyan, 1991) and manuals, which have been successfully tested for high interrater reliability (Luborsky, 1984; Luborsky & Crits-Christoph, 1990). These manuals are helpful for research, in order to establish that the treatment being studied is actually being conducted.

GATHERING PSYCHOANALYTIC DATA SCIENTIFICALLY

The scientific study of psychoanalytic psychotherapies and psychoanalysis goes on at many levels, in a rational scientific sequence. Over the last hundred years, a cumulative scientific literature of thousands of individual psychoanalytic case histories has been published in scores of international journals, and it is through these individual cases that observations and hypotheses are most often generated. The major journals which contain case histories are now indexed (Mosher, 1991).

Case histories and studies of archival materials are supplemented by other forms of empirical validation to test the generalizability of hypotheses. Fonagy and Moran (1993) have described how group-based designs, naturalistic designs, and single-case methods that use quantitative measures all have contributed to the empirical assessment of psychoanalytic treatments and hypotheses. Experimental designs also have a place in examining core concepts, and are dealt with below, in Part II. Researchers have found that, in investigations of core concepts, a variety of designs, including single-case studies, are helpful. When studying outcome (i.e., how effective a treatment is) there is a tendency to use group designs. The methodological background of large-group designs is discussed at the beginning of Part III. Though much of this chapter deals with large-group designs, it is important to give small-group designs and single-case studies their due, for they are often overlooked and can often reveal things that cannot be accessed in other studies.

Fonagy and Moran (1993) have argued that

the belief that knowledge based upon groups of individuals is somehow more likely to be generalizable (that is, applicable beyond the specific locus of its discovery) than is the case for knowledge based upon individual cases is fatally flawed. The belief derives largely from the remarkable achievements of the statistician A.R. Fisher, who worked in the 1920's and 1930's; through the development of the theory of sampling he made it possible for scientists, including psychologists, to make inferences about the populations they were studying on the basis of information gained from relatively small groups. As the criteria for the drawing of a genuinely random sample are very rarely, if ever, met by clinical investigations, the issue of what inferences may be drawn from a finding becomes primarily logical rather than statistical (Edington, 1966). Information must be made available to permit the readers of a research report to make inferences about the applicability of findings concerning how conditions were specified, as well as the characteristics of the patient(s) in treatment. This constraint should apply equally to group and invdividual studies. Wherever possible and whatever the research question, large numbers need to be studied to ensure generality. This injunction implies the need for studies of large numbers of individuals, not large groups. Individual case studies attempt to establish the relationship between intervention and other variables of interest through repeated systematic observation and measurement. (Fonagy & Moran, 1993, p. 65)

Control studies may randomly assign members of a clinic to a treatment or no-treatment control group. However, if the patients who apply to a depression clinic and meet the inclusion and exclusion criteria of these studies represent a subpopulation of depressed patients, they are not necessarily a representative sample of depressed patients, and one cannot apply findings related to them to the population at large.

INDICATIONS FOR PSYCHOANALYSIS AND PSYCHOANALYTIC PSYCHOTHERAPY

Indications for a treatment can be based upon a number of factors. These include: (1) the consensus of clinical literature and expert opinion; (2) established patterns of practice in which large numbers of trained and experienced clinicians express consensus opinions as to what seems efficacious; (3) patient satisfaction studies; and (4) group empirical studies showing that the therapy is efficacious for the conditions treated. It is reasonable to take each of the above factors into account, as each has its strengths and limitations. As well, each of these factors frequently takes the others into account, up to a point.

CONSENSUS OF CLINICAL LITERATURE, EXPERT OPINION, AND PATTERNS OF PRACTICE

In terms of the clinical literature, psychoanalytic psychotherapies are routinely cited in major psychiatric textbooks as the preferred treatment for a number of significant character disorders and symptom disorders or neuroses (Kaplan & Sadock, 1985, 1995; Gabbard, 1994, 1995; Michels, 1991; Ursano & Silberman, 1994). At one extreme, this form of treatment can be helpful in one or two visits in consultation liaison work, or in crisis intervention in the emergency room. At the other extreme, psychoanalysis, at four or five sessions a week for a number of years, may be prescribed for treatment of long-standing character disturbances or symptom disorders. Thus, there is much flexibility in terms of appropriate dose and frequency of sessions.

Knight (1941) reviewed the early (pre-1950) statistical studies of psychoanalysis, which included 951 patients from different settings. These studies were retrospective, and began to establish who would and would not benefit from psychoanalysis. He concluded that psychoanalysis was most effective in treating character disorders, some psychosomatic conditions, and a number of the neuroses.

These early studies corroborated the general clinical impression that unmodified psychoanalysis is not generally an effective treatment in psychoses. (This is not to say that modified supportive psychoanalytic psychotherapy does not play an adjunctive role to medication in the treatment of some psychoses; see below.) The early studies established psychoanalysis as the treatment for a number of repetitive, long-standing, maladaptive problems involving personality or character, and chronic, repetitive behavioural, affective, or mental disturbances.

Chronicity is an important indicator for analysis. If someone who is upset at the death of a spouse becomes depressed for three months, psychoanalysis proper is not the indicated treatment. In some cases, a briefer psychoanalytically oriented treatment to deal with the grief may be indicated. But if an unmarried person in his thirties finds that every time he becomes involved with a woman he becomes nasty, distant, suffers premature ejaculation, is ultimately rejected, and becomes depressed and suicidal, analysis might be indicated. Considerable motivation is required by an individual to invest the time needed for analysis, and only certain types of people have the kinds of psychological ego strengths to endure it and benefit from it (i.e., to be 'analysable'; see Bachrach & Leaff, 1978, and Gabbard, 1994). It should be noted that the presence of these ego strengths does not mean that these people are simply healthy, any more than having a healthy heart guarantees the absence of illness in all other organ systems. These stringent criteria – particular types of chronic disorders, high motivation, and particular strengths – yield the result that most patients assessed by psychiatrists who are also psychoanalysts are not referred for analysis; of the 9,000 applicants who were referred to the Columbia University Psychoanalytic Clinic, fewer than 10 per cent were referred on for analysis (Weber, Solomon, & Bachrach, 1985; Weber, Bachrach, & Solomon, 1985a, 1985b; Bachrach, Weber, & Solomon, 1985).

The American Psychiatric Association peer review guidelines (1985) integrated a number of the findings of the early outcome studies into their set of indications for psychoanalysis. These are described fully in chapter 3, 'Guidelines for the Practice of Individual Psychodynamic Psychotherapy.'

PSYCHIATRIC MORBIDITY, CHILDHOOD TRAUMA, AND PREVIOUS TREATMENT ATTEMPTS IN PSYCHOANALYTIC PATIENTS IN ONTARIO

What kinds of patients are currently in psychoanalysis, and what kinds of character or symptom disorders do patients currently in psychoanalysis generally have? Data from a study of patients in psychoanalysis in Ontario show that 59 per cent of those receiving psychoanalysis are women, and 41 per cent are men. Patients present with a mode of two psychiatric disorders, and a mean of approximately four current psychiatric diagnoses (Doidge, Simon, Gillies, & Ruskin, 1994). As expected, character diagnoses are prevalent, with a mean of one *DSM-III-R* (APA, 1987) personality disorder per patient. While this study is limited by the survey methodology, its findings are fairly consistent with personality findings in psychoanalytic patients in other studies using structured interviews (see Doidge et al [1994] for discussion of related studies). Recent studies of the symptoms of applicants for psychoanalysis in New York show that 32 per cent of these patients have mood disorders, 32 per cent have anxiety disorders, and 12 per cent have substance abuse disorders (Hyler, Skodol, Oldham, Kellman, & Doidge, 1992; Oldham et al, 1995).

In the Ontario study, the most common Axis I diagnoses made were of mood (48 per cent had dysthymia), anxiety, and sexual dysfunction disorders. Dysthymia has been found to have a prevalence of 36 per cent in general outpatient populations (Markowitz, Moran, Kocsis, & Frances, 1992). As noted in the text of *DSM-III-R*, dysthymia is frequently associated with personality disorders, and has a poor prognosis (Wells, Burnam, Rogers, Hays, & Camp, 1992). Axis II disorders were also prevalent, with a predominance of some cluster-B (narcissistic, histrionic, and borderline personality disorders) and some cluster-C (obsessive–compulsive, dependent, avoidant, and passive–aggressive personality disorders).

Many of the diagnoses seen in analytic patients, such as sexual dysfunction disorders, dissociative disorders, sleep disorders, and post-traumatic stress disorders, are not specifically asked about in the current Structured Clinical Interview for *DSM-III-R* that was used in the Oldham study cited above, though the interview includes screening for these items.

The levels of childhood trauma in these patients are significant. Doidge et al (1994) found that 23 per cent suffered traumatic separation in childhood; 23 per cent of psychoanalytic patients in Ontario have been sexually abused; 22.2 per cent were physically abused; 21.3 per cent have had parents or siblings die in childhood or during the teen years; and a significant number have suffered some other kind of overwhelming point trauma. These findings of high rates of trauma are consistent with rates reported in psychoanalytic case histories. The authors point out that these high rates do not mean that all patients with character neuroses have had childhood traumas.

The vast majority of patients (82 per cent) attempted previous treatments (including use of medication and briefer forms of therapy), and resorted to analysis only after previous treatments did not resolve existing symptoms. Briefer treatments have a place, but are not the solution for every patient's problems.

These Ontario findings are consistent with the guidelines for psychoanalytic peer review in the American Psychiatric Association's *Manual of Psychiatric Peer Review* (1985), described in table 3.1. The manual notes that information about the Axis I or Axis II diagnosis is not sufficient for determining that analysis is indicated. The manual requires that the patient's difficulties be based upon both chronic intrapsychic conflict and developmental inhibition or arrest. Other, less-intensive treatments cannot be sufficient to resolve the patient's problems. The patients in psychoanalysis in Ontario showed a number of indicators of chronicity, including childhood traumata, previous treatment, and

Axis II pathology. The high number of mood and anxiety disorders is consistent with the Menninger study (Wallerstein, 1986), which found that 88 per cent of patients in psychoanalysis or psychoanalytic psychotherapy had anxiety, depression, or both. Other psychotherapy studies, such as the well-known Penn Psychotherapy Study by Luborsky, Crits-Christoph, Mintz, and Auerbach (1988) found the commonest Axis I diagnoses in patients in psychoanalytic psychotherapy were dysthymia and anxiety disorders.

The findings of Doidge et al (1994) in Ontario are consistent with the findings of the task force report of the American Psychiatric Association entitled *Treatments of Psychiatric Disorders* (1989), which represents a compilation of expert opinion. This document lists, by disorder, the conditions for which psychoanalysis and psychodynamic psychotherapy may be the treatment of choice, or effective treatments, depending upon clinical conditions. The revised *DSM-IV* edition (Gabbard, 1995) represents an important assembly of expert opinion, based upon literature reviews. For a discussion of the indications for psychoanalytic psychotherapy by diagnosis, see chapter 3, 'Guidelines for the Practice of Individual Psychodynamic Psychotherapy.'

As a summary statement, we may say that there is a convergence between existing expert opinion and patterns of practice as to the indications for psychoanalytic psychotherapy. The third and fourth factors, indications as determined by efficacy and patient satisfaction, are dealt with in Part III.

Part II: Core Concepts and Empirical Evidence for Them

TRANSFERENCE AND UNCONSCIOUS CONFLICT

Transference is the unconscious tendency of all human beings to transfer relationship scenes of the past onto situations in the present. Though transference is an unconscious process, its derivatives, including the tendency to repeat certain themes rather rigidly, or to see other people in certain predictable ways, can be measured by independent, manual-trained judges. A review of these measures can be found in Luborsky, Barber, et al (1993). The following techniques have been developed for measuring transference: the Core Conflictual Relationship Theme Method, the Plan Formulation Method, the Configurational Analysis and Role-Relationship Models, the Frame Method, the Cyclic Maladaptive Pattern Method, the Idiographic Conflict Formulation Method, and the Consensual Response Method. Most of these methods examine the patient's self-and-other representations, unconscious conflicts, wishes, interpersonal goals, and anticipated responses from others. Five studies comparing these measures consistently revealed a core of similarity among the different measures. Perhaps the best-investigated transference-derivative measure is that of Luborsky, the Core Conflictual Relationship Theme (CCRT). This measure rates relationship episodes in therapy for three components: (1) wishes in relationship to another person; (2) the expected responses of the other person; and (3) the responses of the self. The CCRT is manual-based, with good interrater reliability. Clinicians rate the emergence of these core conflictual-relationship themes in sessions. There are both tailor-made versions of the CCRT, which allow extensive clinical leeway in rating wishes, and standardized versions based upon common transference patterns. In successful therapies, components 2 and 3 of the CCRT change towards more adaptive responses as they are made conscious. Luborsky has shown that the transferences that people unconsciously attribute to others in their daily lives begin to be attributed to their clinicians. Ratings using the standard categories show good reliability, and the weighted kappa for wish and response from others was .61 ($p < .01$), and for the negative response from others .70 ($p < .001$).

Clinically, transference and unconscious conflict usually go together. One of the reasons that transference is thought to be an unconscious process is that it expresses wishes that have been repressed, for various conflictual reasons. The conflict may be between the wish and some fear, or between two opposing wishes. Because the wish stirs up counter-wishes or fears, it is repressed. Usually the wish has to do with the satisfaction of a desire with respect to another person, and, for this reason, the wish constellation may stir up the image of that other person. The image may be one from the past transferred onto someone in the present. At times, one 'defence transference' (Greenson, 1967) can be used to ward off another more disturbing transference.

In a review of the CCRT literature on transference, Luborsky and Crits- Christoph (1990) have found that the following Freudian ideas which form the basis of psychoanalytic psychotherapy can be corroborated in a statistically significant way, using the CCRT method of rating psychotherapy sessions.

1 Transference involves the expression not just of images of others, but of wishes. Core wishes are repeated in 60 per cent of interactions.

2 Wishes that are important in therapy involve conflict with other wishes that one has, or conflict with other people (pp. 117, 132, 254).

3 The transference pattern is partly beyond awareness. Though the issue has not yet been systematically studied, some data suggest that therapists pick up these patterns more quickly than do patients. (But it is a common clinical finding that, once it is pointed out, patients begin to see the pattern in many interactions.)

4 There is initial evidence that ratings of CCRTs in sessions can be matched with early memories of parents. In addition, how adults remember childhood predicts how they will treat their own children. Main and Goldwyn (1984), in a controlled study, used the reliable Adult Attachment Interview to measure attachment styles and found that mothers who distorted recollection of their childhood relationship formed attachments to their own children that were similar to the ones they subjectively experienced with their own mothers.

5 There are extensive CCRT data to show that the main pattern in relation to significant others is also repeated with therapists (Fried, Crits-Christoph, & Luborsky, 1990, pp. 145–157). CCRT ratings describing significant others from therapy sessions paralleled Relationship Episodes involving the therapists, as rated by blind judges (inter-judge reliability ranged from .55 to .75, which is adequate, $p = .001$).

6 The CCRT tends to be consistent over time, but, as the unconscious is made conscious, it is altered. Luborsky and Crits-Christoph (1990) have shown the wishes do not alter, but how the patient reacts to them, or expects others to react to them, alters significantly.

7 Symptoms may emerge with the activation of the transference. The appearance of symptoms typically follows or co-occurs with the appearance of the CCRT (Luborsky & Crits-Christoph, 1990, p. 260; for more detail, Luborsky, 1993a, p. 7). The transference derivative appears in patient narratives, dreams, and fantasies.

Table 4.1 summarizes the CCRT data concerning Freud's various hypotheses about transference.

Weiss, Sampson, and the Mount Zion Psychotherapy Research Group (1986) have developed a sophisticated measure of transference that involves accurately measuring not just particular transference images, but how the patient seeks to put the entire transference plan into effect, in an attempt to repeat, and possibly disconfirm, the pathogenic beliefs behind it. As already mentioned, *one* of the reasons patients are thought to repeatedly and unconsciously transfer past scenes is in an attempt to master, both cognitively and emotionally, situations that were over-

Table 4.1: Freud's 'Transference Template' Observation and the CCRT Evidence

Freud's Observation	CCRT Evidence
1 Wishes toward people are prominent	Study with positive results
2 Wishes conflict with responses of self and other	Study with positive results
3 Is especially evident in erotic relationships	Study with positive results
4 Is partly out of awareness	Preliminary study, positive results
5 Originates in early parental relationships	Preliminary study, positive results
6 Comes to involve therapist	Study with positive results
7 May be activated by therapist's perceived characteristics	Remains to be studied
8 May distort perception	Remains to be studied
9 Consists of one main pervasive pattern	Preliminary study, positive results
10 Subpatterns appear for family members	Preliminary study, positive results
11 Is distinctive for each person	Preliminary study, positive results
12 Remains consistent over time	Study with positive results
13 Changes slightly over time	Study with positive results
14 Shows short-term fluctuations in activation	Remains to be studied
15 Interpretation changes expression of pattern	Study with positive results
16 Insight into pattern can benefit patient	Preliminary study, positive results
17 Can serve as a resistance	Remains to be studied
18 Symptoms may emerge during its activations	Preliminary study, positive results
19 Is expressed in and out of therapy	Preliminary study, positive results
20 Positive vs. negative patterns are distinguishable	Study with positive results
21 Is expressed in multiple modes (dreams and narratives)	Study with positive results
22 Innate disposition plays a role	Study with positive results

Source: Luborsky & Crits-Christoph, 1990, p. 264

whelming or traumatic. Independent raters assessed the patient's plan in intake sessions, and then taped therapy sessions are rated to see whether the therapist's interpretations accurately addressed the plan in a case-specific way. Whereas the Luborsky group studied large and small samples, the Weiss et al group performed thousands of measurements of a small number of treatments, in an attempt to examine when interpretations work and when they do not. This group has produced numerous studies (see Weiss et al, 1986, and Weiss, 1993, for bibliography). Fretter, Bucci, Broitman, Silberschatz, and Curtis (1994) studied several different patients in therapy, including some who did well and some who did poorly. Patient sessions were independently rated to determine the patient's transference plan. Next, a separate group of blind independent judges rated whether the therapists' interpretations addressed the transference plan. In all cases, when therapists' interpretations accurately addressed the plan, there were signs of increased progress, as measured by the patient's immediate response to the interpretation on the Patient Insight Scale, which evaluates emotional insight according to seven sets of criteria, and the Referential Activity Scale, a well-known linguistic scale that predicts good working sessions as opposed to resistant sessions. Judges were manual-trained to acceptable reliability in all cases.

DEFENCES, REPRESSION, AND THE UNCONCSCIOUS

Researchers have begun to measure what might best be called 'defence contents' (Gillett, 1987), which are the conscious mental contents that result when particular defences are employed. While many defensive operations are complex, multilayered, and difficult to discern, others are so chronically and rigidly employed that they give rise to relatively stable defence contents. The more stable defense contents are measurable. The development of new and more reliable instruments puts us in a position to further explore Freud's (1896/1962a) proposal that a number of the defences have specific correlations with specific diagnostic categories.

The reviews by Perry (1993a) and Perry and Cooper (1986, 1987) are a good introduction to the burgeoning literature on defences. Other valuable texts include Vaillant's *Empirical Studies of Ego Mechanisms of Defense* (1986) and Vaillant's (1977) longitudinal study of defences and their relation to health and disease. Defences have been reliably rated, with good interrelater reliability, when interviews and transcripts are studied by blind raters. In addition, self-report of defence categories correlate with ratings of audio and video interviews of the same patients by blind raters (Vaillant & Vaillant, 1986). Defences have been studied longitudinally and experimentally. On the strength of these data, the defences are one of the axes which have been inserted into the *DSM-IV* (APA, 1994) appendix for further study. There are also a number of studies which correlate particular defences and diagnoses (Perry & Cooper, 1986). Vaillant and Drake (1985) have shown that patients with Axis II disorders tend to make use of immature defences, unlike those without Axis II disorders. They have also shown that the paranoid patients make use of projection, as Freud proposed. That study also demonstrates that maturer defences correlate with higher ratings on the Health–Sickness

Rating Scale (r = .78). This finding is to be expected, because psycho-analysis and psychoanalytic psychotherapy are thought to promote bet-ter functioning by pointing out and making conscious maladaptive or immature defences.

One of the core psychoanalytic hypotheses is that, in many cases, a patient's symptoms and character problems are related to his or her spe-cific unconscious conflicts. An up-to-date review of the psychoanalytic literature on repression undertaken by Shevrin and Bond (1993) describes the current approach to an area that presents many method-ological challenges. In current studies, both clinical assessments and objective measures of brain function are used.

Shevrin (1988) and Shevrin et al (1992) studied patients diagnosed with social phobias and pathological grief reactions. The subjects were evaluated in depth, using four taped clinical interviews, the Wechsler Adult Intelligence Scale (WAIS), the Rorschach test, and the Thematic Apperception Test (TAT). Psychodynamically oriented clinicians then examined the taped interviews and tests to arrive at a psychodynamic formulation outlining each patient's core unconscious conflicts. Key phrases from each formulation were extracted, and these words were put on tachtiscopic slides. In addition, control words, not based upon the formulation, were put on other slides. Words could be presented to each patient both subliminally (for 1 millisecond) and supraliminally (for 30–40 milliseconds). The briefer subliminal flash is not consciously registered, but the longer supraliminal flash is. Each time words were flashed, brain activity was measured by event-related potentials. Event-related potentials are objectively measured EEG brain responses that are used in subliminal-perception research as markers showing that the brain has recognized a subliminal or supraliminal stimulus. The investi-gators found that, *when words related to the patient's presumed unconscious conflicts were flashed subliminally (too fast for conscious registration), the patient's brain discriminated them early,* within 400 milliseconds. When the control words were flashed, there was much slower discrimination. *When the words related to the patient's conflicts were flashed supraliminally (permitting more conscious registration), the discrimination came very late.* These findings suggest that some kind of inhibitory process is operating when conflict-related words are presented supraliminally (closer to con-sciousness) compared with control words, whereas another kind of thought, unconscious thought, rapidly discriminates and recognizes them.

Currently, there are ongoing studies of changes in defence style over the course of psychodynamic psychotherapy at various centres, including Austen Riggs Hospital, a Harvard-affiliated inpatient unit in Stockbridge, Massachusetts; Columbia University, New York; McGill University, Montreal; and the Clarke Institute, Toronto. Preliminary data from the author's studies of the Defensive Functioning Scale (*DSM-IV*, p. 751) show that, in patients in psychoanalysis, maladaptive defences decrease, and defences from the high adaptive level increase. Perry and Cooper (1987) reviewed the studies relating maturity of ego defences to overall mental health. Mature defences correlated positively with such measures of mental health as Loevinger's Ego Development (Jacobson, Beardslee, Hanser, Noam, & Powers, 1986; Jacobson, Beardslee, Hanser, Noam, Powers, Houlihan, & Rider, 1986); the Global Assessment Scale (GAS) (Perry & Cooper, 1986; Battista, 1982), and the Health–Sickness Rating Scale (HSRS) (Valliant, 1976).

RESISTANCE

Resistance is simply the patient's use of defences against cognitive and emotional insight, either in the treatment situation or outside it. Fonagy and Moran (1993) make use of a time-series analysis, which is an application of the single-case method well suited to analysis. Following a single case of treatment that takes place over many sessions, the investigators take a large number of measurements at roughly equal intervals. Careful observation of changes in variables over time are used to investigate relevant relationships.

Fonagy and Moran report on their use of this technique to test clinical hypotheses and psychodynamic formulations. In a single case study of a brittle diabetic who recurrently transgressed her treatment regimen, they tested Moran's earlier hypothesis that recurrent transgressions of a diabetic regimen are related to underlying unconscious conflicts about anxiety and guilt. A time-series analysis of this patient's treatment was able to show that, as interpretations linking her regimen transgressions to unconscious anxiety and guilt were made, the patient improved her diabetic control. Time-series analysis also showed that, as the improved diabetic control increased, so did the likelihood of manifest guilt and anxiety one to three weeks later.

Resistance has been studied by a number of researchers (Fonagy & Moran 1993; Luborsky, 1993b; Bucci & Miller, 1993; Fretter et al, 1994). Time-series analysis was used by Graff and Luborsky (1977) to study the course of transference and resistance in four psychoanalyses of varying success. In the successful psychoanalyses, both transference and re-sistance were high in the early phases. In mid-phase, transference stabilized and resistance ratings fell. In the unsuccessful analyses, trans-ference and resistance were initially high, and, as treatment progressed, resistance ratings did not fall. This is consistent with the general clinical axiom that, when resistance occurs, it must be interpreted in order for treatment to proceed effectively. There is evidence from Weiss et al (1986) that, when such interventions occur, resistance decreases and pre-viously repressed material comes into session.

Resistance may manifest itself as subtle cognitive disturbances or forgetting during sessions. In studies by Luborsky's group, audio- or videotaped treatments are transcribed, and instances of forgetting are located in sessions (Luborsky, 1993b). Fifty-word units before and after the forgetting are blindly rated for the presence of Core Conflictual Rela-tionship Themes and compared with control units where forgetting does not occur. A study of thirteen such instances in the analysis of Ms A. showed a statistically significant activation of CCRTs, references to the therapist, and a sense of helplessness (such as expectation of rejection) in the forgetting segment versus that of control segments. According to psychoanalytic theory, one would anticipate that resistances (defences against insight) such as repression would emerge when conflicted mate-rial which has not been worked through emerges.

THE THERAPEUTIC ALLIANCE AND RESISTANCE
INTERPRETATION

The concept of therapeutic alliance, which is now used in many forms of treatment, derives from Freud's notion that a rapport is required to con-duct the work of psychoanalysis and psychoanalytic psychotherapy. The therapeutic alliance is a necessary, but not sufficient, condition for therapeutic change, and its development is often best promoted by accu-rate interpretations (Hanly, 1994). There are currently numerous studies showing that a therapeutic alliance is a predictor of positive treatment response in psychoanalytic and other forms of therapy. The empirical literature on the therapeutic alliance has been reviewed most recently by Horvath, Gaston, and Luborsky (1993); see also Marziali, Marmar, & Krupnick [1981].

There are a number of key alliance measures, including the CALPAS, Pen Helping Alliance, Therapeutic Alliance Scale, Vanderbilt Therapeu-tic Alliance Scale, and the Working Alliance Inventory. These measures have in common the measurement of personal attachments to the therapist and the tendency of patient and therapist to collaborate. The reliability of the major therapeutic alliance scales is about .86. 'Instruments rated by therapists are the most reliable, at .93, but the client's scales are also stable, at .88. The average interclass correlation reported for observer's ratings is a respectable .82' (Horvath et al, 1993, p. 255). Horvath et al go on to note that, 'in general, the alliance measures appear to be better at predicting outcomes tailored to the individual client, such as the Target Complaint (TC) measure, than assessments of symptomatic change, such as the Symptom Checklist (SCL 90)' (p. 258). The same authors also point out that there is evidence showing that patients who have difficulty maintaining relationships or who have poor family relationships are less likely to develop strong alliances. These findings are clinically relevant since psychoanalytic psychotherapists often treat patients with relationship difficulties. On the other hand, there is evidence that, when maladaptive patterns are pointed out, the therapeutic alliance can frequently be improved. Luborsky (1993b) points out that the alliance research has clearly shown:

- A positive early therapeutic alliance is correlated with positive outcome.
- An initially negative alliance is not correlated in any way with outcome.
- This means that a patient who starts with a largely negative alliance may not or *may* be improved at the end of treatment.

DEVELOPMENTAL INHIBITIONS AND PSYCHOPATHOLOGY

Freud (1910/1957) argued at the turn of the century that psychic conflict at times could be so intense that normal development is inhibited, delayed, or fixated, or fails to run its course completely. These hypotheses gave rise to new studies of infant and child observation, and to the development of child psychoanalysis and child psychiatry.

The study of childhood trauma is undertaken largely by naturalistic, longitudinal methods, since the scientific community has been sufficiently persuaded by anecdotal evidence of case histories and large-group natural disasters that childhood trauma is, by definition, obviously devastating, and that control experiments designed to bring it about and compare it with control conditions would be unethical.

This field is too vast to review here; however, a few naturalistic studies will be noted. A. Freud and Burlingham (1944), Spitz (1946, 1965), Robertson (1953), and Bowlby (1980) have all studied the effects of the separation of children from parents, and how these lead to later difficulties with attachment. The deprivation of empathic care has been studied in a large number of children by Weil (1992), as have the effects of excessive stimulation of children (Weil 1989a, 1989b). Early parent death and its effect in inhibiting normal development is reviewed by Altschul (1988) and Dietrich (1989). The inhibition of the normal development of autonomy is studied extensively by Mahler, Pine, and Bergman (1975). The effects of family breakdown and divorce in inhibiting the normal development of the ability to trust and make commitments in intimate relationships is studied longitudinally by Wallerstein and Blakeslee (1989).

The operationalized assessment of the level of psychological developmental and its inhibition is extremely complex, because there are so many aspects to development and there appears to be an interactive effect among various developmental lines. Hartley (1993) has reviewed existing measures. There are measures of object relations (the internal representations of the object of a subject's interest), cognitive function, and autonomy; Rorschach measures of development; and epigenetic hierarchies. A scale developed by Piper, Azim, McCallum, and Joyce (1990) has been used to measure interpersonal development in therapy.

THE BENEFITS OF ACCURATE INTERPRETATION

Crits-Christoph, Barber, Baranackie, and Cooper (1993) have reviewed the literature on assessing interpretations. Assessing interpretation means taking into account not only the number of interpretations made, but also the accuracy, dose, depth, timing, effect on outcome, and alliance of any interpretive intervention. Speisman (1959) found some corroboration for the fairly mainstream idea that, in order to achieve a minimal level of resistance, interpretations cannot be too deep or too superficial. Marziali (1984) studied audiotaped psychotherapy sessions and demonstrated that the frequency of transference interpretations correlates positively with a number of positive-outcome indicators, including the capacity for intimacy and using emotional support.

A typical strategy for assessing accuracy of interpretation is to have independent judges rate a number of sessions and score them in terms of Core Conflictual Relationship Themes (CCRTs) and then examine the therapist's interventions to see if they address these conflicts or transference derivatives. Using this method, Luborsky and Crits-Christoph (1990) found that higher levels of CCRT accuracy correlate with better outcomes. Especially important were the accurate depictions of the patient's wishes towards others, and the anticipated response of others. The study (reviewed in Crits-Christoph et al, 1993, p. 376), also showed that accurate interpretations work not only in the context of a positive therapeutic alliance. This is an extremely relevant finding because it underlines that, at least in that sample, the common clinical belief that a background of a positive alliance is essential for interpretive work is a simplification. Earlier work by Luborsky, Crits-Christoph, Alexander, Margolis, and Cohen (1983) had shown that 'accurate interpretations served to both improve a poor alliance and maintain an initially positive one' (discussed in Crits-Christoph et al, 1993, p. 379). Studies by Weiss et al (1986) and Fretter et al (1994), as well as those by Siberschatz, Fretter, and Curtis (1986), show that accurate interpretations correlate with progress in therapy.

TECHNICAL NEUTRALITY, ANONYMITY, NON-JUDGMENTAL LISTENING, ABSTINENCE

The procedures of technical neutrality, anonymity, non-judgmental listening, and abstinence all serve to promote free association in an environment where transference can be examined. The major psychoanalytic psychotherapy manual for severe personality disorders by Kernberg et al (1989) describes technical neutrality this way: 'Technical neutrality is crucial because interpretation of the transference is ineffective without it. Only the therapist who is both participant and yet a neutral observer, aligned with the patient's observing ego, is able to diagnose, clarify, and interpret the principle active transference paradigm. Neutrality does not signify indifference: rather it expresses concerned, objective, even-handed interest in helping the patient develop self-understanding, without a personal investment in any one aspect of the patient's behavior or interactions' (p. 23). The therapist doesn't suggest, incite, coax, or use praise or blame as major motivational strategies. Non-reliance on advice giving is central to the most widely used manual (Luborsky, 1984), as is listening with a high degree of openness to what the patient is saying. Abstinence is neutrality with respect to the patient's wishes towards the therapist. Warme (1994) discusses the dangers of deviation from technical neutrality.

The work of Weiss et al (1986), which involved hundreds of measurements of interventions on a few cases, found that, at times, technical neutrality, if it is in keeping with the patient's plan, is therapeutic, but, on occasion, it can be counter-therapeutic.

The development of psychotherapy manuals, and rating scales which allow researchers to measure adherence by clinicians to the various techniques, has been a methodological move forward, and may help to clarify this kind of issue in the future. Psychoanalytic psychotherapy research manuals have been recently reviewed by Butler and Strupp (1993). The review of Luborsky, Diguer, et al (1993) is based upon a number of manual-guided measures of adherence to various techniques.

METHOD OF CHANGE

Change in psychoanalytic psychotherapy occurs in many ways. Luborsky's recent review of the empirical literature concludes that 'the main curative factors in dynamic psychotherapy come about through working toward three changes: achieving a helping relationship, achieving understanding, and incorporating the gains of treatment. Each of these is fostered by a corresponding technical ability of the therapist' (Luborsky, 1993b, p. 520). Empirical studies of changes in the CCRT in treatment brought about by accurate interpretation show that, as the unconscious is made conscious, aspects of the CCRT are altered. Luborsky and Crits-Christoph (1990) have shown that, while the wishes do not alter, how the patient reacts to them or expects others to react to them alters significantly. As mentioned above, Weiss et al (1986) have developed a measure of transference that involves accurately measuring not just particular transference images, but how the patient seeks to put the entire transference plan into effect, in an attempt to repeat, and possibly disconfirm, the pathogenic beliefs behind it, in a totally case-specific way. This group has produced numerous studies (see Weiss et al, 1986, and Weiss, 1993, for bibliography). Fretter et al (1994) showed that, in all cases, when therapists' interpretations accurately addressed the patient's wish-plan, there were signs of increased progress.

Luborsky (1993b) found that early insight correlates with good outcome. While therapist insight or understanding of the patient correlates with patient progress, it is not the only therapeutic factor, and evidence at this point does not show that patient insight has a simple one-to-one correlation with outcome. But the fact that improvement in patient insight does not appear to have a direct correlation with outcome does not mean that accurate interpretation is not essential to promote cure.

The psychoanalytic notion of insight contains both cognitive and affective components, and the latter are difficult to measure.

Indeed, it has been argued, since mid-century, that many of the curative factors operate at an unconscious level of learning. Strachey (1934) argued that in treatment existing unconscious identifications, including the superego, are modified. Loewald (1960) showed how new positive identifications with the therapist are formed slowly. Instruments to measure how patients identify with the therapists have been reviewed by Orlinsky and Geller (1993).

Operationalization of this complex measure has begun. Studies show that patients think of their therapists as guiding and supportive between sessions and that these therapist representations persist long after the termination of treatment (Geller, Cooley, & Hartley, 1981; Wzontek, 1990). Geller et al (1981), using the Therapist Representation Inventory, found that patients evoke the image of the therapist to mitigate painful feelings.

Follow-up studies show that in many cases, patients develop an analysing function, or the ability to reflect on themselves with critical distance (Schlessinger & Robbins, 1975, 1983). Thus far, however, these studies, which are very costly, have been done only on a small number of patients.

Part III: Outcome Research in Psychoanalytic Psychotherapies and Psychoanalysis

GENERAL METHODOLOGICAL CONSIDERATIONS

Seligman (1995) describes the typical psychotherapy efficacy study or randomized clinical trial. This type of study design has evolved over time, and hundreds of such studies have been performed. It is often taken as the gold standard for proving that a treatment works.

1 A control group is used, to which patients are randomly allocated.
2 Controls receive attention that contains non-specific elements that might substitute for a patient's hopeful expectations or for the benefits of sympathetic attention.
3 The treatments tested follow manuals, so that one can be certain that the treatment, and not a variant, is being adhered to.
4 Treatments are videotaped to make certain the clinician is adhering to the manual.

5 Treatment occurs for a fixed number of sessions so that 'doses' can be determined.
6 The symptoms are all operationalized (defined) according to a standardized system.
7 The patients suffer from a single well-defined disorder. Thus the whole idea is to examine a discrete intervention for a discrete disorder in a large-enough sample so that the results can then be generalized to larger populations.
8 Ratings are made serially, even after the end of treatment, to see whether the gains are maintained.
9 Raters of the outcome are blind to whether the patient comes from the treatment or the control group.
10 Generalizability to the population is sometimes compromised. These studies are expensive, and so inclusion and exclusion criteria, which try to help lower costs by keeping the study small and focused on a single question (e.g., Is this form of treatment good for major depression?), may lead to a non-representative, non-random sample. For instance, if a study on patients with depression excludes all those who also have personality and substance abuse disorders, it may have limited relevance to the treatment of depressed patients in the field, who often have these disorders. This defeats the purpose of the random clinical sample, which is to choose a smaller group that represents a larger population. Fonagy and Moran (1993) have addressed this in detail.

One can see that the efficacy study design is not a senseless carbon copy of the double-blind model used, for example, in drug studies; reasonable adaptations to the matter investigated have been made. Good drug studies are, for instance, double blind. In double-blind drug studies, the raters, the clinicians, and the patients are blind to the drug administered. It would obviously be impossible to be blind to the type of psychotherapy one is administering. As well, it is hard to find a patient 'blind' enough to be unable to distinguish between psychoanalysis on the couch and behaviour therapy.

The typical ideal efficacy study or clinical trial has its limitations as well as its advantages. 'Even though clinical trials test treatments under clinic conditions, generality of the results to clinical settings may still be a relevant concern. Clinical trials often introduce special features into the situation to meet the demands of research that depart from most clinical applications of treatment' (Kazdin, 1986, p. 36; see Kazdin for futher discussion of this). Some go as far as Seligman (1995), a former champion of the typical manualized efficacy study, who now argues that 'the efficacy study is the wrong method for empirically validating psychotherapy as it is actually done, because it omits too many crucial elements of what is done in the field' (p. 966). 'While the random clinical trial is an incredibly valuable instrument, it has in some quarters gained a kind of mystique (Streiner, 1995), rather than remaining a helpful instrument that is an important component of the investigation of outcome. The deficiencies of the randomized clinical trial stem from the fact that the practice of psychotherapy *in the field* differs from the way it is practised in efficacy studies, in the following important ways (Seligman, 1995).

1 In the field, therapists are not randomly assigned, but chosen actively by the patients. Patients actively shop for therapists and screen out those they feel they cannot talk to. In psychotherapy studies with random assignment, as they are currently done, the patient is rendered basically passive in this important process.

2 In the field, the patient's pre-treatment condition, not other control patients, is the baseline against which improvement is judged.

3 In the field, flexibility and nuance are prized. If an approach is not working, the therapist is self-correcting. In manualized studies, clinicians are expected to conform with a particular technique, and to make sure that the therapy being tested is actually being applied.

4 In the field, confidentiality is highly valued, and third-party listening discouraged. Psychodynamic psychotherapy may deal with material about which the patient feels vulnerable, ashamed, or guilty. Audio- or videotaping of sessions inevitably affects the clinical process.

5 In the field, the frequency and number of sessions must be matched to patient need, since each person requires a different dose of therapy. In efficacy studies, there are usually a fixed and limited number of sessions.

6 Symptoms can be operationalized in the field as they are in efficacy studies. However, clinicians often note that the patient may present with one problem (e.g., depression) and, as time goes on, reveal other problems (e.g., a narcissistic style of relating that is subtle and emerges clearly only in the relation with the therapist), which turn out to be core difficulties that are not easy to operationalize.

7 Patients typically present with co-morbid (i.e., multiple) types of problems or disorders, and they are not excluded from treatment in

the field. As well, as Seligman (1995) notes, 'psychotherapy in the field is almost always concerned with *improvement in the general functioning* of patients, as well as amelioration of a disorder and relief of specific, presenting symptoms. Efficacy studies usually focus on specific symptom reduction and whether the disorder ends' (p. 967). Despite these differences, ratings are possible without interfering significantly with what goes on within therapy.

8 Serial ratings are possible at the beginning, during, at the ending, and at follow-up in the field.

9 Independent raters (i.e., not the clinician or the patient) of patient outcome are possible in studies in the field.

OTHER METHODOLOGICAL DIFFICULTIES SPECIFIC TO
LONG-TERM STUDIES: ETHICAL PROBLEMS, CONTROL GROUPS,
CO-MORBIDITY, AND ATTRITION RATE

Hawton (1992), in reviewing some of the special challenges that face investigators of long-term as opposed to shorter-term treatments, points out that long-term studies are far less feasible and far more expensive if comprehensive. In addition, in long-term studies, ethical problems emerge if treatment in the control group is restricted over a period as long as the treatment itself.

Control Groups

'True no-treatment control groups are impossible to set up as contrast groups for psychotherapy efficacy studies. Distressed human beings do not sit still like rats in cages waiting for an experiment to end. They act to relieve their distress' (Lambert, Shapiro, & Bergin, 1986, p. 181). Therefore, waiting lists as controls are possible only for short-term therapies. Clinicians are unwilling to refer patients to long-term studies if there is a risk that they would be assigned to a control group.

Co-morbidity

Long-term treatments are far less specific to a single diagnosis and, like antibiotics, are used for a broad spectrum of disorders. In fact, this is one of the strengths of the psychodynamic approach: it is widely applicable. Co-morbidity is a common clinical problem, if not the rule, in psychoanalytic psychotherapy settings (Doidge et al, 1994). This means that there is always a lot of variation in the sample. To adequately assess the effects of this variation, one would require multiple studies and measures. In addition, statistical power requires large samples

Cost

Many measures and multiple sites may be required to get a large enough sample, raising the cost of the study. Some important designs call for studies that would be so expensive that they have not been performed. Thus, treatments that are often found to be beneficial in practice await empirical validation. Another alternative is to assess the use of psychoanalytic psychotherapies for specific disorders. Manuals have recently been written for the psychoanalytic treatment of depression, panic disorder (Milrod, Busch, Cooper, & Shapiro, 1997), drug abuse, and the borderline personality disorder. However, disorder-specific manuals will not address the problem that patients in these therapies more often than not suffer from a number of disorders, or a pattern of Axis I (symptom) and Axis II (personality) co-morbidity. In other words, disorder-specific manuals are, in a way, at odds with the notion that individual treatments, by definition, are tailored to individuals with co-morbidity problems. Of course, therapists, facilities, and research assistants are employed in the study for a much longer period, increasing costs as well.

Attrition Rate

If only 10 per cent of patients per year drop out of a short-term treatment that lasts one year, at the end of the study 90 per cent of the sample remains. The same low drop-out rate in a long-term treatment, taken over five years, would leave just over half the sample. Yet the initial battery of measures has to be done on all patients. Thus one must double the number of patients to offset the attrition rate, increasing the cost.

Given these limitations, prudence or moderation is called for when assessing data. *In practice, this means reviewing all available data: random clinical trials (which, because they are so expensive, have more often been confined to only very brief therapies), qualitative studies, and single-case studies, as well as examining naturalistic studies.*

In naturalistic studies, the patient is his or her own control, and change is assessed on well-known measures. Researchers measure outcome against their knowledge of the natural history of character disorders, which are by definition chronic and unremitting. Luborsky et al

(1988) argue that there are now in fact so many psychotherapy studies using standardized measures that one can assess psychotherapies with adequate precision without a comparison group. Luborsky, Crits-Christoph, Mintz, and Auerbach (1988) have developed the method of comparing *similar study controls* on well-known measures, and in their study of psychodynamic psychotherapy, Luborsky, Diguer, et al (1993) found that 'the treated group's effects sizes were larger than those from the set of somewhat similar studies' *control* groups' (p. 60). Indeed, one of the purposes of having such well-established measures is for use in such situations.

RESEARCH INTO PSYCHOTHERAPY IN GENERAL

There are so many different types of psychotherapy to evaluate that, for almost fifty years, a popular strategy in evaluating them has been to lump studies together, a strategy called 'meta-analysis.' Whereas in the 1950s Eysenck[*] applied arbitrary standards for what constituted a study worthy of evaluation, researchers in the 1970s and 1980s have addressed these methodological difficulties in recent meta-analyses of psychotherapy outcomes. The first large meta-analysis was done by Smith, Glass, and Miller (1980). Their meta-analysis found that the average person who underwent psychotherapy was better off on outcome measures than were 85 per cent of those who did not undergo it (Smith et al, 1980). The weakness of that analysis was that it included good and bad psychotherapy studies. Hence, only studies that showed methodological rigour were included in a number of recent and prominent meta-analyses that improved on the original work of Smith et al. These new meta-analyses showed that 80 per cent of a number of types of psycho-

---

[*]In the 1950s, Eysenck argued that many psychotherapy response rates were no higher than the rates of spontaneous remission. His charges made their way into many introductory psychology textbooks. However, in the 1960s, 1970s, and 1980s, Eysenck's conclusions were refuted on a number of counts because they were based upon, among other things, 'non-comparable comparison groups, a multitude of arithmetic errors and misinterpretations of the original data, lack of comparable outcome criteria, diagnostic ambiguity and variations on the amount of therapy received' (McNeilly & Howard, 1991, p. 74). It was pointed out that, in his studies, he made the error of assessing outcome before the patients' psychotherapies were completed (APA, 1982). A recent re-evaluation of Eysenck's own data actually shows that, 'according to his [Eysenk's] % improvement estimates, psychotherapy accomplishes in about 15 sessions what spontaneous remission takes two years to do. Thus, Eysenck's data reveal that psychotherapy is very effective' (McNeilly & Howard, 1991, p. 74).

analytic, cognitive, and behavioural psychotherapy are efficacious (Melt-zoff & Kornreich, 1970; Luborsky, Singer, & Luborksy, 1975; Lambert, Shapiro, & Bergin, 1986). Whereas some early opponents of psycho-therapy argued that the rates of improvement were 'modest,' these findings turn out to be equivalent to reducing an illness or death rate from 66 to 34 per cent – a very significant improvement (Rosenthal & Rubin, 1982). Shapiro and Shapiro (1982) found that the mean effect size of a psychotherapeutic treatment is one standard-deviation unit.

The *effect size* is the standard measure of improvement used for com-parative psychotherapy studies, where a number of outcome measures are used. The *effect size* represents the pre-treatment score mean on a measure minus the post-treatment score mean divided by the standard deviation of the pretreatment scores.

COMPARISON OF PSYCHODYNAMIC PSYCHOTHERAPIES WITH OTHER WELL-ESTABLISHED THERAPIES

Do the psychodynamic psychotherapies contribute to the overall posi-tive findings seen in the meta-analyses? Luborsky, Diguer, et al (1993) have reviewed the existing empirical evidence for the efficacy of psy-choanalytic psychotherapy in comparison with other treatments. As stated, the major meta-analyses of psychotherapeutic efficacy have shown that psychotherapy in general works, and the effect size on a number of well-validated measures is equivalent to increasing the suc-cess rate of a treatment from 34 to 66 per cent. However, these meta-analyses lump together a number of treatments, including behavioural, cognitive, psychoanalytic, and other therapies. The authors reviewed studies in which psychoanalytic psychotherapy was compared with other treatments. To be included in the review, the comparison studies had to meet at least 6½ of the inclusion criteria in table 4.2. Judges had good agreement on determining which studies were to be included. That left thirteen comparative studies, but since some of the studies compared several treatments, a total of seventeen comparisons were made. Psychodynamic therapies were compared with the following non-dynamic ones: experiential, behavioural, cognitive, cognitive/behavioural, group, and hypnosis. These studies were compared *only* on well-known outcome measures that had been used in most of the stud-ies. The measures included: general scales such as the Health–Sickness Rating Scale (HSRS), the Global Assessment Scale (GAS), the Brief Psy-chiatric Rating Scale (BPRS), the Symptom Checklist 90 (SCL-90);

Table 4.2: Inclusion Criteria for Comparative Psychotherapy Studies

---

1 There is random assignment of patients (or stratified assignment on prognostic variables).
2 Real patients are used, not actors or student volunteers.
3 Therapists for each group are equally competent.
4 Therapists are not inexperienced; they are knowledgeable about the form of therapy they do.
5 Treatments are equally valued by the patients and therapists in each group.
6 The outcome measures take into account the target goals of the treatment. (weight 1/2)
7 Treatment outcome is evaluated by independent measures.
8 Information is obtained about the patients' concurrent use of treatments other than that intended, both formal and informal. (weight 1/2)
9 Samples of each of the compared treatments are independently evaluated for the extent to which therapists adhere to the manual designated treatment. (weight 1/2)
10 Each of the compared treatments is given in equal amounts in terms of length and frequency.
11 Each treatment is given in an amount that is reasonable and appropriate to the form of treatment.
12 Sample size is adequate.

Source: Luborsky, Barber, et al, 1993, in Miller et al, 1993, p. 498

depression scales such as the Beck Depression Inventory (BDI) and the Hamilton Rating Scale for Depression (HRSD); and the Social Adjustment Scale (SAS). Effects sizes were calculated. Next, Luborsky, Diguer, et al (1993) reliably rated these studies using the box-score method, which divides all improvement into 'significantly better,' 'significantly worse,' and 'no significant change.' Fourteen of the seventeen comparisons showed no significant difference between dynamic treatments and the comparison groups – in other words they were equivalently efficacious. In the remaining three, one psychodynamic therapy was better, and two non-dynamic therapies were better. The studies included are listed in table 4.3.

What do these findings mean? The earlier study by Luborsky et al (1975) had shown that approximately 80 per cent of patients benefit from these psychotherapies. This study showed that dynamic therapies contributed to these high rates of benefit.

It is important to keep in mind that many of these measures are symptom-based and that psychoanalytic treatments commonly also deal with Axis II (personality) pathology or the interactions of symptom and personality or character pathology (Doidge et al, 1994). What these stud-

Table 4.3: Significance of Differences in Effect Sizes, Dynamic versus Other Psychotherapies

Study	Dynamic Versus	Quality Ratings	Termination Cohen's r	Termination Z	Termination N	One Year Follow-Up Cohen's r	One Year Follow-Up Z	One Year Follow-Up N	Box Score T	Box Score FU
Beutler & Mitchel, 1981	Experiential	10.5	-0.41	-2.59	40				-	
Brodarty & Andrews, 1983	Family Doctor	6	0.03	0.18	24	-20	-1.13	32	0	0
Brom et al., 1989	Desensitization	9.5	.12	0.93	60				0	
	Hypnotherapy		0.19	1.45	58				0	
Cross et al., 1982	Behavior	7	.08	0.44	30	-0.40	-1.65	17	0	0
Elkin et al., 1989	Cognitive[b]	11	.08	0.73	84				0	-
Gallagher & Thompson, 1982	Cognitive-behavior Behavior	8	-3.3	-1.92	20	-1.57	-1.44	18	0	
Marmar et al., 1988	Group	7	-0.20	1.56	61	0.17	1.33	61	0	0
Patterson et al., 1971	Behavior	6.5	-2.5	-1.82*	53	0	0	20	-a	0
Pierloot & Vinck, 1978	Desensitization	8	0.12	0.56	60				0	
Sloane et al., 1975	Behaviour	10	0.07	0.54	60	0	0	60	0	0
Thompson et al., 1987	Cognitive-behavior	10	-0.01	-0.08	61				0	
	Behavior		-0.07	-0.54	60				0	
Woody et al., 1983	Cognitive-behavior	10	0.24	2.02*	71				0	
	Drug Counselling		0.26	2.19*	71				+	+
Zitren et al., 1978	Behavior	9.5	0.13	1.37	111				0	

Overall results

Termination	Uncorrected	$r = 0.008$	$Z = 0.40$	$p = 0.40$
	Corrected	$r = 0.01$	$Z = 1.17$	$p = 0.24$
Follow-up	Uncorrected	$r = -0.14$	$Z = -1.43$	$p = 0.15$
	Corrected	$r = -0.19$	$Z = -1.85$	$p = 0.06$

Box score: Dynamic better = +; Nonsignif. diff. = 0; Dynamic worse = -; a = worst in 1st period; same in 2nd period.

* = Z was significant at p < 0.05
b = IPT was the therapy instead of dynamic

From Luborsky, Diguer et al. (1993) in Miller et al. (1993), p. 502. Reprinted with the kind permission of Basic Books, New York, NY.

ies have not examined is whether the analytic therapies have advantages in terms of long-term characterologic benefits and adjustment.

THE PENN STUDY: A NATURALISTIC STUDY WITH OPERATIONALIZED MEASURES AND INDEPENDENT RATERS

The Penn study (Luborsky et al, 1988) was launched in 1968 and lasted five years, seeing seventy-three patients through to completion. Evaluations were performed at the first session, on termination, and on a sample at five years after termination to see if gains were maintained. The most common *DSM-III* (APA, 1985) diagnoses were the following: dysthymia, 22; generalized anxiety disorder, 21; schizoid personality disorder, 10; compulsive personality, 7. The initial Health–Sickness Rating Scale (a global severity measure) was 59.5, meaning that patients could function moderately well without hospital support.

Patients had to complete at least eight sessions of therapy to be included in the study. Of the 111 patients screened, 73 were included. Most drop-outs (15) occurred after one to seven sessions. Sixteen patients were still in therapy at the cut-off point, and so they were not included in the data analysis. Of the therapists in the study, 22 were supervised psychiatry residents, and 20 psychiatrists on staff. The orientation was psychoanalytic. Independent observers conducted pre-treatment and post-treatment prognostic interviews and rated taped sessions. The average length of treatment was thirty-two sessions. The Luborsky manual had not been completed but was used retrospectively to rate the sessions for compliance with the manual. The mean rating of compliance with the manual was only slightly less than that for those who were formally trained in the manual. This was not surprising since the manual codified treatment approaches at that centre. Outcome measures included independent clinician raters, treating clinician ratings, and patient ratings.

Some of the changes on common measures included observer ratings of changes on the Health–Sickness Rating Scale, equivalent to a .69 effect size. (For comparison, the change on the same measure in the Menninger study, discussed below, was .77.) Patient ratings on the Hopkins Symptom Checklist showed effect size changes of .80 (Luborsky et al, 1988, p. 266).

Patients also showed significant decreases in physical as well as psychological symptoms, and these changes correlated with general outcome. Overall improvement rates, according to therapist ratings, were

92 per cent (22 per cent large improvement, 43 per cent moderate improvement, 27 per cent some improvement, 7 per cent no change, and 1 per cent worse). If one excludes the 'some improvement' category and looks at the combined categories of 'moderate' and 'large' improvement, therapists rated 65 per cent of patients falling into either the moderate or large improvement categories, while independent raters found 56 per cent of patients as having made a moderate or large improvement. These improvements were still in place at the seven-year follow-up (Luborsky et al, 1988). In fact, a majority of patients continued to improve after their psychoanalytic psychotherapy was completed. This may occur because internal blocks and developmental inhibitions have been undone in treatment, placing development back on track.

RECENT NON-COMPARISON STUDIES OF PSYCHOANALYTIC
PSYCHOTHERAPY FOR PERSONALITY DISORDERS

Stevenson and Meares (1992), in a study conducted in New South Wales, Australia, evaluated the effectiveness of a psychodynamic psychotherapy based upon object-relations and self-psychological principles in the treatment of patients with borderline personality disorder. All patients had at least six months of unsuccessful treatment prior to the study. Patients were independently rated with the Diagnostic Interview for Borderlines. Treatment was twice weekly for twelve months, and supervised for adherence. It should be kept in mind that, in the field, treatment for this condition continues for a much longer time.

Investigators found a reduction from a mean of 17.40 to 10.50 in the number of *DSM-III* (APA, 1985) criteria fulfilled at follow-up as well as reductions in impulsivity, affective instability, anger, and suicidal behaviour. Seventy per cent fulfilled criteria for borderline personality disorder at follow-up, compared with 100 per cent at intake. There was a marked clinical improvement on the behavioural measures, including a reduction in medical visits, from 3.50 per patient per month to 0.47; a decrease in incidents of self-harm, from 3.77 episodes per year to 0.83; a reduction of hospital admissions, from 1.77 per year to 0.73; and a decrease in months spent as an inpatient, from 2.87 months to 1.47. The mean score on the Cornell Index fell from 42.63 to 28.63. While it is extremely probable that these patients require more therapy if they are to move towards a life that more closely approximates normal functioning, the progress they made is very significant.

Monsen, Oldland, Fangli, Dare, and Eilersten (1995), of Norway, recently reported on a prospective study of twenty-five patients with personality disorders treated with psychodynamic psychotherapy, based on object-relations and self-psychological principles, for a mean period of 25.4 months. The mean follow-up period was 5.2 years. The majority of patients, as in the Stevenson and Meares study (1992), had previously tried less-intensive forms of treatment. Patients were given self-reports, and rated at the beginning of treatment, at termination, and at five years post-termination. Defences, consciousness of affect, symptom scores, and Minnesota Multiphasic Personality Inventories (MMPIs) were obtained. At the five-year follow-up, 68 per cent of the patients no longer met criteria for personality disorder. Seventy-five percent of patients who carried an Axis I (symptom) diagnosis no longer had one on completion.

A CONTROLLED STUDY OF THE USE OF PSYCHODYNAMIC PSYCHOTHERAPY IN PATIENTS WITH PANIC DISORDER

Though the symptoms of panic are often alleviated by medication, the relapse rate remains as high as 75 per cent. Wiborg and Dahl (1996) conducted a controlled study that randomized well-diagnosed panic patients to treatment with clomipramine, versus treatment with clomipramine and fifteen weekly sessions of brief psychodynamic psychotherapy. They found that, at the end of treatment, all patients in the psychotherapy-plus-medication group were free of symptoms, as compared with 75 per cent of those on medication only. All patients were panic-free at the six-month follow-up. Medication was stopped at nine months. By the eighteen-month follow-up, there was a big difference between groups. The relapse rate (defined as satisfying *DSM-II-R* panic disorder criteria) for the medication-only group was 75 per cent, compared with only 20 per cent for those treated with medication and psychotherapy. At the nine-month follow-up, the medication-plus-psychotherapy group had significantly lower scores on most anxiety measures. This is consistent with the findings of Milrod (1995) and others who argue that psychoanalytic psychotherapy or psychoanalysis can reach the underlying vulnerabilities that predispose patients to panic disorder (Milrod, Busch, Cooper, & Shapiro, 1997).

PSYCHOANALYTIC PSYCHOTHERAPY FOR PSYCHOSES

While studies in the first half of this century showed that psychoanalysis is not generally effective in psychotic conditions, modified psychoanalytic psychotherapy has been shown to be helpful in some cases. Stanton et al (1984) assigned non-chronic schizophrenics to a more supportive psychodynamic psychotherapy or to a more expressive psychodynamic psychotherapy, and followed them. The supportive group did better in terms of recidivism and role performance, and the expressive group did better in terms of ego functioning and cognitive improvements. In addition, patients of therapists who were rated as skilled in dynamic exploration showed greater reductions in their global psychopathology and began to show less denial of illness and less apathy. Another study, by McGlashan (1983), from Chestnut Lodge, followed 163 patients who received psychoanalytically oriented psychotherapy for fifteen years. One-third of the patients had moderate to good outcomes, and they fell into two groups: those who attempted to integrate and understand the meaning of their psychosis and those who sealed it over. The first group had a slightly better outcome.

SHORT-TERM VERSUS LONG-TERM PSYCHODYNAMIC PSYCHO-
THERAPIES FOR PATIENTS WITH PERSONALITY PROBLEMS

Short-term psychoanalytic therapies (which focus on target symptoms as opposed to characterological difficulties) have also been meta-analysed, and 'in terms of target symptoms the average brief dynamic therapy patient was better off than 86 per cent of waiting list patients. In terms of general symptoms (SCL-90), the average brief dynamic therapy patient was better off than 79% of the waiting list patients' (Crits-Christoph, 1992, p. 154). Anderson and Lambert (1995) also meta-analysed short-term treatments and had similar results. They found that short-term psychodynamic treatments 'outperformed alternative treatments at follow-up assessment when measures of personality were used or when assessment took place 6 or more months posttreatment' (p. 512). Thus far, short-term psychotherapies seem more effective in relieving symptom distress than in improving patients' adaptive functioning (Horowitz, Marmar, Weiss, Kaltreider, & Wilner, 1986).There is solid evidence that both short- and long-term psychoanalytic psychotherapies are efficacious. However, it is wrong to conclude from these studies that short- and long-term psychotherapies have been shown to be equally efficacious in all cases. *We lack long-term studies that compare long and short-term treatments over the long term.* But there is mounting evidence that, for those with character disorders and symptoms (Axis I and Axis II co-morbidity), short-term treatment is not adequate.

A large literature demonstrates that patients with character or personality disorders have a much poorer prognosis in all sorts of treatments than do patients without them (Gabbard, 1994).

The National Institute of Mental Health Collaborative Study of Depression (Shea et al, 1990) is considered a state-of-the-art investigation that overcame a number of the earlier methodological objections about psychotherapy research. It demonstrated that, for mild to moderate depressions in outpatient populations, there was no significant difference between a form of short-term psychotherapy called 'interpersonal psychotherapy' (a much-shortened offshoot of interpersonal psychoanalysis), cognitive therapy, and medication. The NIMH study randomized patients to four different short-term (sixteen-week) treatment conditions, and then compared outcome on standardized measures by blind raters. When the subsample of those who didn't respond to the sixteen weeks of treatment was analysed, it was found that 'patients with personality disorders (74% of the sample) had significantly worse outcomes in social functioning than patients without personality disorders and were significantly more likely to have residual symptoms of depression' (Shea et al, 1990, p. 711). These careful studies document that the clinical practice of addressing underlying character difficulties to alleviate residual and future outbreaks of symptomatology not only makes sense, but is empirically advisable.

EFFICACY STUDIES OF PSYCHOANALYSIS SINCE 1950

A number of systematic studies of psychoanalysis outcome and efficacy have been performed on large groups of patients and have confirmed that, with the properly chosen patient, psychoanalysis yields significant benefits in terms of quality of life, symptom reduction, and character change. Moreover, these studies have allowed analysts to identify the kind of patient that they can help and many of those that they are unlikely to help. The improvement rates (efficacy) for psychoanalysis have been shown, in various studies, to be in the 60–91 per cent range for those who stay in treatment, depending on the way improvement was measured (Bachrach, Galatzer-Levy, Skilnikoff, & Waldron, 1991). If one does not include the data from patients for whom psychoanalysis is a heroic treatment (i.e., those patients for whom all other treatments failed *and* who had only a guarded prognosis in analysis at the onset of the analysis), the improvement rates for psychoanalysis are in the

75–90 per cent range for those who stay in treatment for at least three years, with the highest rates for those who stay in treatment until its natural termination. These high rates show a selection bias, because they include only those who stay in treatment, and it may be that those who stay in are the ones who are doing well. *But it is precisely this kind of selection bias that operates in the field.* What those high figures mean is not that psychoanalysis is for everybody but, rather, that those who are in a long treatment are likely to be benefiting.

THE MENNINGER PSYCHOTHERAPY RESEARCH PROJECT

The Menninger Foundation Psychotherapy Research Project (Kernberg et al, 1972; Wallerstein, 1986) was the first prospective study of psychoanalysis and psychoanalytic psychotherapy. It aimed to determine precisely what factors are therapeutic in psychoanalysis and what kind of patients are most or least likely to benefit from analysis. The study began in 1954 and traced subjects for a thirty-year period. The Menninger study included patients known to have *brief* psychotic episodes, called 'borderline' patients. In the 1940s, the new diagnostic category of 'borderline' emerged, consisting of patients who were on the borderline between psychoses and neurotic characters (Stern, 1938). Fifty per cent of the psychoanalytic patients in the Menninger study had borderline ego functioning. In addition, 35 per cent were severely alcoholic or drug-addicted, and 33 per cent had strongly paranoid traits. The average Health–Sickness Rating (a measure that was developed in the course of this study) of these analytic patients was about 50, which is significantly below the neurotic range, or that of most outpatients. (Lower scores indicate increased pathology.)

The Menninger study was conducted at a time when a number of analysts were seeking to widen the scope of analytic treatment beyond Freud's recommendations (Stone, 1954). Psychoanalytic researchers wished to see whether their procedures could help the sickest-possible patients who seemed unable to improve in other therapies. The Menninger Hospital, located in Topeka, Kansas, was ideal for studying these severely ill patients because it often functioned as a tertiary-care centre, taking in those who were unmanageable on a solely outpatient basis (Shane, 1988; Wallerstein, 1986). Many of these patients had failed to improve in previous therapies. In fact, one-third had to be hospitalized in the course of analysis. Only 45 per cent of the patients in analysis were actually suitable for analysis by today's criteria, and 27 per cent were accepted on the basis of heroic indications (i.e., psychoanalysis as a treatment of last resort, with a guarded prognosis).

Intake assessment included ten psychiatric interviews, psychological testing, interviews of family members, and physical examination. Progress was assessed in many ways, including examination of process notes and supervisory records. At termination, each patient was re-evaluated by senior clinicians. Forty-two cases were randomly selected for study. Patients were largely analysed by psychoanalysts in training (a drawback of the study).

Independent blind raters used a complex double-matched-pair method for thousands of blind ratings of sessions (early and late in treatment), including ratings on well-known measures such as the Health–Sickness Rating Scale, and even IQ changes. Overall, on global ratings, 25 per cent failed to improve, 14 per cent showed equivocal results, 23 per cent showed moderate improvement, and 36 per cent had very good improvement. In other words, *even among these very ill patients, about 60 per cent improved*. This is an impressive figure, when one considers that half the patients had borderline ego functioning or carried a borderline personality organization, and had multiple co-mor-bid diagnoses, and that most of the analysts were in training. The average improvement on the Health–Sickness Rating was thirteen points.

This study also showed that therapists' skills were related to global improvement. Strengths of the study included the development of a standardized outcome measure (the Health–Sickness Rating Scale, developed by Luborsky, is the precursor of Axis V in *DSM–IV*), the multiple investigations and clinical assessments by blind raters, and a thirty-year follow-up. The study included patients who failed all other treatments. Of course, this study was conducted before the development of standardized criteria for disorders or standardized symptom ratings.

The Menninger study has also given rise to other important findings. For instance, Blatt (1992) analysed the data to see if the responses to psychotherapy differed from those to psychoanalysis. Blatt found that patients whose pathology related primarily to disruptions of interpersonal relatedness and who use primarily avoidant defences (anaclitic patients) did better in psychotherapy. Patients whose pathology relates primarily to issues of self-definition, autonomy, and self-worth, and who use primarily counteractive defences (introjective defences), did better in psychoanalysis.

PERFECTIONISTIC, SELF-CRITICAL, INTROJECTIVE PATIENTS
AND LONG-TERM PSYCHOANALYTIC TREATMENT

More recent work by Blatt, Quinlan, Pilkonis, and Shea (1995) analysed
data from the NIMH Collaborative Study of Depression and found that
these self-critical introjective patients, in fact, did not get better in any of
the treatment conditions, all of which were short-term (medication,
interpersonal psychotherapy, cognitive behavioural therapy, and clinical
management). These patients are also more likely to make suicide
attempts. Blatt and Ford (1994) showed that inpatients who are introjective and received four-times-a-week psychodynamic psychotherapy
actually had a better prognosis after fifteen months of treatment than
their anaclitic counterparts receiving similar treatment. In summary,
data from these sources show that, although 'perfectionistic patients do
poorly in brief treatment for depression, they are significantly more
responsive to long-term, intensive psychoanalysis and psychoanalytically oriented inpatient treatment' (Blatt et al, 1995, p. 130).

MORE RECENT STUDIES OF PSYCHOANALYTIC EFFICACY

There have been five other major quantitative studies of psychoanalytic
efficacy since 1950. The majority of these have been prospective studies,
or have had prospective components.

The Columbia University Research Project

In 1959, the Columbia University Department of Psychiatry Center for
Psychoanalytic Training and Research launched its study of the characteristics and outcomes of 295 cases of psychoanalysis and psychotherapy. The best summaries of the Columbia data were published in
1985 (Weber, Solomon, & Bachrach, 1985; Weber, Bachrach, & Solomon,
1985a, 1985b; Bachrach et al, 1985).
   Of those who continued analysis at least past their analyst's gradua-
tion (and who hence had full-length treatments), 91 per cent were
judged improved (56 per cent much improved, 35 per cent improved).
Of those who switched from psychoanalysis to psychoanalytic psychotherapy when their analyst graduated, 86 per cent were judged
improved (36 per cent much improved, 50 per cent improved). Forty-
three per cent of patients developed an analytic process (the unique
state in which transferences of past experiences emerge onto the analyst,

at which point the patient can observe them and learn from them). The Columbia study showed that a therapeutic benefit could occur even if an analytic process did not develop. However, of those who were deemed to develop a full analytic process, 89 per cent terminated with maximum benefit. This confirmed that, while the analytic process is only one factor in therapeutic benefit, the psychoanalytic hypothesis that the psychoanalytic process is essential to maximum improvement was supported. In short, the Columbia study demonstrated that treatment length correlated with therapeutic benefit and analysability, and that analysis led to a good result. The weakness of the study was that it occurred before an era of agreed-upon symptomatic measures, so the scales used are not well known.

The Second Columbia University Study

Thirty-six analytic patients were involved in the second Columbia study (Weber, Solomon, & Bachrach, 1985), which employed detailed questionnaires, including rating scales, which were distributed to the patients, analysts, and supervisors. The sample was drawn from 112 patients on whom information regarding termination was complete. Only cases where analyst raters could express high degrees of confidence in ratings (confidence ratings) were used. One hundred and twenty-five psychotherapy patients were also studied. These patients tended to be somewhat sicker than the analytic patients. Of those analytic patients who stayed on through to termination, 96 per cent were judged improved (52 per cent much improved, 44 per cent improved), and effect sizes were large. One-third of those had maximum benefit. Among the 125 psychoanalytic psychotherapy patients, the overall improvement rate on all measures was 79 per cent, and all but three reported they were satisfied or very satisfied. The methodological weakness of this study is that treating analysts rated patient outcome.

In this study, analysability was associated with therapeutic benefit (78 per cent of analysable patients were much improved, and 75 per cent terminated with maximum benefit); 'treatment length, was substantially and consistently associated with therapeutic benefit and the development of the analytic process' (Weber, Bachrach, & Solomon, 1985b, p. 260).

The Boston Psychoanalytic Institute Prediction Studies

The Boston studies, conducted from 1959 to 1966 by Sashin, Eldred, and

Van Amerrowgen (1975), observed 130 patients who were treated by supervised analysts in training. All patients had been judged by experienced analysts to be functioning in the neurotic range. Their diagnoses were as follows: 39 hysteric neuroses, 37 obsessive compulsive neuroses, 17 mixed neuroses, and 17 other diagnoses. Outcomes were reported retrospectively by the treating analysts according to global change, situation at termination, and six clinical scales, including measures of: (1) symptom restriction; (2) symptom discomfort; (3) work productivity; (4) sexual adjustment; (5) interpersonal relations; and (6) insight. In addition, all analysts completed both a structural questionnaire of overall change (a seven-point scale) and the six-point Knight scale. Twenty-seven per cent of the cases terminated prematurely. Of the 130 who started analysis, 75 per cent were judged to have improved at least moderately, 4 per cent to be unchanged, and 6 per cent to be worse, and, again, treatment length was associated with a more favourable outcome, with the highest improvement among those who terminated by mutual consent. The study was limited by the use of the student analysts making assessments of their own treatments.

The New York Psychoanalytic Institute Studies

Researchers at the New York Psychoanalytic Institute (Erle, 1979; Erle & Goldberg, 1979) studied the outcomes of a total of eighty-two analytic cases, forty of whom were treated by student analysts, and forty-two by graduate analysts in private practice. The patients carried diagnoses of mixed character neuroses, obsessional neuroses, and hysterical neuroses. The results corroborated those of the Columbia group. Eighty-two per cent of cases who stayed in treatment longer than four years improved.

A second retrospective study by the same group (Erle & Goldberg, 1984) examined the work of 160 cases in treatment with sixteen experienced analysts. This study is still under way, but initial results show a positive correlation between treatment length and outcome, with 76 per cent of those who have completed analyses of at least three years' length having a 'good–excellent' therapeutic result.

OTHER FOLLOW-UP STUDIES OF PSYCHOANALYSIS

Long-term follow-up studies of psychoanalytic patients parallel the findings of Luborsky et al's (1988) follow-up studies of patients in psychoanalytic psychotherapy. Four studies employing four to six in-depth interviews several years after termination (Pfeffer, 1959, 1961, 1963; Schlessinger & Robbins, 1974, 1975, 1983; Norman, Blacker, Oremland, & Barrett, 1976) suggest that the patients achieve significant mastery over their conflicts and difficulties. This is consistent with Luborsky's quantitative findings in patients in psychoanalytic psychotherapy: patients become aware of their core conflictual relationship themes and of previously unconscious pathological dispositions or relationship patterns, and are less prone to enact the maladaptive components of them.

SUMMARY OF EFFICACY STUDIES OF PSYCHOANALYSIS

Bachrach et al (1991) have done the most extensive review and critique of the literature on psychoanalytic efficacy in terms of methodology, design, and results. They conclude that the six systematic studies of a total of 550 patients at four different centres point to the following conclusions: 'Patients who are suitable for psychoanalysis derive substantial therapeutic benefit ... improvement rates are typically in the 60–90% range, and effect sizes, when they have been calculated, are significant' (p. 904). The Columbia, New York, and Boston studies showed a correlation between length of treatment and therapeutic benefit, with improvement rates of 75–90 per cent in those who remained in treatment longer; therefore, psychoanalysis cannot be shortened without detracting from its effect.

Despite repeated efforts over the years to shorten it, psychoanalysis is a long-term intensive treatment requiring on average four sessions per week for a period of typically three to seven years, to produce a positive outcome (Panel, 1992). When one considers that the chief indications today for psychoanalysis are chronic conditions, the three-to-seven-year period is not an unreasonable amount of time to treat conditions associated with significant morbidity.

Longer Is Better – for Some Patients

Doidge et al (1994) found that 82 per cent of psychoanalytic patients had already tried briefer forms of treatment or medication before attempting psychoanalysis. These particular patients did not get sufficient symptom resolution in the briefer treatments.

Psychoanalysis is now, and seems destined to remain, a long-term intensive treatment that works best with four to five weekly sessions for a period of time that likely is no shorter than three years and that can extend to seven years, and, on rare occasions, for the treatment of patients with severe personality disorders or patients with histories of extreme trauma, even longer (Panel, 1992). This may seem like a very lengthy treatment, but it is not when compared with other medical treatments applied by physicians to other kinds of chronic illness. However, data from Doidge et al (1994) show that analysis typically lasts for approximately five to six years. Many chronic conditions, diabetes, for example, call for lifelong medical attention. Analysis is long, but not forever.

Clearly, short-term therapies have an important place in a rational system of health care, and, in fact, psychoanalysts such as Alexander, Beck, Davanloo, Malan, Mann, and Wolpe have pioneered their development. However, at present, most short-term therapies are not used to treat chronic psychic conflict, developmental inhibitions, or character disorders, but, rather, to address particular symptoms. So, short-term therapies and the long-term ones are generally not competitors, but complementary – each, when properly applied, answers the needs of a different patient population. Short-term dynamic and behavioural therapies generally concentrate on focal, or circumscribed, symptomatic problems, and, typically, patients with the more severe character disorders are excluded (Ursano, Sonnenberg, & Lazar, 1991; Gabbard, 1994). Yet, as short-term psychoanalytic researchers Strupp and Binder (1984, p. 275) note, the patients for whom short-term therapies are indicated are 'the least problematic cases. By contrast, patients falling short of optimal suitability for short-term approaches (according to the criteria mentioned earlier) represent by far the largest segment of the patient population.' They go on to write that 'the extensive contemporary literature dealing with borderline conditions and narcissistic personality disorders is almost entirely devoted to long-term intensive therapy' (p. 276). Thus, it doesn't make sense to set up an efficacy horse race between therapies that treat different conditions, and such comparisons should be taken with a grain of salt. This is especially so if characterological problems underlie the symptoms (Binder, Henry, & Strupp, 1987).

Short-term treatment may not always be adequate for depression. Data from the NIMH Collaborative Study of Depression (Shea et al, 1992), *while showing initially good results at sixteen weeks, have had very disappointing results at the eighteen-month follow-up.* Klerman and Weissman (1992), who originally championed an interpersonal short-term approach used in the study, wrote: 'The percentage of patients who had recovered during acute treatment, but who remained well over the 18-month follow-up, was disappointingly low, ranging from 19% to 30%. The rate of relapse for those who recovered – 30% to 50% – was disappointingly high. These rates were not significantly different between [the NIMH] treatment groups' (p. 832). Shea et al (1992) conclude: '16 weeks of these specific forms of treatment is insufficient for most patients to achieve full recovery and lasting remission' (p. 782). The best research from the NIMH is beginning to show what clinical practitioners have found in a century of treatments: brief psychotherapy or medication is not the answer to many depressed patients' needs. Many cognitive and interpersonal psychotherapists now argue for the need to lengthen their treatments, or to have longer-term maintenance treatments.

Dose and Frequency of Sessions

Dose of Sessions: When personality difficulties are present, longer-term therapies are better. In a study of 845 patients in five different outpatient sites, most of whom (71 per cent) were in psychodynamic treatments, using various versions of the well-known Symptom Checklist 90, acute and chronic distress symptoms improved faster than characterological symptoms (Kopta, Howard, Lowry, & Bentler, 1994).

Kopta et al also criticized how their previous attempts to define improvement led to an overestimation of the effects of low doses of treatment (Howard, Kopta, Kranse, & Orlinsky, 1986). In that 1986 paper, which is often quoted as evidence of the efficiency of short-term treatment, they showed that patients with symptoms often improve in a statistically significant way after twenty-six sessions, but beyond that number improvement rates did not increase significantly. In the later critical review of their earlier attempts, they noted that a patient can improve in a highly statistically significant way (e.g., go from having six hours of compulsive rituals to five hours) without having *really* recovered clinically. What their earlier dose studies left out was that long-term treatment gains often occur only after long-term working through. Thus, Kopta et al (1994) switched to calling a patient improved when a patient's scores were 'more similar to [those of] normal functional persons than to [those of] his or her dysfunctional peers' (p. 1009). They point out that their own earlier findings, which estimated fairly quick improvement rates, 'investigated general improvement that did not require a return to normal functioning. Thus it makes sense that fewer sessions are needed to simply improve rather than recover' (p. 1016). Investigators are increasingly finding that clinically relevant measures and definitions are more important than just demonstrating statistical significance. In addition, short-term studies of long-term therapies, by definition, cannot be the final word on long-term efficacy.

Along with length of treatment, frequency of sessions per week appears to be essential for transference analysis in depth. Although there have been no completed randomized studies comparing five-times-a-week to four-times-a-week psychoanalysis, for instance, three studies have compared analysis (at four or five times a week) to psychoanalytic psychotherapy (typically, once or twice a week). In all three studies, two prospective and one retrospective, the analytic patients did better. The Columbia group found that analytic patients who voluntarily switched to psychotherapy did not do as well as those who remained in analysis (Weber, Bachrach, & Solomon, 1985a). The poorer outcome may have been related to poorer motivation, or these patients may not have been doing as well anyway, or it may have been related to a lower dose of treatment.

The Psychotherapy Research Project of the Menninger Foundation compared twenty-two patients in analysis and twenty patients in expressive supportive psychotherapy. 'Patients with good ego strength tend to improve with the entire range of psychoanalytically oriented treatments (that is, psychoanalysis, expressive and supportive psycho-therapies), although improvement is greatest with psychoanalysis proper' (Kernberg, 1982, p. 7; see also Kernberg et al, 1972, for fuller discussion).

One might wonder if this better result in analysis applies only to neurotic patients. Waldinger and Gunderson (1984) did a retrospective review of treatments of seventy-eight patients with borderline personality disorder. They studied patients treated in psychoanalysis (which was more frequent and longer) and in psychoanalytic psychotherapy and found that, 'at the end of treatment, patients who have been in analysis had better object relations [interpersonal relations] and sense of self than patients who had been in psychotherapy. The fact that the two groups began treatment with the same levels of impairment in these areas means that the analytic patients improved more' (p. 195). While the analyses went on longer, which may be a confounding factor, it is important to keep in mind that the psychotherapies were not restricted in time. They conclude: 'A surprising number of these patients profited from psychoanalysis. We found that the longer the patients stayed in treatment, the more they improved' (p. 199). This is not to argue that analysis is the treatment of choice for all borderline patients, but, rather, to point out that analysis is a good treatment for *some* patients with very poor initial ego strength. (For an in-depth portrait of such a treatment, see Volkan, 1987.)

Høglend (1993) of Norway reported on a sample of forty-five out-patients treated with brief to moderate-length, manual-based, psycho-dynamic psychotherapy in from nine to fifty-three sessions. The design employed experienced therapists, who were monitored for adherence to the clinical focus. A manual based on modified principles stemming from the work of Malan and Sifneos was used. Audiotaped sessions were used for peer supervision by the group of participating clinicians, and adherence to the clinical focus was analysed. Patients were rated on the Global Assessment Scale (patients presented with a mean score of 61.9), target complaints, and a psychodynamic scale. *DSM-III* diagnoses were assessed used the LEAD (long-term evaluation of all data) stan-dard technique. For the patients with personality disorders, the number of sessions of treatment correlated with the degree of insight they had developed two years after therapy, and the degree of dynamic change at four years after therapy. No such correlation was noted for patients without personality disorders. Høglend concluded that, for personality-disordered patients, 'length of treatment seemed more essential for long-term dynamic improvement than patient characteristics such as suitability, cluster category, or initial health-sickness' (p. 168). Høglend also noted that 'very small, long-term dynamic changes were observed after a brief, focused treatment approach for patients with personality disorders, but significant long-term dynamic changes were observed after those treatments that last 30 sessions or more' (p. 168). Among fif-teen patients with personality disorders, those seven in longer psycho-dynamic treatments that were less focused (i.e., more typically free-associative, as opposed to using the short-term technique of treating associations outside the dynamic formulation as a resistance) did better. There were no major outcome differences between *DSM-III* clusters B and C.

Frequency of Sessions: The frequency of sessions is related to the overall number or dose of sessions. If number of sessions appears to correlate to outcome, it is reasonable to ask if increasing the frequency of sessions can hasten a good result, and thus help patients to overcome their difficulties and suffering, rather than dragging it out. Bannon, Perry, & Ianni (1995) have recently done a meta-analysis of published studies on personality disorders that used acceptable methods to make diagnoses and acceptable operationalized outcome measures, including observer ratings and self-reports. They reviewed studies from those that made use of daily inpatient psychoanalytic psychotherapy and those that used once-a-week outpatient psychoanalytic therapy. Three psychodynamic studies met their methodological criteria. Mean effect sizes for outcome on the self-reports and observer ratings were 1.04 and 1.00 for the patients versus 0.25 for 0.50 for the waiting list of control cases. Patients in these studies had a remittance of their personality-disorder at a rate of 11.57 per cent a year. None of the treatment patients continued to meet criteria for personality disorder diagnosis at 8.33 years of follow-up. This can be compared with the natural remission rate of, for example, the borderline personality disorder, which is only 3.71 per cent per year (Perry, 1993b). *This means that patients with therapy remit three to four times faster than they might without treatment.* For a 100 per cent remission 384 sessions were required. Patients in once-a-week treatment took 8.7 years for 100 per cent remission, and 2.45 years for a 50 per cent remission rate. *This length of time for remission was halved if patients were in twice-a-week treatment, to 4.3 years for 100 per cent patient remission, and 1.22 years for 50 per cent patient remission.*

Work with children is also showing that the frequency of sessions (sometimes called the 'intensity of treatment') is an important factor for a number of conditions. Target and Fonagy (1994a, 1994b) did a retrospective study of child psychoanalysis and psychotherapy at the Anna Freud Centre. They reviewed the extensive data base of 763 cases of children who met *DSM-III-R* criteria for emotional disorders, including depression and anxiety disorders. Two hundred and fifty were treated in psychoanalysis, and the remainder one to three times weekly. Intensity of treatment (i.e., analysis versus less-intensive psychotherapy) led to greater improvements (87 per cent improved in analysis versus 67 per cent in psychotherapy) independently of age and treatment length. More frequent sessions were associated with larger changes on the Children's Global Assessment Scale (CGAS). The effect was more pronounced for the more emotionally disturbed children with lower initial CGAS scores. In addition, younger children did better in more frequent treatment. Those who were more disturbed had only a 50 per cent rate of improvement in less-frequent treatment.

This finding is also consistent with the findings of Heinicke and

Ramsey-Klee (1986), who showed that intensive psychoanalytic psycho-therapy (four times a week) was more effective in a group of children than less-intensive (once-a-week) sessions. The children seen once a week showed a greater rate of improvement than their counterparts in the first year of treatment, though they were about even by the last year. However, in the two years after the end of treatment, the children seen four times a week now showed greater improvement, 'characterized by being more flexible in their adaptation and having a greater capacity for relationships at both the end and a year after the end of treatment' (p. 247).

The Tortoise and the Hare

Findings such as those by Heinicke and Ramsey-Klee (1986), of Blatt et al with perfectionists (1995), or of Høglend's study of patients with personality disorders versus those without (1993) suggest that, with some patients, long-term intensive work is like the tortoise, compared with less-intensive work, the hare. In two of the studies, there are suggestions that long-term patients get off to a slow start, and that it is only after treatment is complete, or even often several years later, that the gains become fully apparent. This is consistent with the idea that psychoanalytic therapy is often reconstructive and conducted in stages. At first, maladaptive defences against painful inner material are exposed; next, in a painful part of the treatment, developmental inhibitions are exposed, and internal psychic representations are reworked while the patient is in a regressed state; next, progress and development begin again, in a less maladaptive way. The gains in development take time to manifest themselves.

Adults require a reasonable amount of time to change defensive patterns and undo developmental inhibitions, many of which have existed and been reinforced for twenty to forty years before treatment is sought and were often responses to traumatic situations. Referring patients who require long-term intensive treatment for character difficulties to a short-term treatment may lead to extended suffering and wasted years of potential health, not to mention wasted resources.

A BIOLOGICAL BASIS FOR LONG-TERM PSYCHOTHERAPY

In the 1970s and 1980s, it became fashionable to denigrate traditional psychoanalytic treatment in favour of a more modern 'biological' approach. This still occurs, but less so. Traditionally, the answer to these claims has been that human behaviour is a composite of nature and nurture, that is, our biological predisposition and our life experiences. The pioneering molecular biologist and psychiatrist Eric Kandel has shown that the truth is much more complex and that life experience actually affects biology. Kandel, Schwartz, and Jessel (1991) demonstrated how mental experiences actually change the structure and functions of neuronal synaptic transmission. They have also shown that mental experiences actually lead to structural and functional changes in the brain synapses, but that this process takes time. Kandel (1983) has proposed that psychotherapy ultimately leads to synaptic changes and altered gene expression. We are now starting to understand more about why change takes so long and why the natural developmental processes cannot be rushed. Karasu (1992), reflecting on this, has argued that 'this recognition that alteration in gene expression is the common bio-physiological pathway to bring about change in feelings, thought, and behaviour, in conjunction with the length of time needed for such an alteration to take place, gives the psychotherapist the first scientific support for justification of long-term psychotherapy. Because regulating gene expression requires induction of a new protein kinase to alter synaptic relations, such induction necessitates sustained treatment: certainly a number of months if not years' (p. 4; see also Gabbard, 1994). These ideas are not far-fetched; indeed, a recent PET-scan study of obsessive–compulsive patients who were given ten weeks of cognitive/ behavioural treatment demonstrated that those patients who improved clinically also showed brain changes on their orbital cortex, caudate nucleus, and thalamus, similar to those demonstrated with medication, and not seen in non-responders to treatment (Schwartz, Stoessel, Baxter, Martin, & Phelps, 1996).

HEALTH-CARE COSTS AND PSYCHOANALYTIC PSYCHOTHERAPY AND PSYCHOANALYSIS

Long-term psychotherapies lead to decreased physical morbidity in patients. There is evidence from twenty studies for a 47 per cent incidence of significant physical illness among psychiatric patients (Krupnick & Pincus, 1991).

Duehrssen (1957, 1972) and Duehrssen and Jorswiek (1965) did an extensive follow-up of patients who had psychoanalytic psychotherapy or psychoanalysis in Germany, where these treatments are covered by national health insurance. They followed 845 patients for five years after psychoanalysis or psychoanalytic psychotherapy, with direct interviews, questionnaires, and home visits. The average number of days in hospital per year in West Germany for patients not in psychotherapy was 2.5. Prior to treatment, the psychotherapy patients averaged 5.3 days in hospital per year. Five years after psychotherapy, they averaged 0.78 days. In other words, the common clinical impressions that (1) psychoanalysis and psychoanalytic psychotherapy decrease other medical utilization in the treated patient, and (2) patients who have undergone these forms of psychotherapy make less use of medical care facilities than do the general population are validated by this study. Similar results were seen in studies of HMOs in the United States (Follette & Cummings, 1967; Cummings & Follette, 1968).

The German data have recently been updated by another German group. Dossman, Kutter, Heinzel, and Wurmser (1997) found a one-third decrease in medical visits (of all kinds) in a study of psychodynamic psychotherapy and psychoanalysis, conducted on 666 patients who completed therapy between January 1990 and December 1994. Patients also had a 40 per cent decline in lost work days, a 66 per cent decline in hospitalization, and a 33 per cent decrease in the use of all medications. These declines have been sustained in the 2.5 years since the completion of therapy. Better outcome correlated with the length of treatment.

While the German study shows that psychoanalytic treatment is effective in decreasing medical costs across all sorts of conditions, a recent controlled study of brittle diabetic children in Britain shows its effect in a specific disorder. This study revealed that those diabetic children who received four-times-weekly psychoanalytic psychotherapy had improved blood-glucose levels sustained one year later. The control group with no psychotherapy returned to abnormal profiles within three months of discharge. Such findings are important because poorly controlled diabetes has been shown to have significant and serious consequences (such as blindness, amputation, and vessel disease).

A meta-analysis of similar studies in the United States and elsewhere of psychoanalytic and non-psychoanalytic therapies (Mumford, Schlesinger, Glass, Patrick, & Cuerdon, 1984) shows that 'retrospective analysis of health insurance claims data and meta-analysis of time series studies and prospective controlled experimental studies converge to provide evidence of general cost-offset effect following outpatient psychotherapy' (p. 1156). Further, according to Mumford et al, 'older patients show larger cost-offset effects than younger ones' (p. 1156). There is also evidence that psychoanalysis and long-term psychoanalytic psychotherapy forestall psychiatric hospitalization (Duehrssen & Jorswiek, 1965) and that unlimited coverage of intensive (long-term) psychotherapy does not cause an appreciable increase in the number of people using the treatment (Sharfstein & Magnas, 1975; Group for the Advancement of Psychiatry, 1978). A number of studies show that inclusion of full mental health benefits, including outpatient psychotherapy, actually 'caused reduced medical-surgical utilization' (Krupnick & Pincus, 1991).

Gabbard, Lazar, Hornberger, and Spiegel (1997) have updated the work of Mumford et al (1984) and reviewed all data involving the impact on costs of providing psychotherapy for psychiatric disorders, including all studies with implications for costs. Eighty per cent of the random clinical trials suggested that psychotherapy reduces total costs; 100 per cent of the non-random studies suggested that psychotherapy reduced total costs. These beneficial impacts were on a range of disorders from schizophrenia and bipolar affective disorders to personality disorders such as the borderline personality disorder. The authors found that much of the beneficial impact on costs came from reductions in inpatient treatment and decreased work impairment.

Cost-offset data from a comparison study in Australia and New Zealand, two countries with similar populations, show that unlimited outpatient psychotherapy benefits, including analysis, in Australia led to less overall mental health care expenditures compared with New Zealand, which has limited outpatient coverage. There are also twice as many psychiatrists in Australia as in New Zealand, yet, in the same period, Australia spent $5.17 million per 100,000 population on mental health care expenditures, and New Zealand spent $7 million per 100,000 (Andrews, 1989). In other words, cost offset is often immediate. There are other examples of similar savings. In Canada, the use of psychiatric hospital beds decreased by 10 per cent with the advent of unlimited access to outpatient care (Peel, 1990). In 1975, when the major U.S. insurer AETNA dropped outpatient psychotherapy visits to twenty per year, inpatient visits rose to cancel out all the gains made by the decrease in outpatient visits. The very large U.S. government employee benefits program carrier CHAMPUS, which covers health services to the dependants of U.S. uniformed services personnel, maintained extensive outpatient coverage (which are cost-effective) and reduced overall costs. Zients (1993), who was medical director of

HMS, found that liberal outpatient coverage (which includes five-times-a-week analysis) had the effect of reducing hospital costs by keeping people out of hospital. Overall, mental health costs fell over thirty-nine months, saving $200 million. Because psychiatric patients are a distressed group, they seek out medical assistance no matter how the system is funded. The RAND Corporation study of 4,500 subjects in six different areas of the United States showed that *the probability of receiving care and the intensity of the care are directly related to the amount of psychological distress of the patient, regardless of whether the psychiatric care is free or not covered* (Ware, Manning, Duan, Wells, & Newhouse, 1984). Since these patients will seek out treatment one way or another, and since these treatments are ultimately self-limiting once the condition is treated, the most rational form of funding for outpatient mental health care is that based upon medical need of the individual, as opposed to some arbitrary legislated limit.

One reason why some U.S. health care planners often speak of decreasing or eliminating outpatient psychiatric services is that many insurance companies do not offer portable insurance packages. These companies often cover insurees for only several years, before they change jobs or move. Such companies may not find it in their economic interest to focus on the preventive aspects of good medical care and know that they will not benefit from the long-term savings that go with long-term psychiatric services because some other company will insure the patient in a few years. Conversely, the cost-offset data associated with psychoanalysis and psychotherapy are of great interest to larger insurance companies, such as CHAMPUS in the U.S. or the German and Australian health care systems which cover employees for life and which therefore have to factor in long-term cost-offset effects.

CONSUMER SATISFACTION

In 1995, *Consumer Reports* (Seligman, 1995) conducted a massive study on psychotherapy, sending out a detailed questionnaire to its 180,000 readers, asking anyone who had been in psychotherapy in the previous three years to respond. Seven thousand readers responded to the questions on mental health problems; of these, 3,000 dealt with these problems by talking to friends, relatives, or clergy; 2,900 went to mental health professionals; and the rest to self-help groups and family doctors. Patients were asked to rate their improvement; describe their treatments, including the length of treatment; and describe their problems, the level of severity of their presenting problems, improvement in their problems, and global improvement, among other things.

In summary, long-term treatment, which included those that are psychodynamic or influenced by psychoanalytic principles, 'did considerably better than short-term treatment' (Seligman, 1995, p. 965); patients with mental health professionals did considerably better than those who did not see them or those who spoke to friends; psychotherapy alone was as effective as combined psychotherapy and medication. Results applied to sicker patients as well. Patients with more severe problems undertook the longer-term treatments and still did well, in terms of their symptoms and general well-being. 'Patients whose length of therapy or choice of therapist was limited by insurance of managed care did worse' (p. 965). Were these results an artefact of a selection bias with only those who benefited staying in treatment? If this were the case, one would expect higher drop-out rates for those who did not get better; but drop-out rates were uniform for resolution of the presenting problems across the length of treatment. People tended to remain in treatment until their problems improved.

Conclusion

This chapter reviews some of the special methodological considerations posed by the study of psychodynamic and psychoanalytic psychotherapy studies and reviews randomized clinical trials and naturalistic studies. Data is presented to show the types of patients in psychoanalysis and psychoanalytic psychotherapy. The decision to prescribe this treatment is not based upon the disorder alone. The clinical conditions must be based upon unresolved unconscious relationship conflicts, and or developmental inhibitions, and the patient must be someone who is not likely to get adequate benefit from less intensive forms of treatment. In practice, these patients are a well-defined group. There is considerable experimental and clinical data for the core concepts of psychoanalytic treatment, and for its efficacy. A range of individual psychoanalytic psychotherapies, from short- to long-term are effective in comparison with other effective treatments. Data supporting the correlation between length of treatment and good outcomes, and data on frequency of sessions and outcomes, are examined. Certain patients require more intensive treatments to make gains and maintain them. This process can be speeded up by increasing the frequency of treatment.

References

Abend, S. (1986). Sibling loss. In Rothstein (Ed.) *The reconstruction of trauma: its significance in clinical work.* Madison, CT: International Universities Press.

Altschul, S. (1988). *Childhood bereavement and Its aftermath.* Madison, CT: International Universities Press.

American Psychiatric Association (APA). (1985). *Manual of psychiatric peer review, Peer review guidelines for psychoanalysis* (3rd ed.). Washington, DC: Author.

American Psychiatric Association (APA). (1987). *Diagnostic and statistical manual of mental disorders* (3d ed., revised). Washington, DC: Author.

American Psychiatric Association (APA). (1989). *Treatments of psychiatric disorders.* Washington, DC: Author.

American Psychiatric Association (APA). (1994). *Diagnostic and statistical manual of mental disorders* (4th ed.). Washington, DC: Author.

American Psychiatric Association Commission on Psychotherapies. (1982). *Psychotherapy Research.* Washington, DC: Author.

Anderson, E.M., & Lambert, M.J. (1995). Short-term dynamically oriented psychotherapy: A review and meta-analysis. *Clinical Psychology Review, 15,* 503–514.

Andrews, G. (1989). Private and public psychiatry: A comparison of two health care systems. *American Journal of Psychiatry, 146,* 881–886.

Bachrach, H.M., Galatzer-Levy, R., Skolnikoff, A., & Waldron, S. (1991). On the efficacy of psychoanalysis. *Journal of the American Psychoanalytic Association, 39,* 871–916.

Bachrach, H., & Leaff, L. (1978). Analyzability: A systematic review of the clinical and quantitative literature. *Journal of the American Psychoanalytic Association, 20,* 881–920.

Bachrach, H., Weber, J., & Solomon, M. (1985). Factors associated with the outcome of psychoanalysis (clinical and methodological considerations): Report of the Columbia Psychoanalytic Center Research Project (IV). *International Review of Psycho-Analysis, 12,* 379–389.

Bannon, E., Perry, J.C., & Ianni, F. (1995). The effectiveness of psychotherapy for personality disorders. Presentation at the International Society for the Study of Personality Disorders, Dublin, Ireland. By permission of J.C. Perry.

Battista, J.R. (1982). Empirical test of Vaillant's hierarchy of ego functions. *American Journal of Psychiatry, 139,* 356–357.

Bergmann, M.S., & Hartman, F.R. (Eds). (1976). *The evolution of psychoanalytic technique.* New York: Basic.

Berzins, J., Bednar, R., & Severy, L. (1975). The problem of intersource consensus for measuring therapeutic outcome: New data and multivariate perspectives. *Journal of Abnormal Social Psychology, 84*, 10–19.

Beutler, L.E., & Crago, M. (eds). (1991). *Psychotherapy research: An international review of programmatic studies*. Washington, DC: American Psychological Association.

Beutler, L., & Mitchell, R. (1981). Differential psychotherapy outcomes among depressed and impulsive patients as a function of analytic and experiential treatment procedures. *Psychiatry, 44*, 297–306.

Binder, J.L., Henry, W.P., & Strupp, H. (1987). An appraisal of selection criteria for dynamic psychotherapies and implications for setting time limits. *Psychiatry, 50*, 154–166.

Blatt, S.J. (1992). The differential effect of psychotherapy and psychoanalysis with anaclitic and introjective patients: The Menninger Psychotherapy Research Project revisited. *Journal of the American Psychoanalytic Association, 40*, 691–724.

Blatt, S.J., & Ford, R. (1994). *Therapeutic change: an object relations perspective*. New York: Plenum.

Blatt, S.J., Quinlan, D.M., Pilkonis, P.A., & Shea, M.T. (1995). Impact of perfectionism and need for approval on the brief treatment of depression: The National Institute of Mental Health Treatment of Depression Collaborative Research Program revisited. *Journal of Consulting and Clinical Psychology, 63*, 125–132.

Bowlby, J. (1980). *Attachment and loss* (Vol. 3). New York: Basic.

Brodarty, H., & Andrews, G. (1983). Brief psychotherapy in family practice: A controlled prospective intervention trial. *British Journal of Psychiatry, 143*, 11–19.

Brom, D., Kleber, R., & Defares, P.B. (1989). Brief psychotherapy for posttraumatic stress disorders. *Journal of Consulting and Clinical Psychology, 57*, 607–612.

Bucci, W., & Miller, N.E. (1993). Primary process analogue: The Referential Activity (RA) measure. In N.E. Miller, L. Luborsky, J.P. Barber, & J.P. Docherty (Eds.), *Psychodynamic treatment research: A handbook for clinical practice*. New York: Basic.

Butler, S.E., & Strupp, H.H. (1993). Effects of training experienced dynamic therapists to use a psychotherapy manual. In N.E. Miller, L. Luborsky, J.P. Barber & J.P. Docherty (Eds.), *Psychodynamic treatment research: A handbook for clinical practice*. New York: Basic Books.

Crits-Christoph, P. (1992). The efficacy of brief dynamic psychotherapy: A meta-analysis. *American Journal of Psychiatry, 149*, 151–158.

Crits-Christoph, P., Barber, J., Baranackie, K., & Cooper, A. (1993). Assessing the therapist's interpretations. In N.E. Miller, L. Luborsky, J.P. Barber, & J.P. Docherty (Eds.), *Psychodynamic treatment research: A handbook for clinical practice.* New York: Basic.

Cross, D., Sheehan, P., & Khan, J. (1982). Short- and long-term follow-up of clients receiving insight-oriented therapy and behavior therapy. *Journal of Consulting and Clinical Psychology, 30*, 103–112.

Cummings, N., & Follette, W. (1968). Psychiatric services and medical utilization in a prepaid health plan setting: Part II. *Medical Care, 6*, 31–41.

Dietrich, D.R. (1989). Early childhood parent death, psychic trauma and organization and object relations. In D. Dietrich & P. Shabad (eds.), *The problem of loss and mourning.* New York: International Universities Press.

Doidge, N. (1977). Empirical evidence for the efficacy of psychoanalytic psychotherapies: an overview. In Susan G. Lazar (Ed.), Extended dynamic psychotherapy. *Psychoanalytic Inquiry,* Supplement, 102–150.

Doidge, N., Simon, B., Gillies, L.A., & Ruskin, R. (1994). Characteristics of psychoanalytic patients under a nationalized health plan: DSM-III-R diagnoses, previous treatment and childhood traumata. *American Journal of Psychiatry, 151*, 586–590.

Dossman, R., Kutter, P., Heinzel, R., & Wurmser, L. (1997). The long-term benefits of intensive psychotherapy: A view from Germany. In Susan G. Lazar (Ed.), Extended dynamic psychotherapy. *Psychoanalytic Inquiry,* Supplement, 74–85.

Duehrssen, A. (1957). Die beurteilung das behandlungserfolges in der psychotherapie. *Z. Psychosom Med, 3*, 201–210.

Duehrssen, A. (1972). Katamnestische ergebnisse bei 1004 patienten nach analytischer psychotherapie. [Catamnestic results in 1004 patients after analytical psychotherapy] *Z. Psychosom Med, 7*, 94–113.

Duehrssen, V.A., & Jorswiek, E. (1965). Eine empirisch–statistische untersuchung zur leistungsfähigkeit psychoanalytischer behandlung [An empirical–statistical investigation into the efficacy of psychoanalytic psychotherapy]. *Der Nervenarzt, 36*, 166–169.

Edington, E.S. (1966). Statistical inference and non-random samples. *Psychological Bulletin, 66*, 485–487.

Elkin, I., Shea, T., Watkins, J., Imber, S., Collins, J., Glass, D., Leber, W., Docherty, J., Fiester, S., & Parloff, M. (1989). National Institute of Mental Health Treatment of Depression Collaborative Research Program: General effectiveness of treatments. *Archives of General Psychiatry, 46*, 971–982

Erle, J. (1979). An approach to the study of analysability and analysis: The course of forty consecutive cases selected for supervised analysis. *Psychoanalytic Quarterly, 48*, 198–228.

Erle, J., & Goldberg, D. (1979). Problems in the assessment of analysability. *Psychoanalytic Quarterly, 48*, 48–84.

Erle, J., & Goldberg, D. (1984). Observations on assessment of analysability by experienced analysts. *Journal of the American Psychoanalytic Association, 32*, 715–737.

Etchegoyan, R. (1991). *The fundamentals of psychoanalytic technique.* London: Karnac.

Fenichel, O. (1941). *Problems of psychoanalytic technique* (David Brunswick, Trans.). New York: Psychoanalytic Quarterly.

Follette, W., & Cummings, N. (1967). Psychiatric services and medical utilization in a prepaid health plan setting. *Medical Care, 5*, 25–35.

Fonagy, P., & Moran, G. (1993). Selecting single case research designs for clinicians. In N.E. Miller, L. Luborsky, J.P. Barber, & J.P. Docherty (Eds.), *Psychodynamic treatment research: A handbook for clinical practice.* New York: Basic.

Fretter, P.B., Bucci, W., Broitman, J, Silberschatz, G., & Curtis, J.T. (1994). How the patient's plan relates to the concept of transference. *Psychotherapy Research, 4*, 58–72.

Freud, A., & Burlingham, D. (1944). *Infants without families.* New York: International Universities Press.

Freud, S. (1962a). Further remarks on the neuropsychoses of defence. In J. Strachey (Ed. and Trans.), *The standard edition of the complete psychological works of Sigmund Freud* (Vol. 3.) London: Hogarth Press. (Original work published 1896)

Freud, S. (1962b). The aetiology of hysteria. In J. Strachey (Ed. and Trans.), *The standard edition of the complete psychological works of Sigmund Freud* (Vol. 3). London: Hogarth Press. (Original work published 1896)

Freud, S. (1957). Five lectures on psycho-analysis. In J. Strachey (Ed. and Trans.), *The standard edition of the complete psychological works of Sigmund Freud* (Vol. 11, pp. 000). London: Hogarth Press. (Original work published 1910)

Freud, S. (1957). The dynamics of transference. In J. Strachey (Ed. and Trans.), *The standard edition of the complete psychological works of Sigmund Freud* (Vol. 12). London: Hogarth Press. (Original work published 1912)

Fried, D., Crits-Christoph, P., & Luborsky, L. (1990). The parallel of the CCRT for the therapist with the CCRT for other people. In L. Luborsky & P. Crits-Christoph, *Understanding transference: The CCRT method.* New York: Basic.

Gabbard, G. (1994). *Psychodynamic psychiatry in clinical practice: The DSM-IV edition.* Washington, DC: American Psychiatric Association.

Gabbard, G. (Ed.). (1995). *Treatments of psychiatric disorders: The DSM-IV edition.* Washington, DC: American Psychiatric Press.

Gabbard, G.O., Lazar, S.G., Hornberger, J., & Spiegel, D. (1997). The economic impact of psychotherapy: A review. *American Journal of Psychiatry, 154*, 147–155.

Gallagher, D.E., & Thompson, L.W. (1982). Treatment of major depressive disorder in older adult outpatients with brief psychotherapies. *Psychotherapy: Theory, Research and Practice, 19*, 482–490.

Geller, J.D., Cooley, R.S., & Hartley, D. (1981). Images of the psychotherapist: A theoretical and methodological perspective. *Imagination, Cognition and Personality, 1*, 123–146.

Gillett, E. (1987). Defence mechanisms versus defence contents. *International Journal of Psycho-Analysis, 68*, 261–269.

Giovacchini, P. (Ed.). (1972). *Tactics and techniques in psychoanalytic therapy.* New York: Jason Aronson.

Glover, E. (1955). *The technique of psycho-analysis.* New York: International Universities Press.

Graff, H., & Luborsky, L. (1977). Long-term trends in transference and resistance: A quantitative analytic method applied to four psychoanalyses. *Journal of the American Psychoanalytic Association, 25*, 471–490.

Greenson, R.R. (1967). *The technique and practice of psychoanalysis* (Vol. 1). New York: International Universities Press.

Group for the Advancement of Psychiatry (GAP). (1978). Psychotherapy and its financial feasibility within the national health care system, X, February (100).

Hanly, C.M.T. (1994). Reflections on the place of the therapeutic alliance in psychoanalysis. *International Journal of Psycho-Analysis, 75*, 457–467.

Hartley, D. (1993). Assessing psychological developmental level. In N.E. Miller, L. Luborsky, J.P. Barber, & J.P. Docherty (Eds.), *Psychodynamic treatment research: A handbook for clinical practice.* New York: Basic.

Hawton, K. (1992). Long-term outcome studies of psychological treatments. In C. Freeman & P. Tyrer (Eds.), *Research methods in psychiatry* (2d ed.). London: Gaskell, Royal College of Psychiatrists.

Heinicke, C.M., & Ramsey-Klee, D.M. (1986). Outcome of child psychotherapy as a function of frequency of session. *Journal of the American Academy of Child Psychiatry, 25*, 247–253.

Høglend, P. (1993) Personality disorders and long-term outcome after brief dynamic psychotherapy. *Journal of Personality Disorders, 7*, 168–181.

Horowitz, M., Marmar, C., Weiss, D., Kaltreider, N., & Wilner, N. (1986) Comprehensive analysis of change after brief dynamic psychotherapy. *American Journal of Psychiatry, 143*, 582–589.

Horvath, A., Gaston, L., & Luborsky, L. (1993). The therapeutic alliance and its measures. In N.E. Miller, L. Luborsky, J.P. Barber, & J.P. Docherty (Eds.), *Psychodynamic treatment research: A handbook for clinical practice.* New York: Basic.

Howard, K.I., Kopta, S.M., Krause, M.S., & Orlinsky, D.E. (1986). The dose-effect relationship in psychotherapy. *American Psychologist, 41*, 159–164.

Hyler, S.E., Skodol, A.E., Oldham, J.M., Kellman, H.D., & Doidge, N. (1992). Validity of the Personality Diagnostic Questionnaire – Revised: A replication in an outpatient sample. *Comprehensive Psychiatry, 33*, 73–76.

Jacobson, A.M., Beardslee, W., Hauser, S.T., Noam, G.G., & Powers, S.I. (1986). An approach to evaluating ego defence mechanisms using clinical interviews. In G.E. Vaillant (Ed.), *Empirical studies of ego mechanisms of defense.* Washington DC: American Psychiatric Press.

Jacobson, A.M., Beardslee, W., Hauser, S.T. Noam, G.G., Powers, S.I., Houlihan, J., & Rider, E. (1986). Evaluating ego defence mechanisms using clinical interviews: An empirical study of adolescent diabetic and psychiatric patients. *Journal of Adolescence, 9*, 303–319.

Jones, E., Hall, S., & Parke, L. (1990). The process of change: The Berkeley Psychotherapy Research Group. In L.E. Beutler & M. Crago (Eds.), *Psychotherapy research: An international review of programmatic studies.* Washington, DC: American Psychological Association.

Kandel, E.R. (1983). From metapsychology to molecular biology: Explorations in the nature of anxiety. *American Journal of Psychiatry, 140*, 1277–1293.

Kandel, E.R., Schwartz, J.H., & Jessel, T.M. (1991). *Principles of neural science,* (3d ed.). New York: Elsevier.

Kaplan, H.I., & Sadock, B.J. (Eds.). (1995). *Comprehensive textbook of psychiatry* (6th ed.). Baltimore: Williams & Wilkins.

Karasu, T.B. (1992). The worst of times, the best of times: Psychotherapy in the 1990's. *Journal of Psychotherapy Practice and Research, 1*, 2–13.

Kazdin, A.E. (1986). The evaluation of psychotherapy: Research design and methodology. In S.L. Garfield & A.E. Bergin (Eds.), *The handbook of psychotherapy and behavior change* (3d ed.). New York: Wiley.

Kernberg, O. (1982). To teach or not to teach psychotherapy. In E. Joseph and R. Wallerstein (Eds.), *Psychotherapy: Impact on psychoanalytic training.* New York: International Universities Press.

Kernberg, O. (1984). *Severe personality disorders: Psychotherpeutic strategies.* New Haven, CT: Yale University Press.

Kernberg, O., Burstein, E., Coyne, L., Appelbaum, A., Horwitz, L., & Voth, H. (1972). Psychotherapy and psychoanalysis: Final report of the Menninger Foundation Psychotherapy Research Project. *Bulletin of the Menninger Clinic, 36*, 1–275.

Kernberg, O., & Clarkin, J.F. (1993). Developing a disorder-specific manual: The treatment of borderline character disorder. In N.E. Miller, L. Luborsky, J.P.

Barber & J.P. Docherty (Eds.), *Psychodynamic treatment research: A handbook for clinical practice* (pp. 000). New York: Basic.

Kernberg, O., Selzer, M., Koenigsberg, H., Carr, A., & Appelbaum, A. (1989). *Psychodynamic psychotherapy of borderline patients*. New York: Basic.

Klerman, G., & Weissman, M. (1992). The course, morbidity and costs of depression. *Archives of General Psychiatry, 49*, 831–834.

Knight, R. (1941). Evaluation of the results of psychoanalytic therapy. *American Journal of Psychiatry, 98*, 434–446.

Kopta, S.M., Howard, K.I., Lowry, J.L., & Beutler, L.E. (1994). Patterns of symptomatic recovery in psychotherapy. *Journal of Consulting and Clinical Psychology, 62*, 1009–1016.

Krupnick, J., & Pincus, H.A. (1991). *Cost-effectiveness of psychotherapy*. Discussion paper for the American Psychiatric Association.

Lambert, M.J., Shapiro, D.A., & Bergin, A.E. (1986). The effectiveness of psychotherapy. In S.L. Garfield (Ed.) *The handbook of psychotherapy and behaviour change* (3d ed.). New York: Wiley.

Loewald, H. (1960). On the therapeutic action of psychoanalysis. *International Journal of Psycho-Analysis, 41*, 16–33.

Luborsky, L. (1984). *Principles of psychoanalytic psychotherapy: A manual for supportive–expressive treatment*. New York: Basic.

Luborsky, L. (1993a). Documenting symptom formation during psychotherapy. In N.E. Miller, L. Luborsky, J.P. Barber, & J.P. Docherty (Eds.), *Psychodynamic treatment research: A handbook for clinical practice*. New York: Basic.

Luborsky, L., (1993b). How to maximize the curative factors in dynamic psychotherapy. In N.E. Miller, L. Luborsky, J.P. Barber, & J.P. Docherty (Eds.), *Psychodynamic treatment research: A handbook for clinical practice*. New York: Basic.

Luborsky, L., Barber, J.P., Binder, J., Curtis, J., Dahl, H., Horowitz, L.M., Horowitz, M., Perry, J., Schacht, T. Silberschatz G., & Teller, V. (1993a). Transference-related measures: A new class based on psychotherapy session. In N.E. Miller, L. Luborsky, J.P. Barber, & J.P. Docherty (Eds.), *Psychodynamic treatment research: A handbook for clinical practice*. New York: Basic.

Luborsky, L., & Crits-Christoph, P. (1990). *Understanding transference: The CCRT method*. New York: Basic.

Luborsky, L., Crits-Christoph, P., Alexander, L., Margolis, M., & Cohen, M. (1983). Two helping alliance methods for predicting outcomes of psychotherapy. *Journal of Nervous and Mental Diseases, 17*, 480–491.

Luborsky, L., Crits-Christoph, P., Mintz, J., & Auerbach, A. (1988). *Who will benefit from psychotherapy? Predicting therapeutic outcomes*. New York: Basic.

Luborsky, L., Diguer, L., Luborsky, E., Singer, B., Dickter, D., & Schmidt, K.A. (1993). The efficacy of psychodynamic psychotherapy: Is it true that 'everyone has won and all must have prizes,'? In N.E. Miller, L. Luborsky, J.P. Barber, & J.P. Docherty (Eds.), *Psychodynamic treatment research: A handbook for clinical practice*. New York: Basic.

Luborsky, L., Docherty, J.P., Barber, J.P., & Miller, N.E. (1993). How this basic handbook helps the partnership of clinicians and clinical researchers: Preface. In N.E. Miller, L. Luborsky, J.P. Barber, & J.P. Docherty (eds.), *Psychodynamic treatment research: A handbook for clinical practice*. New York: Basic.

Luborsky, L., Singer, B., & Luborsky, L. (1975). Comparative studies of psychotherapies: Is it true that 'Everyone has won and all must have prizes'? *Archives of General Psychiatry, 32*, 995–1008.

Mahler, M.S., Pine, F., & Bergmann, A. (1975). *The psychological birth of the human infant*. New York: Basic.

Main, M., & Goldwyn, R. (1984). Predicting rejection of her infant from mother's representation of her own experience: implications for the abused–abuser intergenerational cycle. *International Journal of Child Abuse and Neglect, 8*, 203–217.

Malan, D.H. (1976). *The frontier of brief psychotherapy*. New York: Plenum.

Markowitz, J., Moran, M.E., Kocsis, J.H., & Frances, A.J. (1992). Prevalence and comorbidity of dysthymic disorder among psychiatric outpatients. *Journal of Affective Disorders, 24*, 63–71.

Marmar, C., Horowitz, M.J., Weiss, D.S., Wilner, N.R., & Kaltreider, N.B. (1988). A controlled trial of brief psychotherapy and mutual-help group treatment of conjugal bereavement. *American Journal of Psychiatry, 145*, 203–209.

Marziali, E. (1984). Prediction of outcome of brief psychotherapy from therapist interpretive interventions. *Archives of General Psychiatry, 41*, 301–304.

Marziali, E., Marmar, C., & Krupnick, J. (1981). Therapeutic alliance scales: Development and relationships to psychotherapy outcome. *American Journal of Psychiatry, 138*, 361–364.

McGlashan, T.H. (1983). Intensive individual psychotherapy of schizophrenia: A review of techniques. *Archives of General Psychiatry, 40*, 909–920.

McNeilly, C.L., & Howard, K.I. (1991). The effects of psychotherapy: A reevaluation based on dosage. *Psychotherapy Research, 1*, 74–78.

Meltzoff, J., & Kornreich, M. (1970). *Research in psychotherapy*. New York: Atherton.

Michels, R. (Chairman, Editorial Board). (1991) *Psychiatry*. Philadelphia: Lippincott.

Miller, N.E., Luborsky, Barber, J.P., & Docherty, J.P. (1993). *Psychodynamic treatment research: A handbook for clinical practice*. New York: Basic.

Milrod, B. (1995). The continued usefulness of psychoanalysis in the treatment armamentarium for panic disorder. *Journal of the American Psychoanalytic Association, 43*, 151–162.

Milrod, B.L., Busch, F.N., Cooper, A.M., & Shapiro, T. (1997). *Manual of panic-focused psychodynamic psychotherapy.* Washington, DC: American Psychiatric Press.

Monsen, J.T., Oldland, T., Faugli, A., Daae, E., & Eilersten, D.E. (1995). Personality disorders: Changes and stability after intensive psychotherapy focusing on affect consciousness. *Psychotherapy Research, 5*, 33–48.

Moran, G., Fonagy, P., Kurt, A., Bolton, A., & Brook, C. (1991). A controlled study of the psychoanalytic treatment of brittle diabetes. *Journal of the American Academy of Child and Adolescent Psychiatry, 30*, 926–935.

Mosher, P.W. (Ed.). (1991). *Title key word and author index to psychoanalytic journals.* New York: American Psychoanalytic Association.

Mumford, E., Schlesinger, H.J., Glass, G.V., Patrick, C., & Cuerdon, T. (1984). A new look at evidence about reduced cost of medical utilization following mental health treatment. *American Journal of Psychiatry, 141*, 1145–1158.

Norcross, J., & Prochaska, J. (1988). A study of eclectic (and interpretive) views revisited. *Professional Psychology: Research and Practice, 19*, 170–174.

Norcross, J., Prochaska, J., & Gallagher, K. (1989). Clinical psychologists in the 1980's: Theory, research and practice. *Clinical Psychologist, 42*, 45–53.

Norman, H., Blacker, K., Oremland, J., & Barrett, W. (1976). The fate of the transference neurosis after termination of a satisfactory analysis. *Journal of the American Psychoanalytic Association, 24*, 471–498.

Oldham, J.M., Skodol, A.E., Kellman, H.D., Hyler, S.E., Doidge, N.R., Rosnick, L., & Gallaher, P.E. (1995) Comorbidity of axis I and axis II disorders. *American Journal of Psychiatry, 152*, 571–578.

Orlinsky, D.E., & Geller, J.D. (1993). Patient's representations of their therapists and therapy: New measures. In N.E. Miller, L. Luborsky, J.P. Barber, & J.P. Docherty (Eds.), *Psychodynamic treatment research: A handbook for clinical practice.* New York: Basic.

Panel. (1992). Psychoanalysis and psychoanalytic psychotherapy – similarities and differences: Indications, contraindications, and initiation. E.R. McNutt, reporter. *Journal of the American Psychoanalytic Association, 40*, 223–231.

Patterson, V., Levene, H., & Berger, L. (1971) Treatment and training outcomes with two time-limited therapies. *Archives of General Psychiatry, 25*, 161–167.

Peel, R. (1990, December). *Psychiatric News, 21*, 3.

Perry, J.C. (1993a). Defences and their effects. In N.E. Miller, L. Luborsky, J.P. Barber, & J.P. Docherty (Eds.), *Psychodynamic treatment research: A handbook for clinical practice.* New York: Basic.

Perry, J.C. (1993b). Longitudinal studies of personality disorders. *Journal of Personality Disorder* (Suppl., Spring), 63–85.

Perry, J. & Cooper, S.H. (1986). A preliminary report on defences and conflicts associated with borderline personality disorder. *Journal of the American Psychoanalytic Association, 34,* 863–893.

Perry, J., & Cooper, S.H. (1987). Empirical studies of psychological defence mechanisms. In R. Michels (Chairman, Editorial Board), *Psychiatry.* Philadelphia: Lippincott.

Pfeffer, A.Z. (1959). A procedure for evaluating the results of psychoanalysis: A preliminary report. *Journal of the American Psychoanalytic Association, 7,* 418–444.

Pfeffer, A.Z. (1961). Followup study of a satisfactory analysis. *Journal of the American Psychoanalytic Association, 9,* 698–718.

Pfeffer, A.Z. (1963). The meaning of the analyst after the analysis. *Journal of the American Psychoanalytic Association, 11,* 229–244.

Piper, W.E., Azim, H.F.A., McCallum, M., & Joyce, A.S. (1990). Patient suitability and outcome in short-term individual psychotherapy. *Journal of Consulting and Clinical Psychology, 58,* 475–481.

Robertson, J. (1953). Some responses of young children to loss of maternal care. *Nursing Times, 49,* 382.

Rosenthal, R., & Rubin, D.B. (1982). A simple, general-purpose display of magnitude of experimental effect. *Journal of Educational Psychology, 74,* 166–169.

Sashin, J., Eldred, S., & Van Amerrowgen, S.T. (1975). A search for predictive factors in institute supervised cases: A retrospective study of 183 cases from 1959–1966 at the Boston Psychoanalytic Society and Institute. *International Journal of Psycho-Analysis, 56,* 343–359.

Schlessinger, N., & Robbins, F. (1974). Assessment and followup in psychoanalysis. *Journal of the American Psychoanalytic, Association 22,* 542–567.

Schlessinger, N., & Robbins, F. (1975). The psychoanalytic process: Recurrent patterns of conflict and change in ego functions. *Journal of the American Psychoanalytic Association, 23,* 761–782.

Schlessinger, N., & Robbins, F. (1983). *A developmental view of the psychoanalytic process.* New York: International Universities Press.

Schwartz, J.M., Stoessel, P.W., Baxter, L.R., Martin, K.M., & Phelps, M.E. (1996). Systematic changes in cerebral glucose metabolic rate after successful behavior modification treatment of obsessive–compulsive disorder. *Archives of General Psychiatry, 53,* 109–113.

Seligman, M.E.P. (1995) The effectiveness of psychotherapy: The *Consumer Reports* study. *American Psychologist, 50,* 965–974.

Shane, E. (1988). Robert Wallerstein: Researcher, educator, organizer. *American Psychoanalytic Association Newsletter, 22*, 1–15.

Shapiro, D., & Shapiro, D. (1982). Meta-analysis of comparative therapy outcome studies: A replication and refinement. *Psychology Bulletin, 92*, 581.

Sharfstein, S.S. (1978). Third-party payers: To pay or not to pay. *American Journal of Psychiatry, 135*, 1185–1188.

Sharfstein, S., & Magnas, H. (1975). Insuring intensive psychotherapy. *American Journal of Psychiatry, 132*, 1252–1256.

Shea, M.T., Elkin, I., Imber, S., Sotsky, S., Watkins, J., Collins J., Pilkonis, P., Beckham, E., Glass, D., Dolan, R., & Parloff, M. (1992). Course of depressive symptoms over follow-up: Findings from the National Institute of Mental Health treatment of depression collaborative research program. *Archives of General Psychiatry, 49*, 782–787.

Shea, M.T., Pilkonis, P., Beckham, E., Collins, J.F., Elkin, I., Sotsky, S.M., & Doherty, J.P. (1990). Personality disorders and treatment outcome in the NIMH treatment of depression collaborative research program. *American Journal of Psychiatry, 147*, 711–718.

Shevrin, H. (1988). Unconscious conflict: A convergent psychodynamic and electrophysiological approach. In M.J. Horowitz (Ed.), *Psychodynamics and cognition*. Chicago: University of Chicago Press.

Shevrin, H., & Bond, J.A. (1993). Repression and the unconscious. In N.E. Miller, L. Luborsky, J.P. Barber, & J.P. Docherty (Eds.), *Psychodynamic treatment research: A handbook for clinical practice*. New York: Basic.

Shevrin, H., Williams, W.J., Marshall, R.E., Hertel, R.K., Bond, J.A., & Brakel, L.A. (1992). Event-related potential indicators of the dynamic unconscious. *Consciousness and Cognition, 1*, 340–366.

Siberschatz, G., Fretter, P., & Curtis, J. (1986). How do interpretations influence the process of psychotherapy? *Journal of Consulting and Clinical Psychology, 54*, 646–652.

Sifneos, P. (1979). *Short-term dynamic psychotherapy*. New York: Plenum.

Sledge, W. (1997). Resource document on medical psychotherapy. *Journal of Psychotherapy Practice and Research, 6*, 123–129.

Sloane, R., Staples, F., Cristol, A., Yorkston, N., & Whipple, K. (1975). *Psychotherapy versus behavior therapy*. Cambridge, MA: Harvard University Press.

Smith, M.L., Glass, G.V., & Miller, T.I. (1980). *The benefits of psychotherapy*. Baltimore, MD: Johns Hopkins University Press.

Speisman, J. (1959). Depth of interpretation and verbal resistance in psychotherapy. *Journal of Consulting Psychology, 23*, 93–99.

Spitz, R. (1946). Anaclitic depression: An inquiry into the genesis of psychiatric conditions in early childhood, II. *Psychoanalytic Study of the Child, 2*, 313–342.

Spitz, R. (1965). *The first year of life: A psychoanalytic study of normal and deviant development of object relations.* New York: International Universities Press.

Stanton, A.H., Gunderson, J.G., Knapp, P.H., Frank, A.F., Vannicelli, M.L., Schnitzer, R., & Rosenthal, R. (1984). Effects of psychotherapy on schizophrenic patients. I: Design and implementation of a controlled study. *Schizophrenia Bulletin, 10,* 520–563.

Stern, A. (1938). Psychoanalytic investigation of and therapy in the border line group of neuroses. *Psychoanalytic Quarterly, 7,* 467–489.

Stevenson, J., & Meares, R. (1992). An outcome study of psychotherapy for patients with borderline personality disorder. *American Journal of Psychiatry, 149,* 358–362.

Stone, L. (1954). The widening scope of indications for psychoanalysis. *Journal of the American Psychoanalytic Association, 2,* 567–594.

Strachey, J. (1934) The nature of the therapeutic action of psycho-analysis. *International Journal of Psycho-Analysis, 38,* 140–157.

Streiner, D.L. (1994, 16 June). RCT: Randomized controlled trial or rigidly constrained thinking? Keynote address, 20th Annual Harvey Stancer Research Day, University of Toronto, Department of Psychiatry. 1994.

Strupp, H., & Binder J. (1984). *Psychotherapy in a new key: A guide to time-limited dynamic psychotherapy.* New York: Basic.

Target, M., & Fonagy P. (1994a). Efficacy of psychoanalysis for children with emotional disorders. *Journal of the American Academy of Child and Adolescent Psychiatry, 3,* 361–371.

Target, M., & Fonagy, P. (1994b). The efficacy of psychoanalysis for children: Prediction of outcome in a developmental context. *Journal of the American Academy of Child and Adolescent Psychiatry, 8,* 1134–1144.

Tasman, A. (1993). Setting standards for psychotherapy training. *Journal of Psychotherapy Practice and Research, 2,* 93–99.

Thomä, H., & Kächele, H. (1987). *Psychoanalytic practice* (M. Wilson & D. Roseveare, Trans.). Berlin: Springer-Verlag.

Thompson, L., Gallagher, D., & Breckenridge, J. (1987). Comparative effectiveness of psychotherapies for depressed elders. *Journal of Consulting and Clinical Psychology, 55,* 385–390.

Ursano, R., & Silberman, E.K. (1994). Psychoanalysis, psychoanalytic psychotherapy, and supportive psychotherapy. In R.E. Hales, S.C. Yudofsky, & J. Talbott (Eds.), *The American Psychiatric Press textbook of psychiatry* (2d ed.). Washington, DC: American Psychiatric Press.

Ursano, R., Sonnenberg, S., & Lazar, S. (1991). *Concise guide to psychodynamic psychotherapy.* Washington, DC: American Psychiatric Association.

Vaillant, G. (1976). Natural history of male psychological health: The relation of choice of ego mechanisms of defense to adult adjustment. *Archives of General Psychiatry, 33,* 535–545.

Vaillant, G. (1977). *Adaptation to life.* Boston: Little, Brown.

Vaillant, G. (1986). *Empirical studies of ego mechanisms of defense.* Washington, DC: American Psychiatric Press.

Vaillant, G.E., & Drake, R.E. (1985). Maturity of ego defences in relation to DSM-III Axis II personality disorder. *Archives of General Psychiatry, 42,* 597–601.

Vaillant, G.E., & Vaillant, C.O. (1986). A cross-validation of two empirical studies of defences. In G.E. Vaillant (Ed.), *Empirical studies of ego mechanisms of defense* Washington, DC: American Psychiatric Press.

Volkan, V. (1987). *Six steps in the treatment of borderline personality organization.* Northvale, NJ: Jason Aronson.

Waldinger, R., & Gunderson, J. (1984). Completed psychotherapies with borderline patients. *American Journal of Psychotherapy, 38,* 190–202.

Wallace, E.R. (1983) *Dynamic psychiatry in theory and practice.* Philadelphia: Lea & Febiger.

Wallerstein, R. (1986). *Forty-two lives in treatment: A study of psychoanalysis and psychotherapy.* New York: Guilford.

Wallerstein, J.S., & Blakeslee, S. (1989). *Second chances: men, women and children a decade after divorce.* New York: Ticknor & Fields.

Ware, J.E., Manning, W.G., Duan, N., Wells, K.B., & Newhouse, J.P. (1984). Health status and the use of outpatient mental health services. *American Psychologist, 39,* 1090–1100.

Warme, G. (1994) *Reluctant treasures: The practice of analytic psychotherapy.* Northvale, NJ: Jason Aronson.

Weber, J., Bachrach, H., & Solomon, M. (1985a). Factors associated with the outcome of psychoanalysis: Report of the Columbia Psychoanalytic Center Research Project (II). *International Review of Psycho-Analysis, 12,* 127–141.

Weber, J., Bachrach, H., & Solomon, M. (1985b). Factors associated with the outcome of psychoanalysis: Report of the Columbia Psychoanalytic Center Research Project (III). *International Review of Psycho-Analysis, 12,* 251–262.

Weber, J., Solomon, M., & Bachrach, H. (1985). Characteristics of psychoanalytic clinic patients: Report of the Columbia Psychoanalytic Center Research Project (I). *International Review of Psycho-Analysis, 12,* 15–26.

Weil, J.L. (1989a). *Instinctual stimulation of children* (Vol. 1). Madison, CT: International Universities Press.

Weil, J.L. (1989b). *Instinctual stimulation of children.* (Vol. 2). Madison, CT: International Universities Press.

Weil, J.L. (1992). *Early deprivation of empathic care*. Madison, CT: International Universities Press.

Weiss, J. (1993). *How psychotherapy works: Process and technique*. New York: Guilford.

Weiss, J., Sampson, H., & the Mount Zion Psychotherapy Research Group. (1986). *The psychoanalytic process: Theory, clinical observations and empirical research*. New York: Guilford Press.

Wells, K.B., Burnam, A., Rogers, W., Hays, R., & Camp, P. (1992). The course of depression in adult outpatients. *Archives of General Psychiatry, 49*, 788–794.

Wiborg, I.M., & Dahl, A.A. (1996). Does brief psychodynamic psychotherapy reduce the relapse rate of panic disorder? *Archives of General Psychiatry, 53*, 689–694.

Wiener, J. (1994, 21 October). From the president: On psychotherapy. *Psychiatric News*, 3–16.

Woody, G., Lubursky, L., McLellan, A.T., O'Brien, C., Beck, A.T., Blaine, J., Herman, I., & Hok, A.V. (1983). Psychotherapy for opiate addicts: Does it help? *Archives of General Psychiatry, 40*, 639–645.

Wzontek, M. (1990). *Factors associated with patients' post-termination images of their psychotherapist*. Doctoral dissertation, Department of Clinical Psychology, Teachers College, Columbia University.

Zitren, C., Klein, D., & Woener, M. (1978). Behavior therapy, supportive psychotherapy, imipramine and phobias. *Archives of General Psychiatry, 35*, 307–316.

5. Guidelines for the Practice of Cognitive Behavioural Psychotherapy

Martin M. Antony and Richard P. Swinson

Description of Modality

Cognitive behavioural therapy (CBT) is a model of psychotherapy based on principles derived from learning theory and cognitive science. It includes a variety of strategies that are continually evolving, based on findings from empirical research. CBT differs from traditional psychotherapies in several respects. The main focus of CBT is identifying and changing variables that currently maintain problem behaviours, rather than those factors that may have initially contributed to the onset of a disorder. In addition, CBT tends to be conducted in fewer sessions than other psychotherapies. Treatment typically lasts from as little as one session (e.g., in the treatment of some specific phobias) to several months. For some disorders (e.g., personality disorders), treatment may last longer. Another unique feature of CBT is that it routinely incorporates a variety of behavioural measures (e.g., behavioural tests, self-report measures, interview measures, monitoring forms) to assess the effects of each therapeutic strategy *throughout treatment*. Finally, the strategies used by cognitive and behavioural therapists are continually being tested in controlled research studies and have been subjected to more investigations than have most other treatment modalities.

Theoretical Concepts

The term 'cognitive/behavioural therapy' encompasses a broad range of theoretical perspectives. However, there are several assumptions that are shared by most advocates of CBT. First, CBT is deeply entrenched in a scientific tradition (O'Donohue & Krasner, 1995). There are several aspects of science that are especially relevant to the theory and empirical research underlying CBT. In science, theories are articulated in such a way that they generate specific predictions that can be disproved. Scientists continually attempt to improve theories by exposing them to empirical criticism. Ideally, scientists are aware of their biases in favour of their own views and therefore actively seek out information to disconfirm their theories. In science, research is conducted to compare and contrast the utility of different theoretical perspectives. In addition, theories are considered to be evolving entities. Finally, good science aims to minimize superfluous content in theories, so that, all things being equal, the simplest explanation for a given phenomenon is preferred over more complicated explanations.

Despite the shared view that scientific research is the best way to uncover the truth, cognitive and behavioural therapists differ from one another in a variety of ways. Among cognitive therapists, cognitions (i.e., thoughts, predictions, interpretations) are believed to cause emotional states and various types of psychopathology. For example, Beck, Rush, Shaw, and Emery (1979) proposed that depression stems from a tendency to see oneself, one's experiences, and one's future in a negative way. Beck et al (1979) use the term 'schema' to refer to the stable tendencies among depressed individuals to view events in a negative way. Finally, Beck and his colleagues propose that depressed individuals make systematic errors in thinking that lead to the maintenance of their negative thinking styles. Similar cognitive models have been derived to explain other types of psychopathology. For example, panic disorder is viewed by many cognitive therapists as stemming from catastrophic misinterpretations of harmless physical sensations (e.g., Clark, 1986).

In contrast, traditional behavioural therapists believe that behaviour and psychopathology stem from learning experiences and patterns of environmental reinforcement and punishment. For example, the maintenance of phobias is proposed to stem from the negative reinforcement that occurs when an individual avoids a phobic stimulus. In other words, an individual learns that it feels better to stay away from a feared situation than to confront it. For traditional behaviourists, cognitions (like all behaviour) are simply the product of events in the environment, but do not actually cause behaviour. Therefore, behavioural therapists do not attempt to change thoughts directly. Rather, behavioural therapy aims to change patterns of behaviour, and patterns of reinforcement and punishment in the environment.

Despite differences between the purest forms of cognitive and behavioural therapy, as discussed above, most therapists who conduct CBT view behaviour as determined by a broad range of factors, including biological factors (e.g., genetics, neurotransmitter function), learning experiences (e.g., conditioning, reinforcement from family members), and cognitive factors (e.g., beliefs, attribution). Therefore, most comprehensive treatments that fall under the general heading 'CBT' include a variety of cognitive and behavioural interventions.

Therapeutic Interventions and Mechanisms of Change

Cognitive/behavioural therapy differs from other psychotherapies in that it often involves treatment sessions that last longer than the traditional fifty minutes. For example, a session of exposure therapy for agoraphobia should last long enough for a patient's anxiety to decrease to a mild level. Likewise, therapists who conduct exposure and response prevention for bulimia nervosa usually continue sessions until the patient's desire to purge has abated. Therefore, although most sessions last about an hour, it is not unusual for the therapist and patient to have sessions that last two hours or longer. Furthermore, therapists who conduct CBT occasionally schedule sessions more frequently than once per week, particularly early in treatment. A variety of studies have shown that exposure therapy for phobias works best when sessions are massed (Marks, 1987). In other words, a series of sessions held daily is more effective than the same number of sessions conducted once per week.

Although CBT treatment tends to be briefer than other therapeutic modalities, the duration of treatment varies across patients and disorders. For example, certain specific phobias can often be overcome in one session lasting several hours (Öst, 1989). In contrast, major depression may take up to twenty sessions or more to treat effectively (Rush, Beck, Kovacs, & Hollon, 1977). Finally, because the strategies used in CBT are structured and clearly articulated, programs are now being developed to provide CBT in a self-help format (e.g., Antony, Craske, & Barlow, 1995; Barlow & Craske, 1994).

In addition to differences in the timing and duration of treatment sessions, CBT differs from traditional psychotherapies in that it is conducted in a variety of settings. For example, for a patient with agoraphobia, treatment sessions may be conducted on subways, in cars, at shopping malls, and in a variety of other situations that are avoided by patients. For patients with obsessive–compulsive disorder, treatment may be conducted in the patient's home. There is evidence that exposure is most effective if it occurs in the same context in which the patient's anxiety and fear tend to be triggered (Bouton, 1988). In addition, skills training may work best if it is conducted in the situation where the skills are eventually to be used. Another reason to conduct sessions in the patient's natural environment is for the purpose of assessment. Patient reports are often unreliable. Observing patients in their homes, in feared situations, and in interaction with their significant others can provide valuable information to aid in planning treatment. Also, unlike other treatment modalities, much of the 'work' that occurs during CBT is in the form of homework assignments that are conducted between sessions.

Although most CBT therapists view a strong therapeutic relationship as an important component of effective treatment, CBT tends to pay relatively little attention to the therapeutic alliance, relative to other treatment modalities. Nevertheless, special attention must be paid to boundary issues that arise, especially when CBT is conducted outside of the therapist's office. For example, a therapist treating an individual with an eating disorder may have a meal with the patient in a restaurant to assess the patient's eating behaviour and teach the patient appropriate eating behaviour. Similarly, a therapist treating obsessive–compulsive disorder may visit a patient's house to 'contaminate' particular areas of the home as part of exposure therapy. As with all forms of psychotherapy, CBT therapists must practise according to appropriate ethical standards, which include being aware of the boundaries of professional conduct and not allowing these boundaries to become blurred. Individuals being treated with CBT should fully understand the parameters and purpose of each intervention. In some cases (e.g., when treatment is being conducted in a non-public place, such as a patient's home), the therapist should consider including a co-therapist or chaperone during the session for his or her own protection as well as the protection of the patient.

In addition to being used as an outpatient treatment, CBT is sometimes conducted on an inpatient basis. For example, some investigators (e.g., van den Hout, Emmelkamp, Kraaykamp, & Griez, 1988) have demonstrated the efficacy of an inpatient CBT program for obsessive–compulsive disorder. Inpatient CBT may be a reasonable treatment option for other severe disorders that are often treated on an inpatient basis (e.g., severe depression, eating disorders, schizophrenia).

The mechanism of change in CBT is believed to be related to changes in patients' thoughts and behaviours. For example, a schizophrenic patient who has received social-skills training may interact more effectively with his or her environment and thereby be reinforced for these newly developed behaviours. A patient with anorexia nervosa may learn more appropriate eating behaviours in addition to learning new ways to interpret body image and eating situations. These changes in thought and behaviour are believed to lead to decreased distress as well as to more-effective interactions with others and with the environment.

SPECIFIC THERAPEUTIC STRATEGIES

a. *Functional analysis:* This consists of an exploration of the environmental variables that maintain a problem behaviour. Functional analysis allows for the development of specific strategies to help the patient change his or her environment so that more adaptive patterns of behaviour are reinforced.

b. *Self-monitoring:* Patients are typically required to monitor relevant feelings, thoughts, and behaviours between therapy sessions. Monitoring forces the patient to be more aware of his or her behaviours and provides the therapist with information necessary for choosing strategies that might be effective for a given patient. On-the-spot monitoring has the advantage of not being contaminated by retrospective recall biases.

c. *Psychoeducation:* This refers to the process of teaching the patient about his or her disorder as well as the rationale for CBT. For example, a patient with panic disorder who believes that panic-attack symptoms are a sign of an impending heart attack will usually be provided with corrective information regarding these symptoms and how they relate to cardiac functioning.

d. *Homework assignments:* Patients are required to complete specific homework assignments between sessions. Homework may include monitoring of the person's reactions, reading about the presenting disorder, practising specific therapeutic strategies (e.g., exposure to feared situations, challenging cognitive distortions, using specific social skills, relaxation exercises, engaging in specific activities).

e. *Cognitive restructuring:* This involves identifying cognitive distortions (i.e., unrealistic beliefs that contribute to the problem) and changing these beliefs by examining the evidence that supports and contradicts these beliefs.

f. *Hypothesis testing:* This involves testing the validity of the patient's negative predictions in specific situations.

g. *Exposure:* This involves confronting feared situations repeatedly in a controlled and structured manner until the fear has decreased. Exposure may be conducted *in vivo* or in the imagination. Furthermore, exposure-based treatments vary with respect to therapist involvement and the rate at which treatment progresses to more difficult situations.

h. *Skills training:* This involves teaching a patient skills to compensate for specific behavioural deficits or to decrease specific behavioural excesses. Strategies may be designed to improve the patient's social-interaction skills (e.g., social phobia, depression) or to teach specific skills of daily living (e.g., schizophrenia).

i. *Relaxation training:* This involves teaching the patient specific strategies to decrease stress and anxiety. Strategies may include muscle relaxation, imagery, and breathing retraining.

j. *Biofeedback:* This involves training patients to be aware of and to change bodily cues that indicate changes in blood pressure, body temperature, and muscle tension.

k. *Problem-solving training:* This involves teaching patients a series of steps (e.g., identifying problems, generating solutions, evaluating solutions, implementing solutions) to solve problems that come up in everyday life.

Indications and Contraindications

Cognitive/behavioural therapy strategies have been demonstrated to be effective in controlled clinical trials for a variety of conditions, including major depression, panic disorder, agoraphobia, social phobia, specific phobia, obsessive–compulsive disorder, post-traumatic stress disorder, generalized anxiety disorder, anorexia nervosa, bulimia, schizophrenia, autism, marital distress, psychophysiological disorders, personality disorders, sexual disorders, and substance abuse. (For references, see 'Scientific Basis and Efficacy,' below.) However, despite the broad range of applications for CBT, it appears that certain strategies may be more or less beneficial for particular types of patients. For example, it is generally believed that behavioural techniques (e.g., exposure) are more effective for specific phobias than are cognitive interventions. Also, there are cases in which co-morbidity can complicate the treatment of a particular disorder. For example, although cognitive strategies are often integrated

into specific phobia treatments, behavioural techniques, such as exposure, are believed to be the most important elements of treatment
(Antony & Barlow, 1997; Antony et al, 1995). Finally, patients who are
unable to understand the content of the sessions or complete assignments (e.g., current psychosis, severe substance use, mania, vegetative
depression) are less likely to benefit from CBT.

Scientific Basis and Efficacy

Numerous studies have examined the efficacy of cognitive and behavioural interventions for a broad range of disorders, including anxiety
disorders, mood disorders, schizophrenia, eating disorders, substance
abuse disorders, sexual disorders, and stress-related medical conditions.
For most of these disorders, CBT has been shown to be of some benefit,
and for many of these disorders it may be the treatment of choice.

DEPRESSION

Several literature reviews (e.g., Hollon, Shelton, & Davis, 1993; Robinson, Berman, & Niemeyer, 1990) have found that CBT (e.g., behaviour
therapy, cognitive therapy) is an effective treatment for depression.
Many of the studies reviewed included patients who met diagnostic criteria for a depressive disorder (e.g., major depression, dysthymia),
whereas other studies did not include formal diagnostic evaluations.
However, there appears to be little evidence that CBT is more effective
than certain alternative treatments such as pharmacotherapy and interpersonal psychotherapy. Furthermore, the majority of studies have
examined CBT only for unipolar depression. The utility of CBT for
depression in patients with bipolar disorder is only now being studied.
Finally, for patients with severe depression and prominent suicidal ideation, initial treatment with medication may be helpful to decrease
depression to a level at which patients can benefit from CBT, a psychological intervention that demands attention, motivation, and compliance with homework assignments. In addition, investigators have
recently begun to examine the effectiveness of CBT for preventing
relapse following pharmacotherapy of depression.

PANIC DISORDER AND AGORAPHOBIA

Panic disorder has been successfully treated with a variety of cognitive and behavioural interventions, including cognitive restructuring, inter-oceptive and *in vivo* exposure, and applied relaxation. Across a wide range of studies, an average of 85 per cent of patients treated with CBT are panic-free at post-treatment, and 88 per cent are panic-free at follow-up (Chambless & Gillis, 1993). Furthermore, CBT for panic disorder leads to changes in associated features, including agoraphobic avoid-ance, generalized anxiety and depression. *In vivo* exposure appears to be the most effective treatment for patients with significant agoraphobic avoidance and there is little evidence that cognitive interventions add anything over and above the effects of exposure for these patients (Chambless & Gillis, 1993). Recently, CBT has been successfully used to prevent the development of panic disorder and agoraphobia in patients presenting to hospital emergency rooms with panic attacks (Swinson, Soulios, Cox, & Kuch, 1992).

SOCIAL AND SPECIFIC PHOBIAS

More than twenty-five studies have been conducted to examine the effi-cacy of CBT for social phobia, and dozens more to examine the use of CBT for specific fears and phobias. Heimberg and Juster (1995) reviewed the literature on CBT for social phobia, and concluded that a variety of treat-ment strategies appear to be effective for social phobia, including social-skills training, exposure, applied relaxation, and cognitive therapy. In addition, studies have examined the use of comprehensive treatment packages containing several of these strategies. In almost all studies, CBT has been shown to be more effective than wait-list control conditions and a variety of other comparison treatments (e.g., supportive psychotherapy, beta blockers). CBT for social phobia appears to be equally as effective as phenelzine, and its effects are longer-lasting. In general, treatment gains following CBT tend to be maintained over time. For example, in one study, Heimberg, Salzman, Holt, and Blendell (1993) found that 89 per cent of patients who received CBT (compared with 44 per cent of patients who received supportive psychotherapy) were judged to be clinically improved by independent evaluations conducted on average 5.5 years following treatment. With respect to specific phobias, *in vivo* exposure to the feared stimulus is clearly effective for decreasing fear and avoidance (Antony & Barlow, 1997). In fact, up to 90 per cent of patients with animal or blood/injection phobias are significantly improved or cured in as little as one session of therapist-assisted exposure. Furthermore, these gains tend to be maintained at follow-up (Öst, 1989).

OBSESSIVE–COMPULSIVE DISORDER (OCD)

Several recent literature reviews (Abel, 1993; Foa, Franklin, & Kozak, 1998; Cox, Swinson, Morrison, & Lee, 1993; van Balkom et al, 1994) have concluded that CBT (usually in the form of 'exposure and response prevention') is an effective treatment for OCD. Although there was no consistent difference in efficacy between CBT and a variety of pharmacological interventions (e.g., clomipramine, fluoxetine) on most measures, Abel (1993) concluded that CBT may be most beneficial for compulsive rituals, whereas pharmacotherapy may be especially helpful or patients with prominent obsessions, overvalued ideation, and depression.

GENERALIZED ANXIETY DISORDER (GAD)

Cognitive behavioural treatment of GAD has consisted primarily of cognitive therapy and various relaxation-based interventions. Recent reviews (e.g., Borkovec & Roemer, 1995; Chambless & Gillis, 1993) of more than ten studies examining the efficacy of CBT for GAD suggest that CBT is an effective treatment for GAD. Furthermore, in a variety of controlled studies, CBT appears to be more beneficial than alternative psychological treatments (e.g., non-directive psychotherapy) and treatment with diazepam (Power et al, 1990). Finally, the effects of CBT appear to be long-lasting, with gains being maintained or augmented at six- and twelve-month follow-up. In contrast, long-term studies of benzodiazepine treatment have found relapse rates of up to 81 per cent (Rickels, Case, & Diamond, 1980).

POST-TRAUMATIC STRESS DISORDER (PTSD)

Few controlled studies of CBT exist for the treatment of PTSD. However, the few studies that have been conducted with individuals who have experienced traumas related to combat or rape suggest that CBT strategies (e.g., imaginal exposure, stress management) are effective for overcoming and preventing the development of PTSD (Emmelkamp, 1994; Foa, Rothbaum, Riggs, & Murdoch, 1991; Foa, Herst-Ikeda, & Perry, 1995).

SCHIZOPHRENIA

Several studies have documented the utility of specific behavioural interventions in the management of schizophrenia. In general, it is believed that CBT has little effect on positive symptoms (e.g., hallucinations, delusions). However, there is evidence that CBT may help to improve social skills, self-care, and independent-living skills, and decrease aggressive behaviour among schizophrenic patients. In addition, behavioural treatments may help to decrease the amount of medication needed by patients as well as increase the time between relapses. For example, Hogarty et al (1986) compared four treatment conditions with respect to relapse rate in the first year following treatment with (1) social-skills training, (2) family psychoeducation, (3) social-skills training plus family psychoeducation, and (4) no psychological intervention. All patients received fluphenazine. The one-year relapse rates for the four groups were 20, 19, 0, and 41 per cent, respectively.

SEXUAL DYSFUNCTION

A variety of cognitive and behavioural strategies have been used successfully to treat sexual dysfunction in men and women. These include systematic desensitization, cognitive therapy, masturbation training, and assertiveness training (Emmelkamp, 1994).

BEHAVIOURAL MEDICINE

Recent reviews by Blanchard (1994) and Hollon and Beck (1994) concluded that CBT can be helpful for reducing distress in patients undergoing surgery and patients diagnosed with serious illness such as HIV and cancer. In addition, CBT has been used effectively to decrease high-risk sexual behaviour in adolescents. Finally, CBT strategies are effective for the management of a variety of psychophysiological disorders, including chronic pain, tension headaches, irritable bowel syndrome, obesity, arthritis, and insomnia, and for decreasing type-A (coronary prone) behaviour. CBT may be effective (although evidence is mixed) for treating hypertension and migraine headaches as well.

ALCOHOL ABUSE

Several cognitive and behavioural strategies have been attempted with patients who abuse alcohol. Whereas aversive therapies (e.g., attempting to pair alcohol with nausea or electrical shock) are not especially effective in the long term, other cognitive and behavioural strategies appear to be helpful for treating alcohol abuse (e.g., Sanchez-Craig, 1990). Some of these include social-skills training, communication training, contingency-management training, and cue exposure (Emmelkamp, 1994). Although CBT has been shown to be more effective than traditional therapies for decreasing the frequency of drinking and relapse rates, eventual relapse is still a serious problem, even for patients treated with CBT.

BULIMIA NERVOSA

Wilson and Fairburn (1993) recently reviewed the literature on CBT for eating disorders. Nearly all of the studies reviewed examined the utility of CBT in patients with bulimia nervosa as opposed to other eating disorders. Across a wide range of studies, CBT led to significantly more improvement than did no treatment or treatment with antidepressants (e.g., imipramine). However, CBT tended to be equally effective as other non-behavioural interventions, including supportive psychotherapy, interpersonal psychotherapy, and group therapy. In some cases, CBT was more effective than other approaches immediately following treatment. However, differences tended to disappear during follow-up. According to a review by Wilson and Pike (1993), controlled studies show a mean percentage reduction in binge eating of 73 to 93 per cent, and a 77 to 94 per cent reduction in purging. Mean remission rates for binge eating range from 51 to 71 per cent, whereas purging remits in 36 to 56 per cent of subjects.

PERSONALITY DISORDERS

Although there have been very few controlled studies of CBT for personality disorders, an exception has been the work of Linehan, Armstrong, Suerez, Allman, and Heard (1991), who found that their version of CBT, called 'dialectical behaviour therapy' (including skills training, contingency management, cognitive therapy, exposure to emotional cues), is more effective than traditional psychotherapy for decreasing parasuicidal behaviour, hospitalization time, and premature termination from treatment among patients with borderline personality disorder. Additionally, Linehan's treatment and the traditional therapies were equally effective at decreasing depression, hopelessness, and suicidal ideation. More controlled studies are needed to determine the efficacy of CBT for personality disorders.

Training

Training in CBT is typically conducted in specialty clinics affiliated with university psychiatry and psychology departments. In general, comprehensive training should provide students with an understanding of the theoretical and treatment-outcome literature related to CBT, a working knowledge of how to implement the range of behavioural and cognitive techniques, and experience in using these strategies in a variety of settings and populations. Training usually begins with observation of a trained CBT therapist followed by the opportunity to conduct cotherapy, supervised therapy, and eventually independent practice. Although very little has been published in the area of CBT training, some university departments are beginning to develop specific guidelines for training (e.g., Antony & Segal, 1995).

References

Abel, J.L. (1993). Exposure with response prevention and serotonergic antidepressants in the treatment of obsessive compulsive disorder: A review and implications for interdisciplinary treatment. *Behaviour Research and Therapy, 31*, 463–478.

Antony, M.M., & Barlow, D.H. (1997). Social and specific phobias. In A. Tasman, J. Kay, & J.A. Lieberman (Eds.), *Psychiatry*. Philadelphia, PA: Saunders.

Antony, M.M., Craske, M.G., & Barlow, D.H. (1995). *Mastery of your specific phobia*. San Antonio, Tx: The Psychological Corporation.

Antony, M.M., & Segal, Z.V. (1995). *Post-graduate training objectives in cognitive behaviour therapy*. Report submitted to Department of Psychiatry, University of Toronto.

Barlow, D.H., & Craske, M.G. (1994). *Mastery of your anxiety and panic*. (2d. ed.). San Antonio, Tx: The Psychological Corporation.

Beck, A.T., Rush, A.J., Shaw, B.F., & Emery, G. (1979). *Cognitive therapy of depression*. New York: Guilford.

Blanchard, E.B. (1994). Behavioral medicine and health psychology. In A.E. Bergin & S.L. Garfield (Eds.), *Handbook of psychotherapy and behavior change* (4th ed.). New York: Wiley.

Borkovec, T.D., & Roemer, L. (1995). Cognitive behavioral treatment of generalized anxiety disorder. In R.T. Ammerman & M. Hersen (Eds.), *Handbook of prescriptive treatments for adults*. New York: Plenum.

Bouton, M.E. (1988). Context and ambiguity in the extinction of emotional learning: Implications for exposure therapy. *Behaviour Research and Therapy, 26,* 137–149.

Chambless, D.L., & Gillis, M.M. (1993). Cognitive therapy of anxiety disorders. *Journal of Consulting and Clinical Psychology, 61,* 248–260.

Clark, D.M. (1986). A cognitive approach to panic. *Behaviour Research and Therapy, 24,* 461–470.

Cox, B.J., Swinson, R.P., Morrison, B., & Lee, P.S. (1993). Clomipramine, fluoxetine, and behavior therapy in the treatment of obsessive–compulsive disorder: A meta-analysis. *Journal of Behavior Therapy and Experimental Psychiatry, 24,* 149–153.

Emmelkamp, P.M.G. (1994). Behavior therapy with adults. In A.E. Bergin & S.L. Garfield (Eds.), *Handbook of psychotherapy and behavior change* (4th ed.). New York: Wiley.

Foa, E.B., Franklin, M.E., & Kozak, M.J. (1998). Psychosocial treatments: Literature Review. In R.P. Swinson, M.M. Antony, S. Rachman, & M.A. Richter (Eds.), *Obsessive compulsive disorder: Theory, research, and treatment.* New York: Guilford.

Foa, E.B., Herst-Ikeda, D., & Perry, K.J. (1995). Evaluation of a brief cognitive–behavioral program for the prevention of chronic PTSD in recent assault victims. *Journal of Consulting and Clinical Psychology, 63,* 948–955.

Foa, E.B., Rothbaum, B.O., Riggs, D.S., & Murdock, T.B., (1991). Treatment of post-traumatic stress disorder in rape victims: A comparison between cognitive–behavioural procedures and counselling. *Journal of Consulting and Clinical Psychology, 59,* 715–723.

Heimberg, R.G., & Juster, H.R. (1995). Cognitive–behavioral treatments: Literature review. In R.G. Heimberg, M.R. Liebowitz, D.A. Hope, & F.R. Schneier (Eds.), *Social phobia: Diagnosis, assessment, and treatment.* New York: Guilford.

Heimberg, R.G., Salzman, D.G., Holt, C.S., & Blendell, K.A. (1993). Cognitive–behavioral group treatment for social phobia: Effectiveness at five-year follow-up. *Cognitive Therapy and Research, 17,* 325–339.

Hogarty, G.E., Anderson, C.M., Reiss, D.J., Kornblith, S.J., Greenwald, D.P., Javna, C.D., & Madonia, M.J. (1986). Family psycho-education, social skills training, and chemotherapy in the aftercare treatment of schizophrenia, I: One-year effects of a controlled study on relapse and expressed emotion. *Archives of General Psychiatry, 43,* 633–642.

Hollon, S.D., & Beck, A.T. (1994). Cognitive and cognitive behavioral therapies. In A.E. Bergin & S.L. Garfield (Eds.), *Handbook of psychotherapy and behavior change* (4th ed.). New York: Wiley.

Hollon, S.D., Shelton, R.C., & Davis, D.D. (1993). Cognitive therapy for depression: Conceptual issues and clinical efficacy. *Journal of Consulting and Clinical Psychology, 61,* 270–275.

Linehan, M.M., Armstrong, H.E., Suerez, A., Allmon, D., & Heard, H.L. (1991). Cognitive–behavioral treatment of chronically parasuicidal borderline patients. *Archives of General Psychiatry, 48,* 1060–1064

Marks, I.M. (1987). *Fears, phobias, and rituals.* New York: Oxford University Press.

O'Donohue, W., & Krasner, L. (1995). Theories in behavior therapy: Philosophical and historical contexts. In W. O'Donohue & L. Krasner (Eds.), *Theories of behavior therapy.* Washington, DC: American Psychological Association.

Öst, L.-G. (1989). One-session treatment for specific phobias. *Behaviour Research and Therapy, 27,* 1–7.

Power, K.G., Simpson, R.J., Swanson, V., Wallace, L.A., Feistner, A.T.C., & Sharp, D. (1990). A controlled comparison of cognitive–behaviour therapy, diazepam, and placebo, alone and in combination, for the treatment of generalized anxiety disorder. *Journal of Anxiety Disorders, 4,* 267–292.

Rickels, K., Case, W.G., & Diamond, L. (1980). Relapse after short-term drug therapy in neurotic outpatients. *International Pharmacopsychiatry, 15,* 186–192.

Robinson, L.A., Berman, J.S., & Neimeyer, R.A. (1990). Psychotherapy for the treatment of depression: A comprehensive review of controlled outcome research. *Psychological Bulletin, 108,* 30–49.

Rush, A.J., Beck, A.T., Kovacs, M., & Hollon, S. (1977). Comparative efficacy of cognitive therapy and imipramine in the treatment of depressed outpatients. *Cognitive Therapy and Research, 1,* 17–37.

Sanchez-Craig, M. (1990). Brief didactic treatment for alcohol and drug related problems: An approach based on client choice. *British Journal of Addiction, 85,* 169–177.

Swinson, R.P., Soulios, C., Cox, B.J., & Kuch, K. (1992). Brief treatment of emergency room patients with panic attacks. *American Journal of Psychiatry, 149,* 944–946.

van Balkom, A.J.L.M., van Oppen, P., Vermeulen, A.W.A, van Dyck, R.V., Nauta, M.C.E., & Vorst, H.C.M. (1994). A meta-analysis on the treatment of obsessive–compulsive disorder: A comparison of antidepressants, behavior, and cognitive therapy. *Clinical Psychology Review, 14,* 359–381.

van den Hout, M., Emmelkamp, P., Kraaykamp, H., & Griez, E. (1988). Behavioral treatment of obsessive–compulsives: Inpatient vs. outpatient. *Behaviour Research and Therapy, 26,* 331–332.

Wilson, G.T., & Fairburn, C.G. (1993). Cognitive treatments for eating disorders. *Journal of Consulting and Clinical Psychology, 61,* 261–269.

Wilson, G.T., & Pike, K.M. (1993). Eating disorders. In D.H. Barlow (Ed.), *Clinical handbook of psychological disorders* (2nd ed.) New York: Guilford.

6. Guidelines for the Practice of Brief Psychodynamic Psychotherapy

Howard E. Book

Definition and Goals

The goals of this chapter are to offer guidelines for the practice of brief psychodynamic psychotherapy by defining its goals, contrasting it with other short psychotherapeutic interventions, describing its theoretical underpinnings, summarizing the major schools of brief psychodynamic psychotherapy, detailing elements common to all the brief psychodynamic psychotherapies, focusing on indications and contraindications, précising its scientific basis, and commenting on training and credentialling. These guidelines are generic, and refer broadly to clinical situations where brief psychodynamic psychotherapy is generally recommended, rather than prescribed for any one specific disorder. It should also be borne in mind that, reflecting the paucity of data comparing dynamic therapies with cognitive or behavioural therapies, little research has been done in this area (Barber, J.: personal communication).

Brief psychodynamic psychotherapy (BPP) encompasses a number of psychotherapy models with well-defined, psychoanalytically derived principles and techniques. Goals, which include both symptom relief (Luborsky, Singer, & Luborsky, 1975; Thompson, Gallager, & Breckenridge, 1987; Piper, Azim, McCallum, & Joyce, 1990, Crits-Christoph, 1992; Shefler, Dasberg, & Ben-Shakbar, 1995) and limited but significant character change (Brom, Kleber, & Defares, 1989; Winston et al, 1991; Winston et al, 1994; Anderson & Lambert, 1995), are obtained within a limited number of weekly sessions. Because it is time-limited, and the techniques can be standardized and manual-based, BPP has been extensively studied scientifically. This large body of empirical work provides a strong evidence base for the establishment of practice guidelines. Two key texts (Bauer & Kobos, 1987; Messer & Warren, 1995) review and compare the various models of BPP developed in different centres. These have been essential in moving towards delineating commonalities among the different forms of BPP.

Some models of brief psychodynamic psychotherapy employ a flexible time limit that is not predetermined, but is less than one year (Budman, 1981; Davanloo, 1980; Malan, 1976; Sifneos, 1987; Strupp & Binder, 1984). Other models use a fixed time limit which is communicated to the patient after the evaluation period, but before initiating treatment (Luborsky, 1984; Mann, 1973). For instance, Mann emphasizes a twelve-session time limit, and Luborsky (1984) generally recommends sixteen sessions.

As will be detailed later, the twin goals of symptom relief and character change are attained by the patient's free association and the therapist's persistent empathic focus on one pivotal, circumscribed segment of the patient's maladaptive character style (MacKenzie, 1988). Through this process, small changes in that one crucial area can be associated with large shifts in functioning (Luborsky, 1984).

COMPARISON WITH OTHER THERAPEUTIC CONTACTS

Too often, the term 'brief psychotherapy' is used casually and erroneously to describe any therapeutic contact that lasts for a just a few sessions. Similarly, the goal of brief psychotherapy is often erroneously confused with the goals of emergency psychotherapy or crisis psychotherapy. The following short comparison sharply clarifies differences between these approaches.

Emergency Psychotherapy: The goal of emergency psychotherapy, or emergency care, is symptomatic relief for a patient who is distressed and disorganized in the face of internal or external stress to the point of being unable to cope with it (Marmor, 1979). Character change is not a goal. The therapist practising emergency psychotherapy offsets this regression by functioning as an 'auxiliary' ego on behalf of the patient's overwhelmed ego. To do so, he or she offers primarily supportive, reality-bolstering clarifying activities, with some confrontation and no interpretation. All of this is in the service of ego functioning. Additionally, the therapist provides vital self–object functions, such as offering validation and accepting idealization, to offset further fragmentation. He or she may also function as a 'container' for a patient's 'unacceptable' internal representations which have been projected onto him or her. The patient is seen sitting up, face to face, and the length of contact, and frequency and duration of treatment are not fixed but shift in response to the clinical status and needs of that patient. The patient thus might be seen for five minutes four times daily, and then less frequently as the patient's ego functions re-emerge.

Crisis Psychotherapy: Crisis is defined by Caplan (1964) as a state which is 'provoked when a person faces an obstacle (hazard) to important life goals that is for a time insurmountable through the utilization of customary methods of problem solving (coping behavior). A period of disorganization ensues, a period of upset (crisis) during which many different abortive attempts at solution are made. Eventually some kind of adaptation is achieved which may or may not be in the best interests of that person or his fellows' (quoted in Jacobson, 1979, p. 40). Jacobson (1979) empasizes that the crisis is time-limited and that its outcome may be more or less adaptive.

The goal of crisis therapy, or crisis intervention, is also symptom relief. In this instance, it is for a patient who has not yet disorganized, but is on the cusp of so being (Marmor, 1979). Crises and emergencies are, of course, on a continuum, but in an emergency situation the patient is more disorganized and less able to cope, and may have impaired reality testing. As in emergency psychotherapy, the therapist attains this goal by functioning as an auxiliary ego in order to bolster the patient's faltering ego functions and by performing vital self–object functions to offset regression. Additionally, he or she makes confronting and, at times, interpretive comments in order to improve the patient's adaptive capacity. Although the goal is symptom relief and returning the patient to his or her previous level of functioning, at times some character change occurs as a result of this later expressive activity. Crisis intervention differs from brief psychotherapy in a number of ways. It is of shorter duration, usually four to six weeks, terminating when the crisis is resolved, rather than after a predetermined time limit. Frequency may be from one to four times a week rather than once a week. It tends to be more supportive and directive and deals only with the present, whereas brief therapy includes exploration of past relationships and transference. As well, crisis intervention, like emergency care, may involve work with family and social network, while BPP is an individual therapy. The patient is seen sitting up, face to face, with the duration of therapy being approximately forty-five minutes (unlike emergency psychotherapy, where the length of contact depends on the patient's status), and the frequency is once per week (unlike emergency psychotherapy, where the frequency also varies, depending on the patient's clinical status).

Long-term Psychodynamic Psychotherapy: Long-term psychotherapy and psychoanalysis are broad-spectrum treatments for a number of disorders (see chapter 3, 'Guidelines for the Practice of Individual Psychodynamic Psychotherapy'). Like BPP, these treatments are conceptualized as operating on an expressive–supportive continuum (Luborsky, 1984). At the expressive end of the continuum, significant and substantial character change along a broad perspective is a primary goal. In this circumstance, a certain amount of regression can be utilized therapeutically. However, long-term psychodynamic psychotherapy may also be used for patients who do not have sufficient ego strength to tolerate brief psychotherapy. The goal of long-term psychotherapy or psychoanalysis emphasizes major character reconstruction rather than symptom improvement. In this way, long-term psychotherapy differs from brief psychotherapy – with its emphasis on focal but significant character change – and from emergency and crisis psychotherapies – with their emphasis only on symptomatic relief.

Frequency is generally two to five times a week, duration of sessions forty-five minutes, and length of treatment two to seven years. However, frequency of supportive psychotherapy may be once a week or less, and sessions might be only twenty minutes in length.

Interpersonal Psychotherapy: Interpersonal psychotherapy is a brief, manual-based therapy which has been extensively evaluated in the treatment of depression (Hirschfeld & Shea, 1989; Weissman & Markowitz, 1994). The goal of interpersonal psychotherapy is reduction of depressive symptomatology in patients experiencing unipolar, non-psychotic, ambulatory depression. Although the significance of early developmental issues is acknowledged, in interpersonal psychotherapy the treatment focus emphasizes the connection between depressive symptoms and current (rather than past) interpersonal problems.

The goal of symptom reduction is attained through a psychoeducational approach. Depression is defined as a medical illness, and the patient is encouraged to assume the sick role rather than blaming him- or herself for the illness. The therapist optimistically reviews the course and positive prognosis of treatment. The focus is on helping the patient deal more effectively with current interpersonal problems, particularly in one of the following four areas: grief; interpersonal role disputes; role transitions; and interpersonal deficits. Frequency is once per week, duration of sessions is forty-five minutes, and length of treatment is twelve to sixteen weeks. Interpersonal psychotherapy does not attempt to promote characterological change or emphasize intrapsychic phenomena or transferential issues.

Cognitive Behavioural Psychotherapy: Cognitive/behavioural psychotherapy (CBT; see chapter 6, 'Guidelines for the Practice of Cognitive Behavioural Psychotherapy') is a model of psychotherapy which includes various strategies based on empirical findings. The emphasis is on behavioural and cognitive change-methods for diminishing distress while increasing coping skills of the patient (Bongar & Beutler, 1995). This approach focuses on dysfunctional cognitive structures that maintain unrealistic thoughts and images in specific situations.

CBT does not embrace core psychoanalytic concepts (as defined below, under 'Theoretical Concepts'). Rather, it is informed by the concept that the perception of events mediates the response and ultimately determines the quality of adaptation. Treatment focuses on aiding patients in recognizing perceptual and cognitive errors, instructing them to thus perceive external problems more realistically, and assisting them to cope with these realistically perceived situations.

CBT tends to be brief and is often time-limited. It includes a number of manual-based treatments.

Solution-Focused Brief Therapy: In this model of brief therapy, the focus is not on the patient's presenting problem or on its putative roots in the past. Rather, the therapist focuses on the patient's goal; the times that this goal is attained, even if infrequently; and what the patient does to attain the goal in these situations. This therapy is solution-focused, rather than problem-centred, and future-oriented, rather than past-concerned. Its presuppositions are that problems (or entrance complaints and concerns) have solutions; that solutions can be constructed; that the therapist facilitates the patient's constructing solutions; and that, indeed, solutions are constructed or invented rather than 'discovered' (Walter & Peller, 1992).

Solution-focused brief therapy is based on the work of deShazer (1985) and Berg (1990). The therapy focuses on solution-oriented talk rather than on problem-oriented talk, seeks exceptions to every problem that can be built on to create solutions, builds on small changes, and is rooted in the assumption of non-pathology and wellness. Individuals are viewed as having all they need to solve their problems. The therapist functions at most as a facilitator.

This model of treatment differs from psychodynamic models in that it does not look at past epigenetic roots of difficulties, unconscious determents, the phenomenon of transference, or the problem itself. Rather, it is solution-focused and future-oriented. The duration of treatment is not stipulated prior to beginning treatment; rather, therapy is approached one session at a time: 'Every session is the first; every session is the last' (Walter & Perry, 1992, p. 141).

Very Brief Psychotherapeutic Contacts: In a study of utilization of outpatient psychotherapy in the United States, Olfson and Pincus (1994) found that approximately 70 per cent of patients made ten or fewer visits, with one-third of patients making only one or two visits. Very brief psychotherapy episodes of one or two sessions tended to be delivered by primary-care physicians for treatment of medical conditions such as headache or lower back pain. In his monograph, Talmon (1990) has described the therapeutic value of a single session in affecting symptomatic relief.

Theoretical Concepts

Like all psychodynamic psychotherapies, brief psychodynamic psychotherapy relies on the following five core psychoanalytic concepts (many of which have been discussed in chapter 4, 'Empirical Evidence for the Core Clinical Concepts and Efficacy of the Psychoanalytic Psychotherapies: An Overview'):

1. The Influence of Early-Childhood Experiences on Current Adult Functioning: The experience of the child's early relationship and the resulting conflicts and defects that emerge from this experience have a profound impact on adult functioning. Whether classical Freudian, object-relational, or self-psychological, all dynamic treatments have their theoretical basis in early infant/child–caretaker interactions (Greenberg & Mitchell, 1983).

2. The Power of Unconscious Functioning in Human Behaviour: All psychodynamic theories emphasize the importance of unconscious determinants on current adult functioning. The overarching thesis is that early unresolved conflicts or defects that arose in the child–caretaker relationships exert a powerful, although unacknowledged, influence on current adult relationships.

3. Reliance on Ego Defences: In order to ensure that the impact of early troubled child–caretaker relationships on current function is kept out of awareness, the ego relies on particular automatic manoeuvres – defined as 'ego defences' – to ensure that this material remains unconscious and unremembered. These ego defences lie on a continuum, from the more healthy and adaptive – such as sublimation or humour – to the more reality-distorting – such as denial, projection, or splitting. Despite the use of these defences, this unconscious material returns in disguised ways to affect current relationships.

4. Repetition Compulsion: Repetition compulsion describes a phenomenon whereby an individual behaves in order not to remember. In an unconscious attempt to master the impact of early shortcomings or deprivations, the adult unconsciously attempts to 'right the wrong' through behaviour. For example, a man who experienced the loss of his mother during early childhood may flit from woman to woman romantically, precipitously dropping each as a way of attempting to mask and master the trauma of early loss. Such behaviour unconsciously represents his fear of commitment lest he suffer loss again, and at the same time unconsciously allows him to do to others what was earlier done to him.

5. Transference: The ubiquity of the transference is common to all psychodynamic treatments. Transference, through which an adult responds to others in his or her current environment with feelings and attitudes displaced from, and aimed at, significant people from his or her childhood, is core to all dynamic treatments. Transference is characterized as the mobilization and direction of feelings and attitudes to someone in the present that really befit and are aimed at others from the past.

Models of Brief Psychodynamic Psychotherapy

Since the 1960s there has been a proliferation of new schools of brief psychodynamic psychotherapies. Messer and Warren (1995) have clustered these therapies according to the theoretical models employed by each school.

The 'drive/structural' model encompasses the work of Davanloo

(1980), Malan (1976), and Sifneos (1987), all of whom rely on classical Freudian theoretical concepts of a drive (either sexual or aggressive) striving for gratification, opposed by an ego and/or superego. The tension between the drive and its opposing forces gives rise to a symptom and/or a disturbance in interpersonal behaviour that offers a compromise solution to this conflict. The focus of these schools of brief treatments is usually on an Oedipal conflict.

The relational model encompasses the work of Luborsky (1984), Strupp and Binder (1984), Weiss, Sampson, the Mount Zion Psychotherapy Research Group (1986), and Horowitz et al (1984). The theoretical concept for these models depends far less on a drive straining for discharge and more on the drive as a way of connecting the self with others. The major emphasis of the relational model is on preserving connections and relationships between the self and others. Patterns of maladaptive interpersonal behaviour reflect how the patient repetitively unconsciously anticipates or constructs something going awry in current relationships on the basis of past unremembered ongoing difficulties in child–caretaker relationships. The focus in this school is usually on current and transference relationship issues as they are influenced by early experiences with significant others.

According to Messer and Warren, James Mann's (1973) time-limited psychotherapy integrates the four major constructs (ego, drive, object, and self) contained within the two basic models. In a fourth model, which they describe as 'eclectic approaches,' techniques or concepts from different therapeutic traditions are incorporated within a psychoanalytic brief therapy. Garfield's (1989) brief psychotherapy attempts to incorporate the processes or elements that appear to be common factors across all psychotherapies. Messer and Warren consider Bellak's brief and emergency psychotherapy (Bellak & Small, 1978), which employs technical eclecticism within a six-session framework, to be an example of emergency psychotherapy rather than BPP. Finally, they include Gustafson's (1986) brief therapy as an example of theoretical integration in which the perspectives of psychoanalytic theory are incorporated with a systems approach.

The Defining Characteristics of Brief Psychodynamic Psychotherapy

Although emphasizing differing perspectives – classical/drive, object relation, self-psychology – all forms of BPP share the fundamental psychodynamic concepts of unconscious motivation, the impact of early childhood experiences on adult functioning, the ubiquity of the transference, and the power of repetition compulsion, as described earlier. In addition, all forms of BPP share four elements which constitute its defining characteristics. These characteristics are: careful attention to patient selection; the setting of a time limit; the establishment of a focus; and the therapist's active stance.

SELECTION CRITERIA

According to Bauer and Kobos (1987), BPP is best suited for 'those patients with the capacity to: (1) rapidly enter into a therapeutic alliance, (2) work effectively in an interactional, uncovering treatment, and (3) separate from the therapist once treatment is over with a minimum of distress' (p. 89).

As in long-term psychotherapy or psychoanalysis, patients who benefit most from brief psychodynamic psychotherapy are those that show the ego strengths of:

a. *Psychological mindedness*, evidenced by the capacity to see connections between dream images and waking concerns; and between childhood experiences and current difficulties;
b. *Insight*, evidenced by the capacity to experience oneself as much an agent as a victim; that is, the patient can recognize that he or she plays a role in his or her problems.
c. *Thoughtfulness*, evidenced by the capacity to consider and ponder rather than react impulsively;
d. *High-adaptive defensive levels*, such as anticipation, sublimation, suppression, repression as compared with disavowal (denial, projection) or image-distorting (projective identification, splitting) defences;
e. *Whole–object relationships*, as evidenced by a history of at least one meaningful childhood relationship, and one meaningful current relationship.

Specific to brief psychodynamic psychotherapy and differentiating it from long-term psychotherapy and psychoanalysis are two important criteria:

f. *The capacity to engage quickly*: Because brief psychodynamic psychotherapy is time-limited, it is primarily indicated for those patients who can quickly develop a therapeutic alliance. As a result, patients who have difficulty trusting, or fear loss of self–other boundaries, are not candidates for this modality. Thus, highly suspicious, paranoid patients, or schizoid patients, are usually excluded from brief psychodynamic psychotherapy because of their inability to easily develop a therapeutic alliance.

g. *The capacity to engage without difficulty*: Because brief psychodynamic psychotherapy is time-limited, it is primarily indicated for those patients who can work through termination issues with a minimum of difficulty. As a result, patients with profound dependency problems or significant separation–individuation concerns are usually excluded. Thus, patients with severe dependent personality disorders or those with borderline personality disorders do not do well in brief psychodynamic psychotherapy.

Although patients with this degree of ego strength are the optimal candidates for BPP, in some settings brief therapy has been applied to more difficult patients (Messer & Warren, 1995).

THE TIME LIMIT

The time limit is an essential and defining characteristic of brief psychodynamic psychotherapy. In some models (Malan, 1976; Sifneos, 1987; Davanloo, 1980), the patient is informed of the time limit in a generalized way by stating therapy will be less than a year. Others models use a specific, predetermined time limit. James Mann (1973) strictly adheres to a twelve-session time limit, communicating the date of the last session to the patient during the assessment period and prior to commencing therapy. Similarly, Lester Luborsky (1984) adheres to a sixteen-session time limit which is also communicated to the patient prior to beginning therapy. This time limit serves to promote the patient's motivation, stimulate a sense of appropriate optimism, minimize regression, and offset dependency (Mann & Goldman, 1982).

THE FOCUS

The identification of one, specific, particular, and pivotal circumscribed segment or focus through which small but critical changes result in significant shifts of functioning is the *sine qua non* of all brief psychotherapies. Various models use different terms to describe their focus: Mann

(1973) refers to the 'central issue,' which is a particular sense of chronic and enduring internal pain, with which the patient has constantly wrestled, despite having significant accomplishments in the external world. This 'chronically endured pain' usually reflects issues of self-esteem. Once it has been elicited during the evaluation period, the therapist might couch the central issue in these terms: 'As I listen to your story, it is clear how very successful you have been [such as, in your field, as a breadwinner, as a parent, as a caretaker] but, despite this, for some reason that is not yet clear, you have always had this nagging concern that you are a phony [that you are an impostor, that you have never made genuine contact with another, that no one recognizes difficulties with which you have contended, etc.]. And I think that you and I should meet over the next twelve sessions in order to understand more about why you continue to be plagued by this feeling of being a phony [an impostor, alone, unknown to others, etc.].'

Mann's orientation during therapy centres on the omnipresence of time, separation, and loss, as well as on issues of patient's experience of parental failure, rage, and disillusionment. His style is one of mirroring, empathic attunement, and gentle confrontation.

Luborsky (1984) focuses on the patient's 'Core Conflictual Relationship Theme' (CCRT). This term refers to the ongoing repetitive phenomenon in which the patient has a wish for a particular kind of relationship with the other (such as a wish to be treated respectfully, to have the opportunity of making his or her achievements known, to be assertive) but experiences a powerful transference-fear that, if he or she should act on that wish, the other would respond negatively (such as by neglecting, exploiting, abandoning, mocking) and so the patient responds by characteristically squelching his or her wish, and ends up feeling dissatisfied (unfulfilled, frustrated, silently angry, etc.). After the evaluation period, but before formal treatment begins, the therapist might present the patient's CCRT in the following way: 'From what we talked about, it seems to me that you want to be in a relationship where you can make your needs known, but you feel that, if you do that, others are going to see you as enormously selfish, so what you do instead is keep quiet, not say a thing, but end up feeling overlooked, resentful, and used.' Therapy focuses on identifying and working through the childhood experiences that fuel these transference-driven fears.

Strupp and Binder (1984) use the term 'cyclical maladaptive pattern' (CMP) to describe their focus. Like the Luborsky model, this, too, has a strong interpersonal perspective. It defines the repetitive, cyclical mal-adaptive relationships that are shaped by the manner in which the patient unconsciously presents him- or herself and unconsciously attempts to induce others to behave in ways that reinforce the patient's maladaptive style and negative self-image. The therapist's formulation speaks to the patient's repetitive patterns of relating, particularly to the patient's perception of self and others in their interactions (Messer & Warren, 1995; Barber & Crits-Christoph, 1991). It refers to the interpersonal roles in which the patient unconsciously casts him- or herself and others, and the maladaptive interactions that result. In many ways their model echoes Luborsky's in its concentration on expectations of others, observed reactions of others, and acts of the self towards the self. Treatment focuses on the manner in which the patient fears, or elicits, certain responses from others.

Weiss et al (1986) and Weiss (1990) focus on recurrent unconscious 'tests' with which the patient challenges the therapist. These tests are the ways in which the patient attempts to discover whether the therapist will respond as the patient's significant childhood caretakers did – disappointingly, frustratingly, or frighteningly. When the therapist does not respond in that manner, the patient then feels safe enough to expose more of him- or herself in therapy. As a result, more material enters the therapeutic arena, to be worked on, understood, and resolved.

Although the focus for each of these models is from a slightly different perspective, it is identified and discussed with the patient after the assessment period and prior to initiating therapy. Additionally, although the focus for each is from a slightly different vantage, all are consistent with the basic theoretical concepts outlined earlier and are identified, understood, worked through, and resolved in treatment by use of the supportive and expressive techniques earlier described. It is through small changes in this one pivotal area (the focus) that significant shifts in functioning occur (Høglend & Heyerdahl, 1994; Book, 1998).

THERAPIST ACTIVITY

The therapist's persistent focus on this pivotal circumscribed segment – such as the central issue or CCRT – is another *sine qua non* of brief psychodynamic psychotherapy. The therapist practising brief psychodynamic psychotherapy is far more active than when he or she is carrying out long-term psychotherapy. Being active and directive does not mean shifting from a position of empathic neutrality. Rather, it implies being active and directive in vigilantly maintaining with the patient a continual focus on the pivotal segment, and analysing or discouraging any digressions from that focus (MacKenzie, 1988). Maintaining therapeutic sight only on the focus is one of the major demands and challenges of BPP.

The therapist practising brief psychodynamic psychotherapy is also active in encouraging the patient to attempt new ways of relating (such as facing the phobic object) so that relationship difficulties will be highlighted for clarification and linkage to the pivotal focus.

Indications and Contraindications

As noted in the discussion of selection criteria, above, the greater the patient's ego strengths, the more likely BPP is indicated. Conversely, the weaker the patient's ego capacities, the less likely the patient will be to benefit from BPP. Thus, BPP is contraindicated for patients with impaired reality testing, such as, patients with Axis I diagnosis of psychosis. Similarly, BPP is usually contraindicated for patients with cluster-B personality disorders (antisocial, borderline, narcissistic) because of compromised ego strengths as reflected in their low frustration tolerance, impulsivity, difficulty in modulating affects, and reliance on ego-distorting defences. It is also contraindicated for patients with cluster-A personality disorders (paranoid, schizoid, schizotypal), who also evidence impaired reality testing and permeable self–other ego boundaries.

Generally speaking, patients who benefit from brief psychodynamic psychotherapy are quite similar to those patient who benefit from long-term psychotherapy or psychoanalysis. Because of their ego strengths, patients in these groups have the ego capacities to make use and take advantage of the rigours of treatment. BPP is thus indicated in generalized anxiety disorders (Durham et al, 1984), depressive disorders, both acute and chronic (Luborsky, Diguer, & Cacciola, 1996), phobias, post-traumatic stress disorders, and pathological grief (Crits-Christoph, 1992). It is also indicated for cluster-C personality disorders (such as dependent or obsessional), and some cluster-B disorders (such as histrionic personality disorders).

If patients who benefit from BPP are similar to those who benefit from long-term psychotherapy, when is long-term psychotherapy rather than

BPP indicated? The answer again reflects subtle but meaningful shifts, permeabilities, and weaknesses in ego strengths. The more there exists a history of impulsivity, inability to tolerate aloneness, the use of low-level defences such as projection and denial, problems with whole–object representation, the less the patient can make use of brief psycho-dynamic psychotherapy, and the more the patient requires a longer-term approach. One other grouping for which longer-term therapy is indi-cated is patients who wish a pervasive shift in character structure, rather than focal (albeit significant) changes (Book, 1998).

There are realistic concerns about brief therapy in a managed-care environment. Because profitability is a major concern, there is always the risk that clinicians may be pressured to utilize brief therapy inappro-priately (Book, 1991). Brief therapy is not equivalent to long-term ther-apy and is not the treatment of choice for many patients.

In contrast, health care systems which allow unlimited psychother-apy, as is currently the case in Canada, pose other challenges for brief therapy. Therapists and patients may both be tempted to collude with unconscious resistances to termination where there are no external con-straints.

Occasionally it is necessary to abort a time-limited therapy with a par-ticular patient and move to an open-ended approach. Some patients will become more symptomatic during the course of brief therapy. Although such patients can be advised to see how they manage post-termination, bearing in mind that the process of therapy continues after termination (Horowitz, 1976), occasionally the degree of symptomatic distress may warrant continued therapy. It is important for the therapist to differenti-ate when the option of continued therapy is clinically warranted from those other more frequent times when it is a reflection of the patient's resistance to termination or the therapist's countertransference prob-lems with termination.

Where the time limit has been specified, as with the Mann (1973) twelve-session or the Luborsky (1984) sixteen-session approach, the time limit may also be waived during emergency or crisis situations. For example, if a spouse or child unexpectedly dies, the patient would remain in therapy without 'counting' these sessions, until the crisis has been dealt with and the patient has returned to his or her pre-crisis level of functioning (Book, 1998).

Some patients, pleased with the outcome of brief psychotherapy and the focal change that has been achieved, are interested in embarking on longer-term psychotherapy in order to achieve wider character changes.

It is generally advisable to encourage the patient to take a break of a few months before embarking on a longer therapy.

Technique

Technique is discussed here in terms of assessment, treatment, and follow-up processes.

ASSESSMENT

During the assessment process, the therapist:

1 carries out a history and mental-status evaluation, makes a diagnosis, and utilizes selection criteria to assess whether the patient would benefit optimally from brief psychodynamic psychotherapy;
2 develops a circumscribed focus according to his or her theoretical model, communicates this focus to the patient, and connects it to the patient's presenting symptom;
3 assesses the patient's response to this focus as being primary and meaningful;
4 communicates to the patient that this will be the focus of treatment and obtains the patient's agreement that this is a significant and relevant focus. If the patient does not agree with the focus, the therapist explores with the patient what seems to be a more accurate focus and/or rethinks his or her focal formulation;
5 discusses the frame of therapy. Specifically important is the time limit – be it general ('fewer than fifty sessions') or specified (such as Mann's twelve-session time-limit or Luborsky's sixteen-session time-limit). Discussion of the frame of therapy also involves clarifying meeting times, length of sessions, emergency contacts, billing, missed appointments, and provision for further therapy;
6 discusses the patient's 'job description' in psychotherapy: the patient should attempt to say whatever comes to mind, regardless of whether it seems foolish, irrelevant, or embarrassing; the patient should attempt to bring up any major decisions – such as getting married, getting divorced, quitting therapy – before embarking on them;
7 discusses his or her (the therapist's) 'job description': listening, commenting on themes, communicating to the patient the patient's themes as they inform and illuminate the focus, and interpreting how this focus developed through early childhood experiences.

TREATMENT

As in long-term psychotherapy, treatment is brought about by the therapist's using both supportive and expressive techniques or activities (Luborsky, 1984). The ultimate goal is to allow the patient to feel secure enough in the psychotherapeutic relationship to allow previously repressed conflictual material to emerge into consciousness and be expressed. Change and resolution occur in working through this material and are promoted by the therapist's empathic, clarifying, confronting, and interpretive activities. The difference between brief and long-term psychotherapy is that, in the former, all of these expressive activities occur on the one pivotal circumscribed area that constitutes the focus for that patient.

1 *Supportive techniques*: The activities are carried out by the therapist to allow the patient to feel secure and safe enough in the relationship to tolerate the expressive techniques of the treatment (Luborsky, 1984). Supportive activities include: empathic comments; appropriate hopefulness and reassurance; supporting vital defences; maintaining appropriate self–object transferences; appropriate limit-setting; and noting gains. Luborsky (1984) recommends a number of activities to facilitate the 'helping alliance':

1 Convey through words and manner support for the patient's wish to achieve the goals.
2 Convey a sense of understanding and acceptance of the patient.
3 Develop a liking for the patient.
4 Help the patient maintain vital defenses and activities which bolster the level of functioning.
5 Communicate a realistically hopeful attitude that the treatment goals are likely to be achieved.
6 Recognition, on appropriate occasions that the patient has made some progress toward the goals.
7 Encourage a 'we bond.'
8 Convey respect for the patient.
9 Convey recognition of the patient's growing ability to do what the therapist does in using the basic tools of the treatment. (pp. 82–89)

2 *Expressive techniques*: The therapist also carries out activities whose goal is to encourage the patient to express previously repressed, dis-

avowed, conflictual material in the safety of the therapeutic alliance. According to Luborsky (1984), there are four phases of the therapist's expressive task: listening, understanding, responding, and returning to listening. When responding, the therapist's activity includes empathic comments, confrontation, clarification, and interpretation, the functions of which are to increase the patient's narrative flow and aid him or her in understanding and resolving the unconscious conflicts and/or defects that are fundamental to his or her circumscribed difficulties.

The expressive activities are brought to bear only on the focus chosen by the therapist and agreed to by the patient. Other non-focus material is avoided. Brief psychodynamic psychotherapy is carried out on the focal issue only, with the goal of 'working through' this segment. This focal conflict is illuminated and resolved by expressive techniques as it repetitively emerges in descriptions of past and current relationships, and as it is enacted in the transference.

In brief psychotherapy, termination is always kept in mind, and is actively focused on in the last third of treatment. This offers yet another opportunity of reworking the focus as it re-emerges through termination issues, for the focus always colours the patient's experience of stopping treatment.

3 *Post-treatment follow-up*: Many brief psychotherapists offer a follow-up, at two, three, or six months. This may be communicated to the patient in the last session, or not communicated but triggered by the therapist at the two-month period. The follow-up has two functions: to provide a transitional phenomenon, or 'booster shot,' in order to offset unresolved termination issues, and as a follow-up evaluation.

Scientific Basis and Efficacy

Brief psychodynamic psychotherapy has been extensively studied scientifically. The research has demonstrated that BPP is an effective treatment. Because of its shorter time limits, BPP has also proved to be a useful tool for research on the core clinical concepts of psychoanalytic psychotherapy (see chapter 4, 'Empirical Evidence for the Core Clinical Concepts and Efficacy of the Psychoanalytic Psychotherapies: An Overview').

Piper et al (1990) compared patients randomly assigned to treatment with brief psychodynamic psychotherapy for an average of nineteen sessions with those on a waiting list. Patients receiving BPP had statistically significant increases in their quality of object-relations as measured by an object-relations assessor. The treatment effect was maintained at the five-month follow-up.

Winston et al (1991) compared patients randomly assigned to once-a-week brief psychodynamic psychotherapy for a maximum of forty sessions with a waiting-list control group. Patients receiving psychotherapy showed significant improvement on target complaints and on the SCL-90 Social Adjustment Scale.

In their study on the efficacy of psychotherapy for the treatment of depression in the elderly, Thompson et al (1987) compared elderly patients with major depressive disorder treated for sixteen to twenty sessions in brief psychotherapy with a control group assigned to a six-week delayed treatment in control conditions. Patients in the treatment conditions showed statistically significant improvements on a number of measures, whereas controls did not.

Acknowledging that the research literature consistently supports the superiority of active psychotherapies with respect to no treatment or placebo controls, Carroll, Rounsaville, and Gawin (1991) studied the effectiveness of two brief psychotherapies in cocaine abusers. Patients received either individual weekly relapse prevention therapy (RPT) or weekly interpersonal psychotherapy (IPT). Patients in both treatment groups did better than patients in other reported studies who received either no treatment or placebo treatment. Among a subgroup of more severe users, subjects who received RPT were significantly more likely to achieve abstinence, and be classified as recovered, compared with subjects receiving IPT.

DiMascio et al (1979) compared patients diagnosed with acute non-bipolar, non-psychotic depression along three treatment dimensions. Patients were assigned to one of four treatment groups: the antidepressant amitriptyline alone; individual interpersonal psychotherapy alone; combined amitriptyline and individual interpersonal psychotherapy; and no active treatment. Psychotherapy and amitriptyline were both effective in reducing overall symptoms compared with the outcome in the control group. Amitriptyline and psychotherapy were approximately equal, and the effects of both treatments in combination were additive, compared with the control group.

In a study of adults suffering from post-traumatic stress disorder, Brom et al (1989) compared outcomes of three forms of psychotherapy (trauma desensitization, hypnotherapy, and brief psychodynamic psychotherapy) with those in a control (non-treatment) group. Clinically significant improvements were observed in 60 per cent of the treated patients but in fewer than 30 per cent of those untreated. Within the subgroup treated by short-term psychotherapy, there was evidence for some changes in personality characteristics, in addition to changes in symptomatology.

In his meta-analysis of eleven studies on brief psychodynamic psychotherapy compared with a controlled group, Crits-Christoph (1992) concluded that the average patient receiving brief dynamic therapy was better off, in terms of target symptoms, than 86 per cent of the waiting-list patients. Concerning general symptoms, the average patient receiving brief dynamic therapy was better off than 79 per cent of the waiting-list patients, and concerning social adjustment, the comparative figure was 79 per cent. The largest noticeable effect among patients treated by a brief psychodynamic psychotherapy, compared with patients receiving other treatments, was for target symptoms. Patients in the brief dynamic treatment group attained goals better than 62 per cent of the comparison group. Crits-Christoph notes that the superiority of brief dynamic psychotherapy over other treatments was not consistently shown. However, many of the outcome measures are not directed or sensitive enough to capture subtle but significant shifts attained by patients in brief psychodynamic psychotherapy. Measures addressing dynamic conflicts, transference themes, relationship patterns, and defensive styles have not yet been fully adapted to efficacy studies. He also refers to the study reported by Howard et al (1986) on the importance of the effective 'dose' of psychotherapy, that is, the relative length of treatment required to target symptomatic versus characterological issues.

In their comparative study of models of BPP, Messer and Warren (1995) review the research on the effectiveness of BPP. Among their conclusions, they claim that time-limited therapy is often as helpful as time-unlimited therapy and that its effects can be long-lasting. There is no evidence for the superiority of one form of brief therapy over another. Depressed and anxious patients improve faster than those diagnosed as borderline. Symptoms improve sooner than characterological features.

Other studies have linked outcome to such patient variables as a highly circumscribed conflict (Høglend & Heyerdahl, 1994) to the process in psychotherapy (Luborsky & Crits-Christoph, 1990), and to the helping (therapeutic) alliance (Luborsky, Crits-Christoph, Mintz, & Auerbach, 1988).

Training

A recent survey of American psychologists demonstrated that 40 per cent of respondents spent a considerable portion of their clinical time doing brief psychotherapy. Despite this, one-third of those currently doing brief therapy had little or no training in theory or technique (Levenson, Speed, & Budman, 1995). Although there is no comparable survey of psychiatrists, it is unlikely that the situation is different. Practising BPP is not the same as practising long-term therapy with a time limit. Competent practice of BPP requires both knowledge of theory and specific training.

POSTGRADUATE TRAINING

The following recommendations, proposed by the Brief Psychotherapy Committee of the Department of Psychiatry, Faculty of Medicine, University of Toronto, are given as an example of optimal standards for training in BPP.

1. *Attitude:* Training should promote an attitude that aids trainees in understanding the resistances and mythologies about BPP, and aids them in considering BPP as an increasingly important, first-line therapeutic modality that is efficacious, efficient, and accessible.
2. *Knowledge:* Trainees should study key papers on: common misperceptions of and biases against BPP (Hoyt, 1985a, 1985b); its history; similarities and differences among various dynamic psychotherapies; selection criteria; developing a focus; maintaining the focus; transference and countertransference issues; and termination.

   Additionally, trainees should study one general overview text on BPP and one manual-based text on BPP. Trainees should also be involved in a clinically based seminar on BPP that emphasizes both theoretical and clinical components.

   All teaching should be carried out by credentialled experienced brief psychotherapists with advanced degrees in their discipline.
3. *Skills:* Residents in Psychiatry and PhD candidates should treat in total four patients in weekly brief psychodynamic psychotherapy for which they receive weekly supervision. The supervision should be carried out by credentialled, experienced, brief psychotherapists with advanced degrees in their discipline.

   An objective evaluation form should be used to assess trainees, monitor their progress, and identify and address those trainees with ongoing substandard functioning in learning brief psychodynamic psychotherapy.

CONTINUING EDUCATION (CE)

Practitioners of BPP should have opportunities to update their knowledge and skills in BPP by attending appropriate CE courses, conferences, workshops, and academies. These could be affiliated with universities, hospitals, training programs, and annual discipline meetings (American Psychiatric Association, American Psychological Association, etc.). Similarly, psychotherapists without formal training in BPP should have an opportunity to attain knowledge and skills in the practice of BPP through CE programs associated with universities, hospitals, training programs, and annual discipline meetings (American Psychiatric Association, American Psychological Association) as well as with credentialled, reputable, free-standing programs.

For those who have limited access to such conferences, a cadre of credentialled, experienced brief-psychotherapist supervisors should be available for ongoing telephone supervision.

Credentialling

Leaving aside the question of which body should have the authority to credential, in principle criteria and standards should be developed that define the minimum education and training requirements necessary to define competence in the practice of brief psychodynamic psychotherapy. As well, standards should also be developed to define minimum attendance at continuing-education activities necessary to maintain competence in the practice of brief psychodynamic psychotherapy.

References

Anderson, E.M., & Lambert, M.J. (1995). Short-term dynamically-oriented psychotherapy: A review and meta-analysis. *Clinical Psychology Review, 15,* 503–514.

Barber, J.P., & Crits-Christoph, P. (1991). Comparison of the brief dynamic therapies. In P. Crits-Christoph & J.P. Barber (Eds.), *Handbook of short-term dynamic psychotherapy,* New York: Basic.

Bauer, G.P., & Kobos, J.C. (1987). *Brief therapy: Short-term psychodynamic interven-tion*. Northvale, NJ: Jason Aronson.

Bellak, L., & Small, L. (1978). *Emergency psychotherapy and brief psychotherapy* (2d ed.). New York: Grune & Stratton.

Berg, I. (1990). *Solution-focused approach to family-based services*. Milwaukee: Brief Family Therapy Center.

Bongar, B., Beutler, L.E. (1995). *Comprehensive textbook of psychotherapy: Theory and practice*. New York: Oxford University Press

Book, H.E. (1991). Is empathy cost efficient? *American Journal of Psychotherapy, 45*, 21–30.

Book, H.E. (1998). *How to practice brief psychodynamic Psychotherapy: The CCRT method*. Washington, DC: American Psychological Association.

Brom, D., Kleber, R.J., & Defares, P.B. (1989). Brief psychotherapy for post-traumatic stress disorders. *Journal of Consulting and Clinical Psychology, 57*, 607–612.

Budman, S.H. (Ed.). (1981). *Forms of brief therapy*. New York: Guilford.

Caplan, G. (1964). *Principles of preventive psychiatry*. New York: Basic.

Carroll, K.M., Rounsaville, B.J., & Gawin, F.H. (1991). A comparative trial of psychotherapies for ambulatory cocaine abusers: Relapse prevention and interpersonal psychotherapy. *American Journal of Drug and Alcohol Abuse, 17*, 229–247.

Crits-Christoph, P. (1992). The efficacy of brief dynamic psychothetapy: A meta-analysis. *American Journal of Psychiatry, 149*, 151–158.

Davanloo, H . (Ed.). (1980). *Basic principles and techniques in short-term dynamic psychotherapy*. New York: Spectrum.

deShazer, S. (1985). *Keys to solution in brief therapy*. New York: Norton.

DiMascio, A., Weissman, M.M., Prusoff, B.A., Neu, C., Zwilling, M., & Klerman, G.L. (1979). Differential symptom reduction by drugs and psychotherapy in acute depression. *Archives of General Psychiatry, 36*, 1450–1456.

Durham, R.C., Murphy, T., Allan, T., Richard, K., Treliving, L.R., & Fenton, G.W. (1994). Cognitive therapy, analytic psychotherapy and anxiety management training for generalized anxiety disorder. *British Journal of Psychiatry, 165*, 315–323.

Garfield, S.L. (1989). *The practice of brief therapy*. New York: Pergamon.

Greenberg, J.R., & Mitchell, S.A. (1983). *Object relations in psychoanalytic theory*. Cambridge, MA: Harvard University Press.

Gustafson, J.P. (1986). *The complex theory of brief psychotherapy*. New York: Norton.

Hirschfeld, R.M.A., & Shea, M.T. (1989). Mood disorders: Psychosocial treat-ments. In H.I. Kaplan & B.J. Sadock (Eds.), *Comprehensive textbook of psychiatry/ V*. Baltimore: Williams & Wilkins.

Høglend, P., & Heyerdahl, O. (1994). The circumscribed focus in intensive brief dynamic psychotherapy. *Psychotherapy and Psychosomatics, 61,* 163–170.

Horowitz, M.J. (1976). *Stress response syndromes.* New York: Jason Aronson.

Horowitz, M., Marmar, C., Krupnick, J., Wilner, N., Kaltreider, N., & Wallerstein, T. (1984). *Personality styles and brief psychotherapy.* New York: Basic.

Howard, K.I., Kopta, S.M., Krause, M.S., & Orlinsky, D. (1986). The dose–effect relationship in psychotherapy. American Psychologist, 41, 159–164.

Hoyt, M.F. (1985a). *Brief therapy and managed care* (pp. 219–235). San Francisco: Jossey-Bass.

Hoyt, M.F. (1985b). Therapist resistances to short-term dynamic psychotherapy. *Journal of the American Academy of Psychoanalysis, 13,* 93–112.

Jacobson, G.F. (1979). Crisis-oriented therapy. *Psychiatric Clinics of North America,* 3, 39–54.

Levenson, H., Speed, J., & Budman, S.H. (1995). Therapist's experience, training, and skill in brief therapy: A bicoastal survey. *American Journal of Psychotherapy, 49,* 95–117.

Luborsky, L. (1984). *Principles of psychoanalytic psychotherapy: A manual for supportive–expressive treatment.* New York: Basic.

Luborsky, L., & Crits-Cristoph, P. (1990). *Understanding transference: The CCRT method.* New York: Basic.

Luborsky, L., Crits-Christoph, P., Mintz, J., & Auerbach, A. (1988). *Who will benefit from psychotherapy? Predicting therapeutic outcomes.* New York: Basic.

Luborsky, L., Diguer, L., & Cacciola, J. (1996). Factors in outcomes of short-term dynamic psychotherapy for chronic vs. nonchronic major depression. *Journal of Psychotherapy, Practice, and Research, 5,* 152–159.

Luborsky L., Singer, B. & Luborsky, L. (1975). Comparative studies of psycho-therapies: Is it true that 'everyone has won and all must have prizes'? *Archives of General Psychiatry, 32,* 995–1008.

MacKenzie, K.R. (1988). Recent developments in brief psychotherapy. *Hospital and Community Psychiatry, 39,* 742–752.

Malan, D.H. (1976). *The frontier of brief psychotherapy.* New York: Plenum.

Mann, J. (1973).*Time-limited psychotherapy.* Cambridge, MA: Harvard University Press.

Mann, J., & Goldman, R. (1982). *A casebook in time-limited psychotherapy.* Washington, DC: American Psychiatric Association Press.

Marmor J. (1979). Short-term dynamic psychotherapy. *American Journal of Psychiatry, 136,* 149–155.

Messer, S.B., & Warren, C.S. (1995). *Models of brief psychodynamic therapy: A comparative approach.* New York: Guilford.

Olfson, M., & Pincus, H.A. (1994) Outpaitent psychotherapy in the United States, II: Patterns of utilization. *American Journal of Psychiatry, 151*, 1289–1294.

Piper, W.E., Azim, H.F., McCallum, M., & Joyce, A.S. (1990). Patient suitability and outcome in short-term individual psychotherapy. *Journal of Consulting and Clinical Psychology, 58*, 475–481.

Shefler, G., Dasberg, H., & Ben-Shakhar, G. (1995). A randomized controlled outcome and follow-up study of Mann's time-limited psychotherapy. *Journal of Consulting and Clinical Psychology, 63*, 585–593.

Sifneos, P.E. (1987). *Short-term dynamic psychotherapy: Evaluation and technique* (2d ed.). New York: Plenum.

Strupp, H.H., & Binder, J.L. (1984) *Psychotherapy in a new key: A guide to time-limited dynamic psychotherapy.* New York: Basic.

Talmon, M. (1990). *Single session therapy.* San Francisco: Jossey-Bass.

Thompson, L.W., Gallager, D., & Breckenridge, J.S. (1987). Comparative effectiveness of psychotherapies for depressed elders. *Journal of Consulting and Clinical Psychology, 55*, 385–390.

Walter, J.L., & Peller, J.E. (1992). *Becoming solution-focused in brief therapy.* New York: Brunner/Mazel.

Weiss, J. (1990) Unconscious mental functioning. *Scientific American, 262*, 103–109.

Weiss, J., Sampson, H., & the Mount Zion Psychotherapy Research Group. (1986).*The psychoanalytic process: Theory, clinical observation and empirical research.* New York: Guilford.

Weissman, M.M., & Markowitz, J.C.(1994). Interpersonal psychotherapy. *Archives of General Psychiatry, 51*, 599–606.

Winston, A., Laikin, M., Pollack, J., Samstag, L.W., McCullough, L., & Murran, J.C. (1994). Short-term psychotherapy of personality disorders. *American Journal of Psychiatry, 151*, 190–194.

Winston, A., Pollack, J., McCullough, L., Flegenheimer, W., Kestenbaum, R., & Trujillo, M. (1991). Brief dynamic psychotherapy of personality disorders. *Journal of Nervous and Mental Disease, 179*, 188–193.

7. Guidelines for the Practice of Couple and Family Psychotherapy

Leopoldo Chagoya and Paul Cameron

Couple and family psychotherapy are interventions with two partners, with the nuclear family, or with the extended family. These interventions include therapy models based on different theories. Although couple and family therapy share features and require similar guidelines, differences are significant enough to base this chapter on *Handbook of Psychotherapy and Behavior Change* (Bergin & Garfield, 1994), and discuss them separately.

Couple Therapy

Physicians are frequently consulted by patients who seek help because of relational problems with their partners. The usual medical training provides little preparation for doctors facing these difficulties. Most practitioners use common sense and good intentions to help, but remain unacquainted with the published wealth of theories, techniques, and research on couple therapy (Jacobson & Addis, 1993).

Jacobson and Gurman (1995) describe three trends in the current practice of couple and family therapy: Increased credibility of marital and family therapists; increased utilization of these therapies within psychiatry; and a good fit of these forms of therapy within managed care. They also report significant advances in conceptualization and empirical data regarding efficacy.

Dr L. Chagoya acknowledges the suggestions of C. Chagoya, RN, FTh, in the writing of this chapter.

MODELS OF COUPLE THERAPY

Jacobson and Gurman (1995) list nine models of couple therapy:

1 Bowenian
2 Behavioural (integrative)
3 Cognitive
4 Ego-analytic
5 Emotion-focused
6 Problem- and solution-focused
7 Psychoanalytic
8 Group (of couples)
9 Relationship enhancement

THEORETICAL CONCEPTS

Most models of couple-therapy use systems theory and communication theory. Dyadic interaction is viewed as striving to maintain homeostasis (Constadine, 1986); couples, therefore, resist changes in the patterns they have established. According to communication theory (Watzlawick, Beavin, & Jackson, 1967), the quality of verbal and non-verbal messages between the partners is the origin of dysfunction, and therefore the focus of intervention. In addition, the different models of couple therapy recommend interventions based on their theory. For example, psychoanalytic and ego-analytic models focus on conflict and factors from early life; behavioural and cognitive therapies focus on maladaptive learned patterns; and emotion-focused therapy emphasizes the role of affect. Therapists' choice of treatment models depends on the training opportunities available at the university or agency where the therapist acquired his or her skills. A detailed description of all of the theoretical concepts and technical interventions is beyond the scope of this book, and not necessary to develop basic guidelines for the practice of couple therapy.

Jacobson and Gurman (1995) suggest that couple therapists of all schools have recognized the importance of therapist–patient interaction, therapeutic alliance, and a 'person-to-person connection' as a central therapeutic mechanism.

ASSESSMENT AND SELECTION OF COUPLES FOR THERAPY

Both members of the couple should be assessed thoroughly to determine whether either is suffering from a major psychiatric disorder. Also, the areas of conflict and dysfunction within the couple must be identified. Sager, Slindick, Kremer, Lenz, and Royce (1968) state that 50 per cent of patients seeking psychotherapy do so largely because of problems in their primary relationship. A major task in the assessment phase involves determining how motivated each member of the couple is to improve the relationship (Rosenbluth & Cameron, 1981). When both are motivated, conjoint therapy can be extremely effective. However, as Cameron (1987) states, it may be necessary to combine individual therapy with conjoint therapy if there is significant ambivalence or pathology in one member of the couple. As with individual therapies, a therapeutic alliance must be established with both.

In order to complete the biopsychosocial formulation of any patient, it is useful to interview the partner, either alone or with the labelled patient. Although this assessment may not lead to couple therapy, it facilitates the selection of the most appropriate intervention.

INDICATIONS FOR COUPLE THERAPY

1 *Interactional difficulties in the relationship with a partner* as the primary complaint of an individual: These difficulties may include: problems of commitment; autonomy; attachment; fairness and trust; sexuality; communication; the unconscious matrix of the relationship, its wider relational context, and its vitality (Karpel, 1994).
2 *Developmental crises:* Turning-points in a couple's history may precipitate referral. Typical crises include: separating from the family of origin; negotiating a division of labour; accommodating to the birth of the first child; problems involving parenting; redefining the structure of the relationship when children are in crisis or ill; handling management of the adolescent progeny; and redefining the relationship when the children leave home.
3 *Loss of the original bond or the original life project of the couple:* Common precursors and stressors leading to couple therapy include: career changes in one or both members of the couple, relocation; unemployment; infidelity and disclosure of the affair; and one member of the couple developing an interest that excludes the other.
4 *Psychiatric illness in one member of the couple:* Stress and conflict arise when one member of a couple develops psychiatric symptoms. It is often difficult for partners to understand the nature of depression or organic illness affecting the brain or to cope with a partner suffering from anxiety or psychosis.

5 *Medical illness in one member of the couple:* This can also cause stress and conflict in the couple. Infertility can often pose a significant stress.
6 *One partner adopting a non-traditional life pattern:* For instance, if a partner reveals a bisexual or homosexual lifestyle and the other does not share these preferences (Buxton, 1991), couple therapy may of help.
7 *Conflict about having children:* When one member of the couple is more eager to procreate than the other, severe conflicts and irreconcilable positions may result. Also, technological advances in the treatment of infertility, such as artificial insemination and *in vitro* fertilization, may induce significant stress that may require therapy.

CONTRAINDICATIONS FOR COUPLE THERAPY

1 Couple therapy can lead to a deterioration of function. Certain dynamic patterns may be inflamed through conjoint sessions: for instance, *couples with a severe sadomasochistic pattern of behaviour* or a history of *antisocial personality* with acting out and violence, in one or both partners. In both cases, couple therapy could provoke an increase in rageful behavior.
2 When the *primary motivation for treatment is to seek financial compensation,* or to use the therapist's opinion to settle a legal problem not disclosed at the assessment.
3 Couples with *rigid culture-bound patterns:* In some cultures, the role of each spouse is rigidly defined. When these predetermined values in each spouse clash, the therapist's attempts at establishing equal rights for both alienates at least one of them, and therapy becomes impossible.
4 When one of the partners is *so disabled by psychological or physical illness that he or she is unable to participate constructively in the sessions,* abreactive or expressive therapy be damaging to the weakened partner.
5 *Couples who arouse intense negative countertransference:* For instance, when a couple involves the therapist in murky triangles of secrecy or overwhelms him or her to the point where the therapist feels unable to handle the conflicts and cannot imagine progress or resolution (Karpel, 1994).
6 *Intense and persistent negative or uncomfortable feelings towards the therapist in one or both partners:* When this happens, the lack of a therapeutic alliance makes it necessary to stop the therapy and refer the couple to someone else.

7 *Inability of one partner to examine his or her contribution to the conflicts:* Therapy cannot be effective if a partner is non-committal towards the relationship or to therapy.

8 *The threat of physical violence without legal deterrents* (towards the therapist or towards the spouse): For instance, when the victim of violence refuses to involve the police or press charges against the abuser, it is counterproductive to discuss violence while it continues to occur.

9 *Trust is persistently low or non-existent between the partners* or when there are no positive feelings left in the couple.

PRACTICE GUIDELINES FOR COUPLE THERAPY

All guidelines outlined in Chapter 2, 'General Guidelines for the Practice of Psychotherapy' and in other chapters apply to couple therapy.

Protecting the Boundaries of the Therapeutic Relationship in Couple Therapy

Couple therapists should not have a social relationship with the couple. Although it is possible to treat health professionals who are colleagues, it is advisable that the therapist have only superficial and infrequent extratherapeutic contact with such colleagues. Therapists should avoid playing multiple roles with the patient. Practice in small communities may require some compromise. Even so, with couples known to the therapist, the treatment may be problematic, and require consultation if there is no progress. To avoid conflicts of interest, the therapist must not treat friends, relatives, or business associates. Any previous privileged alliance with one of the partners will complicate couple therapy.

Any sexual entanglement of the therapist with one member of a couple or with both constitutes an extremely serious breach of ethics. Therapy cannot continue under such circumstances.

Maintaining Confidentiality

Before treatment begins, the clinician may warn both partners that privileged confidentiality between him/her and *one* of the partners is incompatible with a constructive process of couple therapy (Scharff, 1978; Karpel, 1980). The therapist must inform each spouse of any individual contact one of the partners makes with him or her. If the secretive partner insists on keeping that contact, or the material therein revealed, confidential, the couple's therapy cannot proceed as of that moment. The therapist has no right to disclose a secret against the wishes of one of the partners. However, if the therapist were to continue the treatment while being the recipient of information he or she cannot discuss, the therapist would become the accomplice of one of the partners' deceit and betray the trust of the other. She or he would be conducting a pseudo-treatment which the secretive partner may detonate at any moment.

In some cases, the couple's therapist may recommend alternating sessions with the couple and sessions with one of the partners alone. Before such a combination is implemented, the three members of the therapeutic process (the therapist and the two partners) must decide conjointly how to handle issues of confidentiality. As a general guideline, it is important for the therapist to preserve the freedom to use his or her clinical judgment about when to discuss material from an individual session in a couple session. The therapist should be aware of the legal danger posed (a charge of breach of confidentiality) by introducing in the couple's session, without previous authorization, a subject one of the partners wishes to keep secret.

Therapeutic Sensitivity

Since sexual matters are frequently part of the material couples in therapy discuss, at all times the therapist must show a scrupulous respect towards both partners and use language the couple will not find offensive. Treatment may require candid openness about sexual practices. The therapist therefore will be well advised to keep verifying both partners' level of comfort with the discussion. Humour may be used, but tact can stem only from the therapist's empathy towards both individuals.

The couple therapist should be aware of how money matters, unequal income, unemployment of one partner, career competition, cultural values, and gender issues influence couple distress and his or her countertransference towards the couple. The triangular situation may revive in him or her conflicts with his or her own parents or spouse (Frelick & Waring, 1987). The therapist should be able to empathize genuinely with both partners, be they heterosexual, homosexual, or bisexual. The therapist's own values, culture and marital situation unavoidably influence his or her stance (Fine & Turner, 1991). Nevertheless, the more the therapist knows about his or her prejudices and blind spots, the more effective she or he will be.

Protecting the Patient's Safety

In cases of sexual or physical abuse, the therapist must ensure that safety measures are in place so the victim is in less danger. It is impossible to calmly practice confidential couple therapy when one partner, or the therapist, fears the sessions will unchain violence. As in general psychiatric practice, the help of the police, of women's shelters, or of other social agencies may have to be sought.

Facilitating Separation

Couple psychotherapy is not designed to keep two persons together at all costs. When love has died (Kayser, 1993), when one of the partners has become attached to someone else (Pittman, 1989) or has unilaterally decided to leave the relationship, or when the couple cannot rekindle the respect, trust, and goodwill they once shared, the therapist may help the two patients separate. The objectives of therapy are then to control the pain, avert potential emotional violence, and minimize the unavoidable hurt both partners will inflict on each other and on their children (if any). In such cases, it may be part of the therapist's work to refer the couple to a mediator or to recommend they seek legal advice in a non-adversarial process, if possible.

When separation is contemplated, the countertransferential prejudices of therapists have to be kept in scrupulous check. The therapist may have gone through a divorce him- or herself or be in the process of one. If she or he is not self-observant and self-critical, his or her own suffering inevitably affects the way he or she conducts divorce or separation therapy (Wallerstein, 1990). When the couple is uncertain about whether to dismantle their relationship or to attempt to reconstruct it, the patience of the therapist is of prime importance; if she or he cannot tolerate the patient's ambivalence for as long as necessary, he or she may impose premature closure on a process that required longer elaboration. Should the wish of the couple to separate arise in treatment, the therapist may help facilitate the redefinition of the therapy with a minimum of destructive communication or behaviour.

Maintaining Awareness of Medical and Psychiatric Disorders

The couple therapist must keep in mind his or her medical training and identify when an individual's medical, neurological, or psychiatric condition affects the couple's interaction. The physician may then prescribe pharmacological agents, or recommend a consultation with another specialist. It is essential to avoid the pitfall of treating individual disorders (such as adult attention deficit disorder) as if they were only psychological reactions to couple stress.

EFFICACY AND OUTCOME RESEARCH

A good outcome in couple therapy is defined as a lessening of relational conflict and distress, and a redefinition of ways to resolve conflicts. Alternatively, another positive outcome is the realization that the relationship is unworkable and both partners' well-being can be achieved only through separation or divorce.

In a critical review of couple-therapy outcome research, Wesley and Waring (1996) concluded that none of four approaches (behavioural, cognitive, emotion-focused, and insight-oriented) proved to be superior over the others. These authors propose a standard for efficacy studies in which a positive outcome for a form of couple therapy would produce subjective and objective improvement in 50 per cent of eligible couples, and this improvement would be maintained for one year. They argue that a waiting-list control group is not appropriate for ethical reasons. Furthermore, they suggest that no marital-therapy outcome study has included enough couples (sixty-three per treatment group) to offer a suitable standard for determining an effect size.

Waring and Patton (1984) reported that depressed women can be helped with marital therapy, and that those who rate intimacy in their marriage as low remain more depressed compared with women who rate intimacy in their marriage as high.

Alexander, Holtzworth-Monroe, and Jameson (1994) reviewed outcome research in couple therapy through its impact on symptoms and couple satisfaction. Studies included self-report of couples and observational scales. Improvement rates varied from 50 per cent to 83 per cent. The most effective modalities of couple therapy included behavioural, cognitive, insight-oriented, and communicational training methods. No approach provided an advantage in terms of effectiveness. Change occurred when couples experienced, not merely understood, the self and the other as different, and fundamentally redefined their relationship in terms of experienced accessibility and responsiveness to each other.

Alexander et al (1994) report also that most couples who accept marital-therapy interventions show more improvement than the controls. Snyder and Wills (1989) compared behaviour-management marital therapy, insight-oriented marital therapy, and a wait-list control group. Both treatment groups produced positive changes at termination, and the effects were maintained at the six-month follow-up. At the four-year follow-up, however, 38 per cent of couples who had received behavioural-management therapy had divorced and had a higher rate of deterioration after improving, compared with those who had had insight-oriented marital therapy, who had a divorce rate of 3 per cent. Johnson and Greenberg (1985), in a study of forty-five couples, reported significant improvement in couples receiving emotion-focused treatment at the two-month follow-up, compared with couples treated with a problem-solving approach, and a wait-list control group.

In their meta-analysis of behavioural marital therapy, Hahlweg and Markman (1988) examined seventeen studies of behavioural marital therapy (613 couples). The average effect size of those receiving behavioural marital therapy versus the control or placebo control group was 0.95. According to Alexander et al (1994), this means that 'the average person who had received behavioural marital therapy was better off at the end of treatment than 83% of the people who had received either no treatment or a placebo treatment' (p. 597).

The effectiveness of couple therapy has been studied in relation to a variety of clinical conditions. It has been shown to be an effective adjunctive treatment for depression (Beach & O'Leary, 1992; Jacobson, Dobson, Fruzzetti, Schmaling, & Salusky, 1991; O'Leary & Beach, 1990) and for agoraphobia (Arnow, Taylor, Agras, & Telch, 1985; Barlow, O'Brien, & Last, 1984). Among alcoholic patients, couples receiving marital therapy do better than controls on both marital and drinking measures (O'Farrell, Cutter, & Floyd, 1985; McCrady, Stout, Noel, Abrams, & Nelson, 1991). In a study of couples where one partner experienced a disorder of sexual desire, Hawton, Catalan, and Fagg (1991) reported an 84 per cent improvement.

In studying unsatisfactory outcomes in couple therapy, Anderson, Atilano, Bergen, Russell, and Jurich (1985) showed that therapies which maintain high intensity, encourage conflict escalation, and emphasize advice giving produce the highest drop-out rate. Allgood and Crane (1991) found that treatment drop-outs from marital therapy had fewer children and tended to present with problems related to individual or family-of-origin issues, rather than problems related to the interaction between the partners.

Family Therapy

Alexander et al (1994) suggest that the complexities in marital therapy are magnified in family therapy. The treatment unit is more variable, and the resistances and affects of multiple individuals, intensified conflicts. Many families presenting for therapy have multiple problems.

MODELS OF FAMILY THERAPY

Kaplan, Sadock, and Grebb (1994) suggest the classification of modalities of family therapy should include:

1 Structural
2 Strategic
3 Behavioural – Social exchange–based
4 Psychodynamic
5 Bowenian
6 Experiential
7 Psychoeducational
8 Integrative

THEORETICAL CONCEPTS

Constadine (1986) suggests that family therapists must be cognizant of communication and systems theories and be aware of the interdependence between interpersonal and intrapsychic factors in relationships. In Canada, psychiatric residencies offer, at best, elementary teaching in the specialty. As a result, some family-therapy failures occur when well-intentioned but poorly trained clinicians do not take into account psychodynamic, interpersonal, or sociocultural issues. Patients flee when they experience the physician imposing on them values and objectives which do not fit the family.

When the therapist knows only one theoretical framework, she or he may try to force the family to fit into it. The more theories and techniques the therapist can integrate in his or her own mind, the more opportunities he or she will have to help different families. Rigid adherence to any set of hypotheses tends to close rather than open the thinking space about the therapeutic relationship. A clinician with relative ideological freedom and the curiosity necessary to integrate different theories enhances his or her potential for helping a wider spectrum of families (Fine & Turner, 1991).

INDICATIONS FOR FAMILY THERAPY

1 *Schizophrenia:* Family psychoeducational programs, integrated with pharmacotherapy, offer a delay in relapse and improved social functioning (Goldstein & Miklowitz, 1995).
2 *Affective disorder:* Keitner, Miller, Epstein, Bishop, and Fruzzetti (1987) found that family therapy plus pharmacotherapy results in improved family functioning and recovery from an adolescent depressive episode. Clarkin et al (1990) showed that inpatient family interventions were effective for bipolar patients but not for unipolar patients. They suggested that patients who are too depressed cannot make use of family psychotherapy.
3 *Anorexia nervosa:* Family therapy can be helpful for adolescent females with anorexia provided the duration of the disorder is less than three years (Russell, Szmuckler, Dare, & Eisler, 1987; Robin, Siegal, Koepke, Moye, & Tice, 1994).
4 *Conduct disorder:* Family therapy can play a positive role in adolescent conduct disorders and adolescent suicide attempts (Roy & Frankel, 1995; Pinsof & Wynne, 1995). In treating adolescents, Henggeler, Borduin, Melton, Mann, and Smith (1995) reported that a flexible, individual, community-based intervention was effective in a large group of delinquent adolescents. Approaches based on social learning and parent-training for parents of aggressive children and pre-adolescents have been shown to be effective (Gurman & Kniskern, 1981; Alexander et al, 1994).
5 *After a suicide:* Family therapy may prove helpful to help a family deal with the aftermath of the suicide of one of its members (Kaye & Soreff, 1991; Brownstein, 1992).
6 Any drastic change, be it medical (e.g., a surgical intervention in the mother), psychological (e.g., a severe neurosis or psychosis in one of the parents), developmental (e.g., a difficult adolescence in a son), socioeconomic (e.g., unemployment or a forced move to a new city due to work), or bereavement (e.g., after the death of a parent or a child), severely disrupts the family system. Therefore, any of these crises is an indication for the family to meet with a therapist, analyse problems, and find second-order solutions for the whole family system.

7 *A pattern of physical or sexual abuse of children:* The severity of the pathology of the perpetrator has to be taken into account.
8 When the complaints of a patient centre on his or her interaction with family members, and not on a sense of inner turmoil.

CONTRAINDICATIONS FOR FAMILY THERAPY

1 Abreactive or cathartic family sessions, where anger is freely expressed, are contraindicated when the target of the aggression is too young or too old, or weakened by a physical or psychological illness. In these cases, a suicide or a psychotic reaction could be precipitated by a family session where everyone tactlessly 'speaks the truth.'
2 Antisocial families whose members collude to deceive the therapist.
3 Families with a rigid hierarchy, where the therapist's attempts to democratize the system are seen as an affront or a blasphemy.
4 Families who evoke in the therapist an intense negative countertransference or a sense of despair. A referral to another therapist solves this kind of impasse.
5 Families anticipating financial compensation after a work-related accident or a malpractice lawsuit. Since attempts at improving go against the financial interest of these families, they are amenable to treatment only after the trial has ended.
6 Families involved in court actions where a charge of sexual or physical abuse has been pressed against one or several members. In some of these cases, members may collude to produce a cooperative pseudo-treatment and thus protect a perpetrator. Others families request therapy so one of the members may gather ammunition for the impending legal fight. Both types of families are amenable to treatment once the trial has ended.

PRACTICE GUIDELINES FOR FAMILY THERAPY

Ethical practice guidelines for family psychotherapy encompass the principles already delineated for individual and couple psychotherapy. The family therapist must have a thorough knowledge of developmental issues to conduct sessions at levels each member of the family will understand, not undermine parental authority when adult failures or mistakes are examined, and not reveal explicit sexual (or other) conflicts of competent individuals without their consent.

Informed Consent and Confidentiality

Informed consent, in family therapy, implies clarifying in whose best interests the therapist will act and what the competing interests of each family member are. The potential positive and adverse effects of therapy must be discussed (Jenson, Josephson, & Frey, 1989).

Confidentiality in family therapy is a complex issue. The therapist has to decide when it is appropriate to respect the boundary of privacy for parents' problems, or for an older adolescent's issues; ethical dilemmas appear when keeping one family member's confidentiality implies danger of death or serious harm for that family member or for others. When in doubt, the therapist can openly discuss such dilemmas with the family, and if possible reach an agreement which will not alienate any member. Therapist and family may decide some private matters can be kept private in the best interest of the entire family system.

In Ontario and most other jurisdictions, physicians have the legal duty to report child abuse (or the suspicion of abuse) to the appropriate social agencies, even if such a report provokes the parents to suspend family therapy.

Some patients seek omniscience in the therapist. By discussing the possibility of difficulties during the treatment, the therapist may dispel his or her own tendency to such omniscience, heighten the patients' realistic anxiety, and paradoxically strengthen the family commitment to collaborate in therapy. By discussing potential distress, the therapist may enhance the patients' trust, establish an empathic link with each one of them, and define the potentiality and limitations of the therapeutic work.

Therapy Objectives

Therapy objectives can take into account the welfare of individuals and the family as a whole, and fit the life-cycle phase of the family. For instance, the therapy for a couple with their first baby has different objectives from the therapy for a family with conflicts among three generations living in one household. It is useful for the therapist to keep in mind the developmental goals appropriate for the age of each family member (AAMFT, 1988; Zygmond & Boorhem, 1989).

The medical and psychiatric training of the family therapist allows him or her to decide when medication, hospitalization, organic treatments, psychopharmacology, tutoring, or combined psychotherapies are indicated in addition to family psychotherapy.

Paradoxical and Expressive Instructions

When the technique of treatment includes paradoxical instructions (pre-scribing the symptom, for instance) or free expression of negative affect, the therapist has to make ethical decisions about how much to manipu-late the process of the family interaction 'for their own good' and how much emotional pain to allow before soothing manoeuvres are attempted (Wendorf & Wendorf, 1985). Some family therapy drop-outs complain of feeling that the therapist was dogmatic or arrogant, played with their emotions, or was guided by a theoretical construct more than by an empathic alliance with the family. Paradoxical and expressive techniques are deceptively simple. The therapist has to possess a clear understanding of psychodynamics, communication, and interpersonal theories before he or she can safely attempt the use of methods that can backfire, hurt the family, or land the therapist in the middle of a mal-practice suit.

Outcome Research

The meta-analysis undertaken by Alexander et al (1994) of twenty years of family therapy showed positive effects compared with no treatment or placebo treatment. However, these authors concluded that the superi-ority of family therapy to other modalities has not been substantiated. Gurman and Kniskern (1981) concluded that 73 per cent of family cases improved during treatment. Recent reviews of the positive impact of couple and family therapy on a clinical population have been published by Lebow (1995), Lebow and Gurman (1995), and Roy and Frankel (1995).

Negative Outcomes

Gurman and Kniskern (1978) report that poor outcomes of family ther-apy are associated with therapists with deficient relationship skills who confront patients bluntly about loaded issues, and therapists who fail to intervene when there is serious confrontation between family members. Coleman (1985) edited a multiauthored volume entitled *Failures in Family Therapy*. It is commendable to publish negative results; therapists could otherwise obtain a false sense of security, unaware of the possibility of doing harm to some patients.

Training in Couple and Family Therapy

The couple or family therapist must obtain training from specialists in these modalities. Canadian psychiatric residencies, owing to a lack of time, usually offer only an overview, and some basic principles to allow the students to start a practice. In most large urban areas, there are two- or three-year programs to train practitioners to become couple and family therapists. Training, awareness of the ever-growing literature about the field, and supervision facilitate the development of a non-hurtful couple/family psychotherapist. Personal psychotherapy for the therapist may also be beneficial. Psychiatrists working in smaller communities, however, must attend workshops, teach themselves through readings and peer discussions, and seek supervision for at least two years. Teleconferences and Internet continuing medical education will help this process.

References

Alexander, J.F., Holtzworth-Monroe, A., & Jameson, P. (1994). The process and outcome of marital and family therapy: Research review and evaluation. In A.E. Bergin & S.L. Garfield (Eds.), *Handbook of psychotherapy and behavior change* (4th ed.). New York: Wiley.

Allgood, S.M., & Crane, D.R. (1991). Predicting marital therapy dropouts. *Journal of Marital and Family Therapy, 17,* 73–79.

American Association for Marriage and Family Therapy (AAMFT). (1988). *AAMFT code of ethical principles for marriage and family therapists.* Washington, DC: Author.

Anderson, S.A., Atilano, R.B., Bergen, L.P., Russell, C.S. & Jurich, A.P. (1985). Dropping out of marriage and family therapy: Intervention strategies and spouses' perceptions. *American Journal of Family Therapy, 13,* 39–54.

Arnow, B.A., Taylor, C.B., Agras, W.S., & Telch, M.J. (1985). Enhancing agoraphobia treatment by changing couple communications patterns. *Behavioural Therapy, 16,* 452–456.

Barlow, D.H., O'Brien, G.T., & Last, C.G. (1984). Couples treatment of agoraphobia. *Behavioural Therapy, 15,* 41–48.

Beach, S.R.H., & O'Leary, K.D. (1992). Treating depression in the context of marital discord: Outcome and predictors of response for marital therapy vs. cognitive therapy. *Behavior Therapy, 23,* 507–528.

Bergin, A.E., & Garfield, S.L. (Eds.). (1994). *Handbook of psychotherapy and behavior change* (4th Ed.), New York: Wiley.

Brownstein, M. (1992). Contacting the family after a suicide. *Canadian Journal of Psychiatry, 37,* 208–212.

Buxton, A.M. (1991). *The other side of the closet.* Santa Monica, CA: IBS.

Cameron, P.M. (1987). Marital therapy: Outcome research – multiple pathways to progress. In L.F. Frelick & E.M. Waring (Eds.), *Marital therapy in psychiatric practice: An overview.* New York: Brunner/Mazel.

Clarkin, J.F., Glick, I.D., Haas, C.L., Spencer, J.H., Lewis, A.B., Peyser, J., DeMane, N., Good-Ellis, M., Harris, E., & Lestelle, V. (1990). A randomized clinical trial of inpatient family intervention, V: Results for affective disorders. *Journal of Affective Disorders, 18,* 17–28.

Coleman, S. (Ed.). (1985) *Failures in family therapy.* New York/London: Guilford.

Constadine, L. (1986). *Family paradigms: The practice of theory in family therapy.* New York/London: Guilford.

Fine, M.F., & Turner, J. (1991). Tyranny and freedom: Looking at ideas in the practice of family therapy. *Family Process, 30,* 307–320.

Frelick, L.F., & Waring, E.M. (1987). *Marital therapy in psychiatric practice: An overview.* New York: Brunner/Mazel.

Goldstein, M.J., & Miklowitz, D.J. (1995). Effectiveness of psychoeducational family therapy in the treatment of schizophrenic disorders. *Journal of Marital and Family Therapy, 21,* 361–376.

Gurman, A.S., & Kniskern, D.P. (1978). Deterioration in marital and family therapy: Empirical, clinical and conceptual issues. *Family Process, 17,* 3–20.

Gurman, A.S., & Kniskern, D.P. (1981). *Handbook of family therapy.* New York: Brunner/Mazel.

Hahlweg, K., & Markman, H.J. (1988). Effectiveness of behavioural marital therapy: Empirical status of behavioural techniques in preventing and alleviating marital distress. *Journal of Consulting and Clinical Psychology, 56,* 440–447.

Hawton, K., Catalan, J., & Fagg, J. (1991). Low sexual desire: Sex therapy results and prognostic factors. *Behaviour Research and Therapy, 29,* 217–244.

Henggeler, S.W., Borduin, C.M., Melton, G.B., Mann, B.J., & Smith, L.A. (1995). Effects of multisystemic therapy on drug use and abuse in serious juvenile offenders: A progress report from two outcome studies. *Family Dynamics Addicts Q.,* 40–51.

Jacobson, N.S., & Addis, M.E. (1993). Research on couples and couple therapy: What do we know? Where are we going? *Journal of Consulting and Clinical Psychology, 61,* 85–93.

Jacobson, N.S., Dobson, K., Fruzzetti, A.E., Schmaling, K.B., & Salusky, S. (1991). Marital therapy as a treatment for depression. *Journal of Consulting and Clinical Psychology, 59,* 547–557.

Jacobson, N.S., & Gurman, A.S. (Eds.). (1995). *Clinical handbook of couple therapy.* New York: Guilford.

Jenson, P.S., Josephson, A.M., & Frey, J. (1989). Informed consent as a framework for treatment: Ethical and therapeutic considerations. *American Journal of Psychotherapy, 43,* 378–386.

Johnson, S.M., & Greenberg, L.S. (1985). Differential effects of experiential and problem-solving interventions in resolving marital conflict. *Journal of Consulting Clinical Psychology, 53,* 175–184.

Kaplan, H.I., Sadock, B.J., & Grebb, J.A. (1994). *Synopsis of psychiatry. Behavioral sciences/clinical psychiatry* (7th Ed.). Baltimore/Philadelphia/Hong Kong/London/Munich/Sydney/Tokyo: Williams & Wilkins.

Karpel, M.A. (1980). Family secrets: I. Conceptual and ethical issues in the relational context. II. Ethical and practical considerations in therapeutic management. *Family Process, 19,* 295–306.

Karpel, M.A. (1994). *Evaluating couples: A handbook for practitioners.* New York/London: Norton.

Kaye, N.S., & Soreff, S.M. (1991). The psychiatrist's role, responses and responsibilities when a patient commits suicide. *American Journal of Psychiatry, 148,* 739–743.

Kayser, K. (1993). *When love dies: The process of marital disaffection.* New York/London: Guilford.

Keitner, G., Miller, I.W., Epstein, N.B., Bishop, D.S., & Fruzzetti, A.E. (1987). Family functioning and the course of major depression. *Comprehensive Psychiatry, 28,* 54–64.

Lebow, J. (1995). Research on assessing outcome in couple and family therapy. *AFTA Newsletter, 64,* 43–45.

Lebow, J., & Gurman, A.S. (1995). Research assessing couple and family therapy. *Annual Review of Psychology, 46,* 27–57.

McCrady, B.S., Stout, R., Noel, N., Abrams, D., & Nelson, H.F. (1991). Effectiveness of three types of spouse-involved behavioural alcoholism treatment. *British Journal of Addiction, 86,* 1415–1424.

O'Farrell, T.J., Cutter, H.S.G., & Floyd, F.J. (1985). Evaluating behavioural marital therapy for male alcoholics: Effects on marital adjustment and communication from before to after treatment. *Behaviour Therapy, 16,* 147–167.

O'Leary, K.D., & Beach, S.R.H. (1990). Marital therapy: A viable treatment for depression and marital discord. *American Journal of Psychiatry, 147,* 183–186.

Pinsof, W.M., & Wynne, L.C. (1995). The efficacy of marital and family therapy:

An empirical overview, conclusions and recommendations. *Journal of Marital and Family Therapy, 21,* 585–610.

Pittman, F. (1989). *Private lies: Infidelity and the betrayal of intimacy.* New York/London: Norton.

Robin, A.L., Siegal, P.T., Koepke, T., Moye, A.W., & Tice, S. (1994). Family therapy versus individual therapy for adolescent females with anorexia nervosa. *Journal of Developmental and Behavioural Pediatrics, 15,* 111–116.

Rosenbluth, M., & Cameron, P.M. (1981). Assessment, commitment and motivation in marital therapy. *Canadian Journal of Psychiatry, 26,* 151–154.

Roy, R., & Frankel, H. (1995). *How good is family therapy? A reassessment.* Toronto: University of Toronto Press.

Russell, G.F.M., Szmukler, G.I., Dare, E., & Eisler, I. (1987). An evaluation of family therapy in anorexia nervosa and bulimia nervosa. *Archives of General Psychiatry, 44,* 1047–1056.

Sager, C., Slindick, R., Kremer, M., Lenz, R., & Royce, J.R. (1968). The married in treatment. *Archives of General Psychiatry, 19,* 205–217.

Scharff, D. (1978). Truth and consequences in sex and marital therapy: The revelation of secrets in the therapeutic setting. *Journal for Sex and Marital Therapy, 4,* 35–49.

Scharff, D.E., Savege Scharff, J.S. (1991). *Object relations couple therapy.* Northvale, NJ/London: Jason Aronson.

Snyder, D.K., & Wills, R.M. (1989). Behavioural versus insight-oriented marital. therapy: Effects on individual and interspousal functioning. *Journal of Consulting and Clinical Psychology, 57,* 39–46.

Wallerstein, J.S. (1990).Transference and countertransference in clinical intervention with divorcing families. *American Journal of Orthopsychiatry, 60,* 337–345.

Waring, E.M., & Patton, D. (1984). Marital intimacy and depression. *British Journal of Psychiatry, 145,* 641–644.

Watzlawick, P., Beavin, J.H., & Jackson, D.D. (1967). *Pragmatics of human communication. A study of interactional patterns, pathologies and paradoxes.* New York: Norton.

Wendorf, D.J., & Wendorf, R.J. (1985). A systemic view of family therapy ethics. *Family Process, 24,* 443–453.

Wesley, S., & Waring, E.M. (1996). A critical review of marital therapy outcome research. *Canadian Journal of Psychiatry, 41,* 421–428.

Zygmond, M.J., & Boorhem, H. (1989). Ethical decision making in family therapy. *Family Process, 28,* 269–280.

8. Guidelines for the Practice of Group Psychotherapy

Molyn Leszcz

Description of Modality

Group therapy encompasses a range of interventions that include focused psychoeducational groups, support groups, time-limited groups, and ongoing psychotherapy groups intended to change behaviour and character structure. This chapter focuses on the standard psychotherapy group for moderately disturbed ambulatory patients, which constitutes the core of group therapy. The principles that emerge from this model provide relevant practice guidelines for all types of group psychotherapy.

According to Yalom (1995), the enormous expansion of group approaches in the past ten years reflects the attempts of practitioners to identify unique patient problems and concerns, to devise suitable models of intervention, and to develop therapeutic mechanisms that can ameliorate patient distress.

A recent text by Alonso and Swiller (1993) gives a useful description of group therapy: 'Group psychotherapy offers the opportunity for purposefully created, closely observed, and skillfully guided interpersonal interaction. Such interactions can positively influence the complex varieties of human distress and malfunction.' The authors comment that this involves a dynamic and exploratory process of the 'vital enactment of the characterological dilemmas of the members, exposure and resolution of shameful secrets; support around the universality of the members' wishes, fears and distress and reintegration of split-off aspects of the self' (p. xxxi).

Dies (1992) surveyed senior practitioners of the American Group Psychotherapy Association (AGPA) to identify the scope of contemporary group therapy. The survey demonstrates a broad field with ten models in three main categories, which include the interpersonal; the psychodynamic, encompassing psychodynamic, group as a whole/systems, object-relations, group analysis, existential/humanistic, and self-psychology approaches; and the actional, including cognitive/behavioural group therapy, transactional analysis/gestalt/redecision therapy, and psychodrama. Although they may appear very different from one another, group models fall within an acceptable practice frame, provided the model is followed in an integral, coherent fashion, respecting patients' need for growth, maturation, and development. Models may be distinguished by virtue of their intervention target, emphasizing the individual, the interaction, or the group as a whole. Group-therapy models can be further distinguished by the therapist's relative activity; non-activity; transparency; opaqueness; posture of gratification/frustration; focus on the past, present, or future; or relative emphasis on affect/cognition or process/content.

Particular therapeutic factors further differentiate the group therapies. For example, virtually all effective group formats encompass universality (a sense of fundamental alikeness with others), cohesion (a sense of belonging and acceptance within a group offering both emotional support and a sense of task effectiveness), altruism (opportunities to elevate one's own self-esteem by giving to others), and the instillation of hope. Other factors, such as self-understanding, are more prominent in psychodynamic models, while interpersonal learning (learning from feedback about the way in which one communicates and relates) more accurately reflects the interpersonal model. Actional groups emphasize cognitive restructuring, education, and role play.

What is striking in the Dies survey (1992) is that the more than 100 respondents agreed that the two most important issues to address in group therapy are therapist countertransference and recognition of the patient's transference. Only in the action-oriented groups were these two factors considered unimportant.

Psychodynamic group therapies emphasize interpretation and group process, aiming to resolve patient transference by searching for the meaning and motivation underlying a person's behaviour and thought. Efforts are made to link present and past. The therapist is a reactive interpreter of unstructured group processes, individual patient exposition, and patient interactions. The interpersonal model emphasizes therapist facilitation, working in the here-and-now, focusing on the interactive process within the group, employing therapist transparency to facilitate patient self-disclosure. Group cohesion and attention to group norms are emphasized to encourage interpersonal learning within the social microcosm of the group. Role play, behavioural practice, and homework are de-emphasized in models that use the here-and-now to access required behavioural practice.

The action-oriented groups emphasize cognitive reframing, goal-setting, feedback, behavioural practice, and role playing, distinguishing these models from the interpersonal and psychodynamic models (which overlap substantially). In the action-oriented models, there is a de-emphasis on interpretation and process commentary. Therapy involves active structuring by the therapist to address dysfunctional thoughts and behaviours directly with a rapid transfer of learning from the group environment to real life.

Group therapy takes place in various settings, with various age groups and diagnostic populations. To illustrate, 50 per cent of acute psychiatric inpatients will participate in group therapy during the course of their hospitalization (McGarrick, Rosenstein, Milazzo-Sayre, & Manderscheid, 1988). That type of group therapy occurs in a rapidly changing milieu with very disturbed patients, thereby requiring its own unique models (Yalom, 1983). However, there is a limit to creativity, and the framework articulated by Gutheil and Gabbard (1993) is relevant. They suggest that each model and each therapist's conduct must be evaluated within its clinical context, clearly articulating the therapist's treatment rationale, in a way that can withstand objective scrutiny. Organizations such as the American Psychiatric Association monitor standards of practice in order to help patients identify and evaluate the treatment received; to help practitioners evaluate their work relative to contemporary practice; to aid clinical decision making; and to ensure ethical and effective treatments of a high standard (Zarin, Pincus, & McIntyre, 1993).

The following guidelines are broad, general, and based on research with moderately disturbed, adult outpatient groups. Much of this work reflects interpersonal and psychodynamic therapy groups with added notation reflecting cognitive/behavioural therapy groups.

Scientific Basis and Efficacy

The pioneering work of Smith, Glass, and Miller (1980) in the meta-analysis of the outcome literature on psychotherapies concluded that group psychotherapy is an effective model of intervention. Preliminary reviews and meta-analyses (Tillitski, 1990; Luborsky, Diguer, Luborsky et al., 1993) confirm that, according to certain outcome measures, patients treated in group therapy improve in a manner equivalent to those treated by individual therapy, and significantly better than controls. Treatment produces durable gains. This finding is confirmed both for time-limited group therapy (Budman et al, 1988) and for longer-term group therapy. Combined therapy is more effective than single therapies, and integration with pharmacotherapy and medical care, when appropriate, enhances effectiveness (Luborsky et al, 1993). Dies (1993) concluded that group therapy offers an effective, cost-effective, relatively low-risk form of treatment, usable in a broad range of different patient populations in a range of settings. Decisions must be individualized regarding treatment matching. As Toseland and Siporin (1986) note, this aspect of the work is still in its infancy. Research is required to evaluate and predict who does best with group therapy as opposed to individual therapy.

The evaluation of treatment and therapist effectiveness also requires attention, which in turn needs evaluation of patient X therapist X group variables. The type of patient, the length of time available for treatment, the developmental phase of the group, the leadership style, and the treatment context (Dies, 1993), all influence the value and evaluation of the therapeutic intervention.

Therapeutic Action and Mechanisms of Change

THERAPEUTIC FACTORS

Therapeutic mechanisms are defined as elements of the group therapy that contribute to patient improvement and depend on action by the patient, therapist, or group (Bloch, 1986). Through humbling clinical experience, the original concept of 'curative factors' has been replaced by 'therapeutic factors,' and occasionally 'putative therapeutic factors' (Bloch & Crouch, 1985; Yalom, 1995). These mechanisms include the following: instillation of hope; universality; altruism; belonging/cohesion; interpersonal learning; self-understanding; self-disclosure/catharsis; vicarious learning (learning about oneself or how to address difficulties by watching and learning from the progress of others in the group); education/imparting information; and coming to grips with responsibility for oneself within the existential realities of living. These factors may be viewed as moving on a spectrum from non-specific, general mechanisms that reflect the early stages of group development (such as instillation of hope, altruism, and feelings of universality) to belonging/ cohesion, giving rise to specific and developmentally mature therapeutic mechanisms. All groups in the ten therapeutic models cited have in common non-specific therapeutic mechanisms that serve to maintain the group, but groups differ in the later, putative therapeutic mechanisms. Interpersonal learning and self-understanding are more mature therapeutic factors that are likely to occur only through specific therapist design.

The factors described do not occur in isolation from one another. For example, group cohesion is a therapeutic mechanism through which patients derive comfort, support, and stability by belonging to a group that is highly valued by the members and that values the individual. Cohesion also facilitates other therapeutic factors. Cohesive groups elicit more patient self-disclosure and a willingness both to be influenced by others and to learn about oneself in ways that can alter behaviour (Yalom, 1995). Similarly, feelings of universality increase the willingness of participants to disclose things about themselves, and thereby to enter into the therapeutic loop that generates interpersonal feedback and cohesion.

Awareness of the desired and achievable therapeutic mechanisms helps to set realistic goals. For example, inpatient groups, which are characterized by rapid turnover and more attention to ill members, do not achieve the same levels of maturity as open-ended outpatient groups or stable, time-limited groups (Leszcz, 1986). Hence, aiming for character change through an affect-intensifying group is likely to overwhelm members of an inpatient group. More realistic aims are to address patient demoralization – by capitalizing on earlier developmental therapeutic factors that emphasize cohesion, universality, instillation of hope, and the benefits of talking one to another – and to ensure that the group is not a 'failure experience.'

Cohesion is vital. It is a complex concept that can be evaluated both for the group as a whole and for the individual (Mackenzie & Tschushke, 1993). The experience of the individual is central. In order to benefit from treatment, patients must feel a sense of belonging to a cohesive group and feel they are valued and accepted members of the group. Hence, patients may evaluate the group as an effective, cohesive, and desirable entity, yet on measures of group relatedness (which reflect personal, individual experience) may feel 'outside the interactive loop'

(Mackenzie & Tschuschke, 1993). Group cohesion parallels the therapeutic alliance in individual therapy, and an early feeling of cohesion is
essential for ultimate therapeutic benefit. The achievement of cohesion
relies on therapist qualities such as genuineness, warmth, empathy, and
a positive regard for patients. Equally important are specific therapeutic
actions that articulate structure, norm-setting, culture-building, and the
safety of emotional disclosure and engagement.

THE THERAPIST'S ROLE

In general, the central functions of the therapist include establishing and
administering the group; gate-keeping for entry and exit to and from the
group; and facilitating the group's session-to-session work. The therapist facilitates activation and illumination of group dynamics, at the levels of affective engagement, cognitive integration, and attribution of
meaning to the experience of patients within the group. Malan, Balfour,
Hood, and Shooter (1975) concluded that an absence of clear structure
leads to regression. Therapists who adopt a posture that is abstinent and
interpret only group-wide processes without attention to individual
needs are likely to produce frustrated, dissatisfied participants who reap
no benefit from their group participation. Yalom (1995), reviewing work
on the outcome of encounter groups, notes that therapists must maintain a balance between activation of affect and attribution of meaning.
Group leaders who emphasize either extreme are likely to trigger
negative outcomes or minimal improvement. Excesses of cognitive
integration or a third dimension – executive function – may generate
boring, subdued groups that fail to achieve independent levels of functioning. Excessive emotional activation may also produce casualties as it
may overwhelm the patient's capacity to integrate the experience.

Attention to the group's developmental stages is equally essential.
Groups do not emerge fully formed. They develop through phases of
apprehension about engagement, to engagement, and on to differentiation, individuation, feelings of mutuality, and genuine intimacy (Mackenzie & Livesley, 1983), as well as to termination. A therapist's facilitation of patient actions at one point in the group's interaction may be
inappropriate at another phase of the group's development. The therapist must be able to identify when to be active or facilitative and,
equally, when activity may increase patient dependence and lead to
avoidance of responsibility for the therapeutic task. The degree of self-
disclosure on the part of patients must match the developmental stage

of the group, avoiding the pursuit of 'instant intimacy' or premature confrontation before the group becomes cohesive. It is vital to build an atmosphere that stimulates progressive self-disclosure and mutual feedback, thereby diminishing the risk of scapegoating or activating unworkable shame and imbalances in self-disclosure that may lead to premature termination of treatment.

Specific actions that identify and forestall negative patient outcomes include proper pre-group preparation and early identification of patient difficulties that may precipitate premature termination from treatment (Bernard, 1989). The therapist's ability to bridge between group members (Ormont, 1990) and to identify patient barriers against intimate engagement with one another (Ormont, 1988) are critical skills that promote respectful, mutual self-disclosure and deepening interaction.

The therapist's attention to clear boundaries around the group, defining the tasks at hand, activation of affect, and attribution of meaning serve to illuminate immediate interpersonal processes in the here-and-now of the group. This process generates a window into the past that may have shaped contemporary patterns, and creates opportunities to modify interpersonal behaviour in the contemporary environment, first within the group, and then in an adaptive spiral leading to change outside the group setting (Leszcz, 1992; Yalom, 1995).

The group members provide feedback that illuminates and modifies interpersonal behaviour. Although feedback is not something group members come to easily and naturally, it is pivotal to successful group therapy. The group therapist must shape norms, and model and reinforce appropriate feedback. Useful guidelines from Rothke (1986) and Yalom (1995) emphasize the use of here-and-now behaviour as a focus for feedback, rather than highly inferential conceptualizations about the past. Non-pejorative language illuminates the impact on the provider of the feedback in a way that shares some emotional risk with the receiver of feedback and invites, but does not demand, change. Linking negative feedback with positive feedback directly or in sequence is more effective than either alone. Of course, feedback must be timely and not exceed the patient's capacity to integrate it. The therapist's articulation of his or her reactions to the unfolding dynamics and interactions within the here-and-now of the group, and therapist transparency play a role in interpersonal interaction and feedback. It should be guided by the principles of responsibility, therapeutic usefulness, timeliness, and maintenance of therapeutic boundaries.

The capacity to work in the here-and-now is a major force for change and essential to understanding the group process and the individual's interplay within it – as reflected by here-and-now behaviour, comments, and expressions. The therapist must be able to activate the here-and-now by creating a group in which members are emotionally engaged with one another and encouraged to reflect upon their feelings and reactions towards one another, recognizing that the group is a 'social microcosm.' Behaviour or relationships outside the group often have an analogous representation within the group. Exploring such connections brings maximum therapeutic benefits. The here-and-now work examines the way in which patients actually relate through what transpires in the group, rather than via the patient's reports of what goes on outside the group. Such reports are inevitably incomplete and accordingly limit the group's ability to achieve therapeutic change. Facilitating the group's self-reflection creates opportunities for cognitive integration and attribution of meaning, promoting maximum growth and change. The leader's ability to intervene at ever-increasing levels of inference, drawing attention to patterns of behaviour, makes the work collaborative, reducing confrontations that are premature, dissonant, and/or excessive.

Indications and Contraindictions for Group Therapy

Group therapy can be useful for a broad range of heterogeneous and homogeneous clinical situations. Group therapists must recognize patient needs, patient capacities, and logistical parameters regarding the time frame and institutional requirements. They must be able to modify traditional techniques and set realistic objectives (Yalom, 1995). The American Psychiatric Association (APA) 1989 task force report notes that group therapy can be applied effectively for victims of sexual abuse and patients with schizophrenia, mood disorders, post-traumatic stress disorder, sexual dysfunction and paraphilia, substance abuse, addictive disorders, eating disorders – in particular, bulimia – personality disorders, somatoform disorders, medical illnesses, and a range of adjustment disorders. For the last-named disorders, groups are useful to facilitate adjustment and to diminish maladaptive stress responses. Group therapy may be a primary modality or an adjunct to other forms of psychiatric or medical treatment. The remarkable finding by Spiegel, Bloom, Kraemer and Gottheil (1989), demonstrating a highly significant survival effect for women with metastatic breast cancer treated in supportive–expressive group therapy, points to the likelihood that groups will in future be used for an increasingly broad range of clinical situations. In fact, virtually all Axis I and Axis II disorders can be treated by one or another form of group therapy. Patients with contraindications for general, heterogeneously composed outpatient groups are often well treated in a homogeneously composed group. To illustrate, a substance-abusing patient would not do well in a standard, dynamic and interactive psychotherapy group, yet might be successfully treated in groups homogeneous for this condition. Suicidal, acting-out patients have similarly been treated effectively in homogeneous, highly structured groups (Piper, 1993).

A group for patients with schizophrenia is very different from one for victims of sexual abuse, and both of these groups will differ substantially from a group for spouses of Alzheimer's patients (Leszcz, 1991). The groups differ as to the role of transference, therapeutic mechanisms, the role of cognitive reframing, and choice of therapeutic factors emphasized. Networking and contact between group patients outside the group is generally discouraged in dynamic psychotherapy groups, yet is an integral part of treatment for certain medical conditions or adjustment disorders. Even within a particular diagnostic population, such as patients with schizophrenia, Cole (1989) notes that there will be a range of group approaches, and that maximum effectiveness may be achieved by treating good pre-morbid, high-functioning patients with an interactional-oriented group therapy, and poor pre-morbid, low-functioning patients with supportive, social learning–oriented therapy.

Although most patients with relative contraindications for standard psychotherapy groups can be treated in a specific homogeneous group, it is essential to set selection criteria for a typical ambulatory group of mixed neurotic and characterologically disturbed patients. Reviewing the literature, Dies (1993) comments that there is little research about clear indications for treatment matching. Although group therapy has been proved effective, it is often viewed by patients as inferior treatment. Toseland and Siporin (1986) suggest group therapy for patients with interpersonal problems, interpersonal distress, and isolation. In addition, Grunebaum and Kates (1977) advocate group therapy for patients who have a tendency towards action, or who demonstrate a need for dilution or activation of the transference. Patients with good ego strengths and focused concerns may do well in a short-term group (Mackenzie, 1990).

The literature suggests that decisions are still made essentially on clinical grounds and therefore patients require a diagnostic interview to make a comprehensive assessment (Salvendy, 1993). Toseland and Siporin (1986), summarizing contraindications, suggest that patients should not participate in group therapy if there are significant barriers to their participation, thereby impairing group cohesion, or a cognitive/ sensory difficulty that will preclude their participation in the life of the group. Personality traits that can make individuals deviant to the group are relative contraindications, as is a tendency to paranoid distortion or an inability to tolerate anxiety. Yalom (1995) opposes group methods for patients who tend to externalize, deny, suffer from severe mistrust, lack internal focus, or are embroiled in an external crisis (again, unless the group is geared to that crisis). The therapist must ask whether the patient can effectively use this group at that particular time. Unlike individual therapy, when a group leader brings a patient into therapy, the therapist not only commits to treat that patient, but simultaneously commits all group members to a relationship with that person.

There must be sufficient incentive for individual patients to develop a working alliance with the therapist and to develop cohesion with the group. The more the patient's concerns meet the group goals, the better the beginning will be. In short, the patient must have the intellectual, logistical, and psychological ability to adhere to the group task.

Melnick and Woods (1976) note that compositional match is never perfect, and what really matters is the overall resonance/dissonance between group members. Compositional mismatches can be offset by more structure and more focused treatment, and, in general, compositional concerns are more relevant in unstructured, longer-term therapies.

The addition of a new member to an ongoing group must be evaluated, assessing how this patient will work with the particular group at this particular time. Characterologically difficult patients with a tendency to act out, blame, and devalue may be very taxing to young, immature groups, but can be better tolerated in mature, stable groups (Leszcz, 1989). Salvendy (1993) recommends that groups be heterogeneous in terms of the central problems patients present, but homogeneous regarding ego function. In addition, certain aspects of interpersonal function, such as ego-syntonic character pathology, that impede group participation may be contained by proper pre-training and early identification of maladaptive patterns to forestall preliminary difficulties. However, as Horner (1975) notes, although groups are excellent vehicles for the illumination of characterological disturbances, some patients may not tolerate interpersonal feedback and may experience it

as a narcissistic injury. A longer period of assessment, allowing comprehensive preparation and collaborative identification of problems, goals,
and targets for treatment, can promote successful treatment (Dies, 1993;
Salvendy, 1993).

COGNITIVE BEHAVIOURAL GROUP THERAPIES

Cognitive behavioural therapy (CBT) is often conducted in a group format. In most cases, groups comprise patients with the same disorder.
Group treatment has several advantages over individual therapy. First,
it is helpful for patients to see others who have similar difficulties. It is
not unusual for a patient to report feeling initially that he or she is the
only person around with a particular disorder. Second, conducting treatment in groups can help to 'normalize' the patient's experience, and
thereby decrease the stigma that a patient might feel about being in therapy. Third, group treatment provides patients with the opportunity to
learn from one another. For example, if a patient is having difficulties
completing a particular homework assignment, group members can
share their experiences and provide suggestions to the patient. Fourth,
CBT lends itself well to a group format. Many of the CBT techniques are
taught through a combination of didactic lessons and Socratic questioning. In many ways, CBT resembles classroom learning and tends to be
easily adapted to a group format. Finally, for certain disorders CBT may
be very difficult to conduct on an individual basis. For example, the
treatment of social phobias involves, among other things, exposing
patients to social situations and teaching patients to communicate more
effectively. A group format provides many natural opportunities for
practising the appropriate CBT strategies to overcome social phobia.

There are several situations in which CBT might be better conducted
on an individual basis. Patients who are likely to dominate a group and
interfere with the progress of other group members are best treated individually. In addition, because CBT tends to be tailored to specific disorders, patients with certain disorders may not benefit as much and
should be treated individually or in groups with similar individuals.
Finally, patients who require extensive individual attention should not
be treated in groups. For example, a patient with very severe agoropho-
bia may need several sessions of therapist-assisted exposure to feared
situations. A group format may not provide the flexibility and time
needed to address such a patient's needs.

Preventing Negative Outcomes in Group Psychotherapy

Dies and Teleska (1985) define negative outcome as occurring when 'a patient becomes worse as a result of treatment as shown by an exacerbation of presenting symptoms, emergence of new ones, misuse of therapy, or disillusionment with treatment' (p. 1187). A negative outcome occurs in about 10 per cent of instances. Groups can exert substantial influence on those group members who wish to belong and be accepted. Excessive pressure to conform and limiting participants' freedom of choice, reflect a potentially coercive, ideologically driven treatment. In overview, difficulties emerge from misunderstanding or misuse of specific group phenomena related to leadership variables, therapeutic factors, and developmental stages and member roles.

LEADERSHIP VARIABLES

Leszcz (1994) notes that a negative outcome in group psychotherapy may reflect frank therapist hostility towards a patient; premature or excessive confrontation; or a countertransferential enactment in which the therapist cannot get disentangled from an interpersonal recapitulation with the patient. When a therapist is unable to examine a patient's difficulties in a systemic fashion within the group, which includes the therapist's contribution, this is a failure of the principle of boundary maintenance in psychotherapy. The therapist's need for security overrides his or her objective ability to assess the reasons for an impasse or deterioration. When the therapist experiences exaggerated emotional stimulation or excessive subjectivity, or allows his or her personal needs to take precedence over those of a patient, negative outcomes may result (Leszcz, 1994). Conversely, therapists who are excessively distant and aloof or develop a *laissez-faire* attitude towards the group are associated with poor therapeutic outcomes (Lieberman, Yalom, & Miles, 1973). Leaders with extremes of emotional stimulation or executive function also may have poor treatment outcomes. In contrast, leaders who actively attribute meaning to their patients' behaviour have more positive outcomes. Hence, the level and nature of therapist activity is crucial to therapy outcomes.

Gutheil and Gabbard (1993) stress that therapists must be able to articulate a rationale for their therapeutic interventions, identify any deviation from their normal practice, and be able to offer objective therapeutic reasons for any variation from the normal posture. Leszcz (1992) comments that, similarly to group patients, the group leader can also become interpersonally engaged, responding emotionally to the behaviour of group members. However, it is essential to know how to regain therapeutic perspective in order to avoid a negative recapitulation, and to provide a learning experience that deepens the patient's understanding of self, rather than a complementary experience that confirms the patient's pathological paradigms of self and others.

THERAPEUTIC FACTORS

Dies and Teleska (1985) comment on the negative outcomes that emerge from the therapist's failure to understand and utilize different therapeutic factors. The therapeutic mechanism of self-disclosure cannot be understood without considering the context in which it occurs. Excessive, premature stimulation of patient self-disclosure, before there is group cohesion, may overstimulate and overwhelm a patient, making the patient feel humiliated and fearful of continuing in the group. The activation must be linked to a patient's ability to integrate and assimilate the therapy experience. Emotional expressiveness is not an end in itself, but a mediator of other therapeutic mechanisms, such as self-understanding and interpersonal learning. Cohesion also acts as a therapeutic mechanism. As noted by Mackenzie and Tschuschke (1993), patients who fail to engage and for whom the group is experienced as a non-accepting environment have poorer outcomes than patients who make an early, positive group connection. In general, poorly cohesive groups will not easily accept feedback and member confrontation, thereby failing to promote change. Conversely, such groups may fragment in the face of confrontation. Hence, maintaining cohesion is essential at every step of group therapy, from selection, preparation, and early developmental stages to the working-through phase. Similarly, any ruptures in cohesion must be identified and directly addressed. Easy-to-use measures are available for therapists to employ and to help evaluate quantitatively the experience of cohesion and group engagement and to help augment clinical impressions (Mackenzie & Tschuschke, 1993).

DEVELOPMENTAL STAGES AND MEMBER ROLES

Another key factor in reducing negative outcomes and facilitating positive ones is attention to group development and member roles. Dies and Teleska (1985) note that a common error occurs when therapists operate as though the group begins fully formed instead of following a developmental course from preliminary engagement, through differentiation, to mutuality and intimacy (Mackenzie & Livesley, 1983). Therapists may need to guide the group through its developmental stages, recognizing that what is appropriate and required for one stage may be regressive or overstimulating for another. Groups may get stuck at an early developmental phase in which universality and cohesion are emphasized at the expense of differentiation and disagreement. More frequently, premature and excessive hostility and confrontation occur.

In institutional settings, the goals of group therapy must be compatible with the goals of the institution. Although these goals need not be identical, they must be complementary and mutually endorsed, in order to protect patients from being caught in territorial battles. Similarly, institutional requirements must be considered within the structure and frame of the group. Different environments and different patient needs translate into different goals and objectives. For example, Yalom (1983) notes that it is inappropriate to attempt personality reconstruction in a short-stay, acute-care inpatient group. In general, the iller the patient and the briefer the intervention, the greater the need for structure within the group and for therapist sensitivity to affective overstimulation.

PREMATURE TERMINATION/DROP-OUTS FROM GROUP THERAPY

Drop-outs from therapy are an inevitable feature of group psychotherapy (Roback & Smith, 1987; Bernard, 1989; Yalom, 1995). The most critical time for drop-outs is in the early stages of group development, usually within the first twelve weeks (Yalom, 1995). Notwithstanding the best selection process and preparation, drop-outs occur at a rate of 10 to 40 per cent (Stone & Rutan, 1984; Yalom, 1995). Premature termination can produce negative consequences. Individuals may feel rejected, demoralized about psychotherapeutic prospects, and confirmed in 'their worst fears' about themselves. There may also be a negative impact on the group that hinders cohesion and inhibits therapy, although Lothstein (1978) suggests that 'dropping out' may be a necessary facet of group development, and can in fact encourage group cohesion.

Roback and Smith (1987) suggest that the phenomenon of drop-outs be conceptualized in terms of an equation of the patient X therapist X group variables. What fails in one equation may work in another (Bernard, 1989). Features associated with premature termination include:

1 *patient variables*, which include patients who take an inordinately deviant position in the group; those who suffer from a serious impairment in the ability to disclose; those who are afraid of engagement; patients with unworkable character defences (Horner, 1975); patients who are unable to share the leader with others; and complications of concurrent individual psychotherapy, such as competition or unresolvable disagreements between group and individual therapists;

2 *therapist variables*, which include a technical failure to assign patients to groups appropriately, with inadequate treatment matching or inadequate preparation;

3 *patient/therapist interaction variables*, which are also pivotal, and may reflect a countertransference impasse and excesses of therapist function along the vector of activity/passivity that either overstimulate or abandon the patient;

4 *group variables*, which include failure to achieve cohesion or to integrate new members (Rosenthal, 1992).

'Scapegoating' is an associated feature that can go unrecognized and unaddressed, resulting in a vulnerable patient who becomes the object of projected, unacceptable emotions, characteristics, and attributes of other group members.

Therapists must be alert to all aspects of the treatment process, beginning with the kind of referral and the patient's motivation. They must recognize the possibility that group therapy may be perceived by the patient as a cheaper, devalued, second-tier type of therapy. Detailed assessment and preparation (Bernard, 1989; Salvendy, 1993; Rutan & Stone, 1993) are essential to evaluate the patient's capacity to make use of group therapy with a particular group at a particular time. Factors to consider are the ability to identify realistic treatment objectives and the establishment of positive relationships upon which a therapeutic alliance, and ultimately, group cohesion depend. Additional aspects of pre-therapy preparation include informing the patient of the nature and rationale of group therapy and of patient and therapist roles, and anticipating some anxiety about group participation. Preparation can include encouraging the patient to bring personal concerns to the group and to anticipate revisiting core interpersonal and psychological issues that might surface. Establishing a treatment agreement, as discussed later, is another crucial aspect of the assessment and preparation phase.

Dies and Teleska (1985) note that, in the initial phases, the therapist must be alert to imbalances in self-disclosure or space-sharing in the group. Extreme outlyers are liable to drop out of treatment. Conflicts and negative reactions within the group must be addressed in a timely fashion. Group norms for open exploration rather than for acting out or hostile confrontation must be promoted.

Occasionally, treatment is stopped on a therapist's recommendation when an unworkable impasse is reached (Rutan & Stone, 1993). In such cases the patient cannot work productively and undefensively, and is untouched by group norms, resulting in personal and group stagnation. Yalom (1995) notes that it might be necessary to ask a patient to leave, in order not to risk further damage to the individual and the group. He emphasizes that this should be done only after reviewing the contributions of patient, therapist, and group to the impasse (Weiner, 1983) and making efforts to resolve it, including obtaining consultation or supervision. Although it would be ideal for the patient to deal with termination within the group, Yalom notes that it is unlikely to happen at this stage of events. He suggests an individual meeting to facilitate closure. The group may view this event with ambivalence, feeling both relief and guilt at the departure of a patient who obstructed the group, and anger at the therapist for the abandonment. Working through this event may be aided by reaffirming group therapy as an effective treatment and pointing out that, like all treatments, when it is no longer useful, alternative arrangements are needed. The therapist must ensure that suitable, alternative therapy is offered to the terminated individual.

The Setting and the Frame of Group Psychotherapy

THE FRAME OF GROUP PSYCHOTHERAPY

The general frame of group psychotherapy is a once-weekly meeting lasting 90 to 120 minutes, with seven to ten patients, generally both male and female. The group meets regularly at an inviolate time in the same location, which is secure and well boundaried. Modifications to this system might be a group that meets twice weekly, or one with a homogeneous composition to deal with particular issues. Shorter sessions reduce available working time, but sessions longer than two hours generally lead to fatigue, and the work will be less well paced because of inertia or through weakened defences (Rutan & Stone, 1993).

There is general consensus (Rutan & Stone, 1993; Yalom, 1995) that a group size beyond ten provides less opportunity for all members to engage successfully. Small groups of fewer than four or five provide less opportunity for interaction and are liable to disintegrate because of absences and illnesses. Smaller groups tend to become preoccupied with their survival, and hence may be less challenging to their members.

In institutional settings, group therapy is best designed as an integral and valued component of the overall treatment provided by the institution. Group meetings may be more frequent, even daily, and held for shorter lengths of time (Yalom, 1995).

PRE-GROUP PREPARATION AND CONTRACT

There is general consensus that preparation and pre-group contracts facilitate effective outcomes in group therapy (Dies, 1993). The objectives are to clarify patient roles and expectations; to reduce dissonance and undue anxiety; to induce patient behaviour that will be appropriate to the group; and to develop a positive connection between the patient and the therapist (Rutan & Stone, 1993). The therapist explains the rationale for group therapy and illuminates unique aspects of the group. These include working in the here-and-now, the group's function as a social microcosm, and the importance of interpersonal learning. In addition to administrative details, the norms, rules, and structure can be set. These include provisions for confidentiality that note patients' mutual responsibility to protect one another's confidentiality and anonymity; rules about extra-group contact; patient permission for open dialogue between collaborating therapists in concurrent therapies; provision of pharmacotherapy; and the boundaries regarding transmission and exchange of information. This process generally requires two individual sessions prior to the beginning of the group. Proper preparation is correlated with improved tenure, task adherence, self-disclosure, reduced anxiety, and fewer drop-outs. However, there is no overall correlation with improved outcome (Piper, 1993; Yalom, 1993). Frequently, patients with interpersonal difficulties dread recapitulating central difficulties within treatment. It is often helpful for patients to understand that this occurrence, although painful, need not be viewed as a sign of their intractability, but rather as a sign that they are bringing themselves as they 'genuinely are' to the group, in order to address core issues. The anticipation of these difficulties may diminish patient distress and early demoralization (Leszcz, 1989).

DURATION OF THERAPY

Surprisingly, there is little documentation on the typical stay in open-ended dynamic group therapy. Time-limited groups generally run from eight to twenty sessions, but there is little research to guide clinicians as to the optimum number of sessions. A meta-analysis of group therapy with bulimics suggest that a minimum of fifteen sessions is required for effectiveness, and shorter time-limited interventions are significantly less effective (Hartmann, Herzog, & Drinkmann, 1992). It is unclear whether this finding applies to other patient populations treated in time-limited psychotherapy groups.

A study of long-term group therapy (Stone & Rutan, 1984) concluded that approximately 65 per cent of patients complete their therapy within two years. About 35 per cent spend longer than two years in group therapy, with 10 per cent of the remaining one-third leaving after each successive year, resulting in 10 per cent of patients staying in group therapy for four years or longer. Prior or concurrent individual therapy is a strong positive predictor for successful tenure in group psychotherapy. The drop-out rate is significantly higher for patients without previous or concurrent individual therapy. It may be that patients with more experience in therapy are better able to tolerate some of the initial difficulties involved in joining a group. Such patients may be more highly motivated. Further, ongoing individual therapy may provide the new group member with support on entering the group. The frequency, timing, and manner of addressing the entry of a new member is critical because of the powerful effect a new member may have on group cohesion and group development (Stone & Rutan, 1984). Hence, groups that are in crisis, unstable, or dealing with intense and new disclosures are less suitable for the entry of new members. As the entrance of a new member is a major event in the life of the group, the therapist must discuss reactions with group members in order to diminish the possibility that the existing members painfully exclude the new member from the group (Rosenthal, 1992).

CONCURRENT GROUP AND INDIVIDUAL THERAPY

Porter (1993) describes a complementary and potentiating effect of individual and group therapy on each other. Each has its strength in the relative emphasis on intrapsychic exploration versus interpersonal exploration. However, concurrent group and individual therapy is not without controversy, and arguments are put forward by separationists, who fear contamination of one treatment by the other, and by integrationists, who advocate the complementary effectiveness of the two modalities.

Group and individual therapy may be offered by the same therapist – as combined therapy, or by two separate group and individual therapists – as conjoint therapy (Ormont, 1981). Proponents of combined therapy cite the potential for difficulties in collaboration between the conjoint therapists, reflecting competition; failure to communicate information; and the capacity of characterologically difficult patients to use the defence of splitting (Porter, 1993). The two therapists must be genuine collaborators, with mutual respect and clear agreements about the nature and goals of treatment. It is essential to obtain the patient's agreement for open communication between both therapists. Advocates of conjoint therapy suggest that the provision of multiple transference objects, multiple observers, multiple interpreters, multiple maturational agents, and multiple therapeutic settings bolsters the psychotherapy (Ormont, 1981). A particular advantage of conjoint treatment is that both group and individual therapists serve as peer supervisors.

On the other hand, problems with splitting may be better contained in combined therapy. When one therapist has access to all the relevant information the patient presents, there is less potential for the patient to resist treatment by addressing group concerns in the individual therapy and focusing on individual concerns in group therapy. At times, individual therapy may be absolutely necessary in order to sustain a patient in group therapy so that the group experience alone is not too overwhelming or depriving to the individual.

The referral process should not reflect a slough. Issues that are unresolved in one treatment may contaminate the other if they are passed on without recognition. When a second modality is added, it is important to secure the first before adding the second. Typically, individual therapy is begun, and group therapy is added, after the therapeutic alliance is stabilized.

Gans (1990) draws attention to the complexity of the decision to add group therapy to individual therapy, commenting on the impact it has on a patient whose individual therapist informs him or her of the need to enter a group. Several factors need attention – including such countertransference factors as therapist demoralization or hopelessness, or patient factors such as dependence and excessive demandingness. Gans cautions against the countertransferential risk that the recommendation serves the therapist's interest in filling his or her own group with patients. The suggestion of adding group to individual therapy may illuminate therapy issues, especially resistance to further exploration owing to shame, fear of sharing, fear of neglect or the inability to refuse the therapist.

Lipsius (1991) articulates a range of interface issues, noting that handling them is critical to the success of combined treatment. He suggests that the therapist clearly explain the patient's responsibility for bridging material from session to session and bringing material back to the appropriate setting. However, the patient must also agree with the therapist that there is no absolute confidentiality binding the therapist. Rather, the therapist must act with maximum discretion and sensitivity to the clinical needs of the patient, cognizant of the necessity to preserve the essence of each modality. Integration should be the goal. On the other hand, the therapist can use ever-increasing levels of inference, based upon knowledge of patient disclosure in the alternative setting, to seize opportunities for exploration that occur naturally. Similarly, the therapist may subtly encourage more elaboration to help the patient face anticipated conflicts. It may even be appropriate to help the patient directly by introducing the material. Lipsius (1991) notes that the greater value is often obtained by working through the resistance at the interface, not just in reaching disclosure.

CO-THERAPY

There is general consensus that co-therapy is a useful model for training, providing an opportunity for a neophyte to work closely with a more experienced therapist, gaining the rare opportunity of witnessing an experienced therapist at work (Roller & Nelson, 1991; Rutan & Stone, 1993). There is, however, much controversy regarding the utility of co-therapy in non-training situations. Critics suggest that co-therapy is an inefficient use of therapist time, and that it hinders the therapist from assuming full responsibility for treatment. It is also criticized as an attempt to address therapist anxiety, rather than offering something unique or advantageous to the group (Rutan & Stone, 1993). Co-therapy may function as 'a group within the group' (McGee & Schuman, 1970), and the dynamics of that relationship must be monitored to ensure that it does not contaminate the group treatment. There should be genuine equality and sharing of clinical responsibility. Co-therapists must demonstrate mutual respect and a readiness to examine their relationship in regard to dependence, competitiveness, rivalry, and differences in their working rhythm. This may involve consultation or supervision in training situations. They must be alert to the risk of developing a neurotic complementarity and role lock in which each assumes a narrow or constricted posture within the group.

Ideally, co-therapy provides the co-leaders with the opportunities to give each other feedback and deepen awareness of each therapist's use of self; to model openness and conflict resolution for members of the group; to validate each other's feedback; to dilute difficult transferences and countertransferences; and to reduce blind spots that could interfere with the progress of treatment. In some treatment populations in which the emotional load on the therapist is taxing, as with HIV patients, terminally ill patients, or very difficult psychiatric populations, co-therapy may offer support to the co-leaders. For full cooperation, therapists must develop a frame or contract for their relationship so that they can openly evaluate their reactions to each other in a way that is not judgmental or dominated by power or rivalry. Co-therapists will generally have opportunities to meet at five separate interfaces – at pre-group meetings; within the group; at a rehash following the group; in supervision; and at social, non-group occasions. All venues influence the development of a good working co-therapy.

COMBINING DRUG AND GROUP THERAPY

(See chapter 11, 'Guidelines for Combining Psychotherapy and Pharmacology.')

It is increasingly common to have patients treated simultaneously in group psychotherapy and with psychotropic drugs. Stone, Rodenhauser, and Markert (1991), in a survey of AGPA members, noted that group and drug therapy are frequently combined in outpatient group therapy, particularly for patients with mood disorders. In this extensive survey, virtually two-thirds of all group leaders had patients who were treated with medication. Salvendy and Joffe (1991) state that this generally proceeds well with little reported impediment in terms of the psychotherapy. The drug therapy is rarely a focus of resistance. Increasing comfort with integration and eclecticism and a less doctrinaire approach enable therapists to prescribe both modalities simultaneously, without viewing medication as a sign of disappointment or failure of psychotherapy. Rather, the addition of medication can be viewed as a way to treat an affective diathesis, enabling the patient to return to a level playing field on which psychotherapy may be better utilized. Effective anti-depressants do not create a new capacity in the patient, but rather reduce obstructions to capacities already present. Salvendy and Joffe (1991) note that depression may be a cause of therapeutic impasse, and treatment with medication may be pivotal in overcoming it. Medication may be prescribed conjointly, or by the treating group therapist, commonly outside actual group time. Process considerations may include patient compliance, the symbolism of ingesting medication, and reactions of other group members.

Group therapy may support a patient while the patient starts on anti-depressants, and serve as a 'holding environment' until the drug takes effect. Alternatively, many patients who have benefited from antidepressant medication enter a group in order to regain interpersonal function that has been undermined by the affective disorder.

ABSENCE OF LEADERS

The literature documents little consensus regarding recommendations to group therapists about dealing with a therapist's anticipated absence. Rutan and Stone (1993) suggest a range of responses, each with advantages and disadvantages. There are five possible choices a leader or group can make: (1) the group can be cancelled; (2) a double session can be offered; (3) an alternate session without leaders can be held; (4) a substitute leader can be found; or (5) a make-up session can be scheduled. No single solution covers all occasions, but guidelines should be consistently employed within each group, and patients can be told at the outset about them as part of the treatment agreement. Additionally, full opportunities must be provided to process and address reactions to the therapist's absence, to work through any feelings of loss and anger, while at the same time providing continuity and integrating the group-therapy experience.

TERMINATION AND OUTCOME

There is little in the literature to guide the clinician regarding evaluation and suitability for termination in open-ended therapies (Mackenzie, 1990; Rutan & Stone, 1993). Guidelines are clearer in time-limited therapy, in particular with closed groups in which an ending date is established at the outset of treatment. Alternatively, a more elastic approach may give adequate time to conclude therapy and deal with feelings of loss and grief, to work through patients' reactions and resistance to ending. Dealing with the ending phase of treatment requires particular emphasis on translating in-group learning to real-life situations. Therapists should inform patients that therapy is a bridge, not a destination, and that it provides translatable skills, some of which may be actualized only after treatment ends.

If a second course of therapy is required in time-limited treatments, it is best that it be separated by a therapeutic holiday and resumed with clear objectives, rather than as a resumption to avoid ending the first treatment (Mackenzie, 1990). In open-ended situations, treatment should move towards resolution and ending rather than taking an unlimited and interminable course. Goals must be identified and progress towards achievement of these goals regularly evaluated. Rutan and Stone (1993) note that ending an ongoing group is permanent, unlike ending individual therapy, in that the group will change and the individual can no longer return at some later point, as it will be a different group.

Criteria for ending therapy reflect the theoretical underpinnings of contributors to the literature. In addition to symptomatic improvement, these criteria include an increased capacity for stable and intimate engagement; broadening and increasing competence of defensive functions with increased flexibility; resolution of transference; acquisition of greater object constancy; and enhanced creativity and empathic capacity. Rutan and Stone (1993) recommend assessing whether there is more that the patient can realistically gain in a particular context at a particular time. Difficulty in ending may reflect an incompletely effective treatment in which the group is still a major social outlet and in which skills have not been effectively translated into the life of the individual. Alternatively, pursuit of a perfect result may reflect the therapist's wish to achieve completion and reflect the therapist's narcissistic needs, or his or her own difficulties with separation and ending. The general consensus is to set a mutually accepted date for ending, and work towards it (Rutan & Stone, 1993; Yalom, 1995). Setting a date allows an appropriate frame to address the grief and feelings of loss, avoiding a sudden flight or, alternatively, letting it slip away in the midst of other issues.

QUALITY ASSURANCE

Therapy should be thought of as a dynamic treatment process. As such, it may be difficult to evaluate its effectiveness in isolation at any particular moment. Therapists should be aware of the general guidelines regarding the duration of therapy and evaluate the progress of patients regularly in a collaborative fashion. This is easier to do if treatment objectives have been clarified, and patient and therapist agree at the outset that this will be a standard component of the treatment.

Ethical and Legal Considerations

In sum, it is the ethical responsibility of a group leader not to exploit the group or patients for gratification of personal needs (Leszcz, 1994). Gutheil and Gabbard's (1993) outline of boundary maintenance and risk management is as essential for group therapists as it is for individual therapists. These considerations are reflected in the standards of ethical practice put forward by the AGPA (1991a) and by others (Lymberis, 1993), and as noted elsewhere in this text. Unique considerations for group therapy that occur because of the multilateral, multipersonal nature of the treatment include:

1 maintaining confidentiality within the constraints of the law. It is the therapist's responsibility to ensure that co-patients also understand the requirement in this regard and agree to maintain confidentiality about one another.
2 prohibiting sexual contact between therapist and patients, and ensuring that patients do not exploit one another sexually or in any other fashion. Sexual activity between patients is invariably a treatment failure.
3 Ensuring an open process of identifying and working through the tension between the individual's needs and the group needs that exists in properly conducted therapy. It is essential to ensure that the group not exert undue or coercive pressure on the individual members of the group or restrict individual freedom of choice regarding participation.

Proper record keeping is essential, including the initial evaluation, diagnosis, indications for treatment, the patient's informed consent, recognition of other treatment options, group session summaries, regular progress notes, and evaluation of the therapy at regular intervals. This is particularly important in those situations in which there is a lack of positive change (Lymberis, 1993). When group therapy is combined with individual therapy or pharmacotherapy, the therapist must obtain the patient's agreement for collaboration between conjoint therapists and the appropriate exchange of information.

Training of Group Therapists

In order to practise effective group psychotherapy, it is insufficient to be an expert in individual psychotherapy. Familiarity with the principles of dynamic psychotherapy and an understanding of personality development and psychopathology are prerequisites, and a solid grounding in individual therapy is invaluable. However, the practice of group therapy requires special training and knowledge about the mechanisms of change in group therapy; group process; group dynamics; group development; and the pressures exerted by groups on the behaviour of their members, as well as on the group therapist. These forces operate at both overt and covert levels, and require considerable conceptual and experiential knowledge (Rosenberg, 1993). The personal attributes considered desirable for a group therapist include the ability to understand oneself; comprehension of the importance of boundary maintenance; the ability to process countertransference; and the capacity to request supervision and consultation when necessary. Consultation can be useful in any protracted treatment, but is generally underutilized.

With respect to the amount of training required in addition to qualities described elsewhere in this report, the AGPA (1991b) recommends 60 clinical hours and 25 hours of supervision as a minimum. The Canadian Group Psychotherapy Association (CGPA) (1986) has much more demanding requirements: 180 hours of clinical work and 120 hours of supervision. In both situations, supervision must be by a trained and experienced group therapist who belongs to a major professional organization. In addition, the supervisor must be someone actively involved in group psychotherapy. Although there is a discrepancy in the amount of training these two organizations recommend, possibly reflecting the degree of prior training their respective members have, there is agreement that training involves certain core components. These include didactic and theoretical lectures, an opportunity for observing experienced group therapists, and an experiential component involving participation in a psychotherapy group or in a training group, in addition to the clinical/supervisory requirements noted above. Although personal therapy is recommended for group therapists, as it is for individual therapists, there is no definitive evidence to date that the therapist's personal therapy translates into more effective psychotherapeutic outcomes (Aveline, 1992).

References

Alonso, A., & Swiller, H.I. (1993). Introduction: The case for group therapy. In A. Alonso & H.I. Swiller (Eds.), *Group therapy in clinical practice*. Washington, DC: American Psychiatric Press.

American Group Psychotherapy Association (AGPA). (1991a). *Guidelines for ethics*. New York: Author.

American Group Psychotherapy Association (AGPA). (1991b). *The official AGPA training program of the American Group Psychotherapy Association*. New York: Author.

American Psychiatric Association (APA). (1989). *Treatment of psychiatric disorders: A task force report of the American Psychiatric Association*. Washington, DC: Author.

Aveline, M. (1992). Training in psychotherapy. *Current Opinion in Psychiatry, 5,* 365–369.

Bernard, H.S. (1989). Guidelines to minimize premature terminations. *International Journal of Group Psychotherapy, 39,* 523–529.

Bloch, S. (1986). Therapeutic factors in group psychotherapy. In A.J. Frances & R.E. Hales (Eds.), *American Psychiatric Association annual review* (Vol. 5). Washington, DC: American Psychiatric Press.

Bloch, S., & Crouch, E. (1985). *Therapeutic factors in group therapy*. Oxford: Oxford University Press.

Budman, S.H., Demby, A., Redondo, J.P., Hannan, M., Feldstein, M., Ring, J., & Springer, T. (1988). Comparative outcome in time-limited individual and group psychotherapy. *International Journal of Group Psychotherapy, 38,* 63–86.

Canadian Group Psychotherapy Association (CGPA). (1986). *National standards for group psychotherapy training in Canada*. Toronto: Author.

Cole, S.A. (1989). Group therapy in schizophrenia. In APA, *Treatment of psychiatric Disorders: A task force report of the American Psychiatric Association*. Washington, DC: American Psychiatric Association.

Dies, R.R. (1992). Models of group therapy: Sifting through confusion. *International Journal of Group Psychotherapy, 42,* 1–17.

Dies, R.R. (1993). Research on group psychotherapy: Overview and clinical applications. In A. Alonso & H.I. Swiller (Eds.), *Group therapy in clinical practice*. Washington, DC: American Psychiatric Press.

Dies, R.R., & Teleska, P.A. (1985). Negative outcome in group psychotherapy. In D.T. Mays & C. Franks (Eds.), *Negative outcome in psychotherapy and what to do about it*. New York: Springer.

Gans, J.S. (1990). Broaching and exploring the question of combined group and individual therapy. *International Journal of Group Psychotherapy, 40,* 123–137.

Grunenbaum, H., & Kates, W. (1977). Whom to refer for group psychotherapy. *American Journal of Psychiatry, 134,* 130–133.

Gutheil, T.G., & Gabbard, G.O. (1993). The concepts of boundaries in clinical practice: Theoretical and risk-management decisions. *American Journal of Psychiatry, 150,* 188–196.

Hartmann, A., Herzog, T., & Drinkmann, A. (1992). Psychotherapy of bulimia nervosa: 'What is effective?' A meta-analysis. *Journal of Psychosomatics, 32,* 159–167.

Horner, A.J. (1975). A characterological contraindication for group psychotherapy. *Journal of the American Academy of Psychoanalysts, 3,* 301–305.

Leszcz, M. (1986). Inpatient groups. In A.J. Frances & R.E. Hales (Eds.), *American Psychiatric Association annual review* (Vol. 5). Washington, DC: American Psychiatric Press.

Leszcz, M. (1989). Group psychotherapy of the characterologically difficult period. *International Journal of Group Psychotherapy, 39,* 311–335.

Leszcz, M. (1991). Group therapy with the elderly. In J. Sadavoy, L.W. Lazarus & L. Jarvik (Eds.), *Comprehensive review of geriatric psychiatry.* Washington, DC: American Psychiatric Press.

Leszcz, M. (1992). The interpersonal approach to group psychotherapy. *International Journal of Group Psychotherapy, 42,* 37–62.

Leszcz, M. (1994). Failure in group psychotherapy: The therapist variable. *International Journal of Group Psychotherapy, 44,* 25–30.

Lieberman, M.A., Yalom, I.D., & Miles, M.B. (1973). *Encounter groups: First facts.* New York: Basic.

Lipsius, S.H. (1991). Combined individual and group psychotherapy: Guidelines at the interface. *International Journal of Group Psychotherapy, 41,* 313–327.

Lothstein, L.M. (1978). The group psychotherapy dropout phenomenon revisited. *American Journal of Psychiatry, 135,* 1492–1495.

Luborsky, L., Diguer, L., Luborsky, E., Singer, B., Dickter, D., & Schmidt, K.A. (1993). The efficacy of dynamic psychotherapies: Is it true that 'everyone has won and all must have prizes'? In N.E. Miller, L. Luborsky, J.P. Barber, & John P. Docherty (Eds.), *Psychodynamic treatment research: A handbook for clinical practice.* New York: Basic.

Lymberis, M.T. (1983). Ethical and legal issues in group psychotherapy. In A. Alonso & H.I. Swiller (Eds.), *Group therapy in clinical practice.* Washington, DC: American Psychiatric Press.

Mackenzie, K.R. (1990). *Introduction to time-limited group psychotherapy.* Washington, DC: American Psychiatric Press.

Mackenzie, K.R., & Livesley, W.J. (1983). A developmental model for brief group therapy. In R.R. Dies & K.R. Mackenzie (Eds.), *Advances in group psychotherapy integrating research and practice*. New York: International Universities Press.

Mackenzie, Y.R., & Tschuschke, V. (1993). Relatedness, group work and outcome in long-term inpatient psychotherapy groups. *Journal of Psychotherapeutic Practice and Research, 2*, 147–156.

Malan, D.H., Balfour, F.H., Hood, V.G., & Shooter, A.M. (1975). Group psychotherapy: A long-term follow-up study. *Archives of General Psychiatry, 33*, 1303–1315.

McGarrick, A.K., Rosenstein, M.J., Milazzo-Sayre, L.J., & Manderscheid, R.W. (1988). National trends in use of psychotherapy in psychiatric inpatient settings. *Hospital and Community Psychiatry, 39*, 835–841.

McGee, T.F., & Schuman, B.N. (1970). The nature of the co-therapy relationship. *International Journal of Group Psychotherapy, 20*, 25–35.

Melnick, J., & Woods, M. (1976). Analysis of group composition research and theory for psychotherapeutic and growth-oriented groups. *Journal of Applied Behavioral Science, 12*, 473–512.

Ormont, L.R. (1981). Principles and practice of conjoint psychoanalytic treatment. *American Journal of Psychiatry, 138*, 67–73.

Ormont, L.R. (1988). The role of the leader in resolving resistances to intimacy in the group setting. *International Journal of Group Psychotherapy, 38*, 29–45.

Ormont, L.R. (1990). The craft of bridging. *International Journal of Group Psychotherapy, 40*, 3–17.

Piper, W.E. (1993). Group psychotherapy research. In H. Kaplan & B. Sadock (Eds.), *Comprehensive group psychotherapy*. Baltimore: Williams & Wilkins.

Porter, K.I. (1993). Combined individual and group psychotherapy. In H. Kaplan & B. Sadock (Eds.), *Comprehensive group psychotherapy*. Baltimore: Williams & Wilkins.

Roback, H.B., & Smith, M. (1987). Patient attrition in dynamically oriented treatment groups. *American Journal of Psychiatry, 144*, 426–431.

Roller, B., & Nelson, V. (1991). *The Art of cotherapy: How therapists work together*. New York: Guilford.

Rosenberg, P.P. (1993). Qualities of the group therapist. In H. Kaplan & B. Sadock (Eds.), *Comprehensive group psychotherapy*. Baltimore: Williams & Wilkins.

Rosenthal, L. (1992). The new number: 'Infanticide' in group psychotherapy. *International Journal of Group Psychotherapy, 42*, 277–286.

Rothke, S. (1986). The role of interpersonal feedback in group psychotherapy. *International Journal of Group Psychotherapy, 36*, 225–240.

Rutan, J.S., & Stone, W.N. (1993). *Psychodynamic group psychotherapy* (2d ed.). New York: Guilford.

Salvendy, J.T. (1993). Selection and preparation of patients and organization of the group. In H. Kaplan & B. Sadock (Eds.), *Comprehensive group psychotherapy*. Baltimore: Williams & Wilkins.

Salvendy, J.T., & Joffe, R. (1991). Antidepressants in group psychotherapy. *International Journal of Group Psychotherapy, 41*, 465–480.

Smith, M.H., Glass, G.V., & Miller, T.I. (1980). *The benefits of psychotherapy*. Baltimore: Johns Hopkins University Press.

Spiegel, D., Bloom, J.R., Kraemer, H.C., & Gottheil, E. (1989). Effect of psychosocial treatment on survival of patients with metastatic breast cancer. *Lancet, 2* (8668): 888–891.

Stone, W.N., Rodenhauser, P., & Markert, R.J. (1991). Combining group psychotherapy and pharmacotherapy: A survey. *International Journal of Group Psychotherapy, 41*, 449–464.

Stone, W.N., & Rutan, J.S. (1984). Duration of treatment in group psychotherapy. *International Journal of Group Psychotherapy, 34*, 93–109.

Tillitski, C.J. (1990). A meta-analysis of estimated effect sizes for group versus individual versus control treatments. *International Journal of Group Psychotherapy, 40*, 215–224.

Toseland, R., & Siporin, M. (1986). When to recommend group treatment: A review of the clinical and the research literature. *International Journal of Group Psychotherapy, 36*, 171–201.

Weiner, M.F. (1983). The assessment and resolution of impasse in group psychotherapy. *International Journal of Group Psychotherapy, 33*, 313–331.

Yalom, I.D. (1983). *Inpatient group therapy*. New York: Basic.

Yalom, I.D. (1995). *The theory and practice of group psychotherapy* (4th Ed.). New York: Basic.

Zarin, D.A., Pincus, H.A., & McIntyre, J.S. (1993). Editorial: Practice guidelines. *American Journal of Psychiatry, 150*, 175–177.

9. Standards and Guidelines for the Practice of Supportive Psychotherapy

Paul C.S. Hoaken and Harvey Golombek

Supportive factors in psychotherapy refer to those attitudes, personal characteristics, and behaviours a therapist presents in his or her ongoing interaction with a patient that enable the development of a real relationship and a therapeutic alliance. In some supportive therapies, a mild transference may emerge but it is not evident in all supportive therapies. Thus, when a patient experiences support in an interaction with a therapist, he or she enters a safe space where change and development can be entertained and optimistically worked towards.

What is clear with experience and consistent with theoretical formulation is that support does not mean 'doing what comes naturally.' An attitude and presentation that may be deemed supportive by one patient can be experienced by another as unempathic and hostile. To be effective, support must be offered within an appreciation (intuitive or trained) of another person's level of personality organization and central conflictual issues. Some patients feel comforted in the presence of a therapist who seems strong, knowledgeable, and authoritative, while others find such a demeanour to be threatening or infantilizing. It is clear that a therapist must adjust therapeutic style and presentation to meet the individual needs of different patients.

All psychotherapies rely on supportive measures. These refer to those aspects of the treatment that lead a patient to experience both the therapist and the therapy as useful. These techniques tend to be non-cognitive in the sense that they are not primarily aimed at improving self-understanding. Many supportive elements derive from the frame and general attitude of therapy, that is, establishing consistent and reliable meeting times, providing an atmosphere in which both patient and therapist are demonstrably interested in the patient's problems and working towards change, continuously showing interest in the patient's symptoms and goals, conveying a hope that change is possible, and allowing common positive transference expectations to develop and motivate the patient.

Definition of Supportive Psychotherapy

HISTORICAL BACKGROUND

Therapists commonly assert that supportive techniques are an important part of the psychotherapeutic enterprise. When asked to define what is meant by 'support,' they offer varied responses. Giving support tends to mean something different to different therapists who adhere to different conceptual frameworks. The literature contains many definitions and descriptions.

Wolberg (1967), in his chapter on supportive psychotherapy, avoids a definition and proceeds to describe indications for 'supportive measures.' He views such measures as 'a short term exigency for basically sound personality structures'; or 'a primary long-term means of keeping borderline and characterologically dependent patients in homeostasis'; or a way of 'ego building,' a prelude to 'more reintegrative psychotherapeutic tasks'; 'a temporary expedient during insight therapy' (pp. 71–72), to allow undue anxiety to subside. Further, Wolberg indicates that these measures include those used 'haphazardly' by the patient's friends. However, those in helping roles, such as general physicians, ministers, nurses, teachers, and correctional workers, use them in a more planned and deliberate way, while social workers, psychologists, and psychiatrists use them most deliberately. Wolberg's concept of supportive psychotherapy is enlarged by his inclusion in the chapter of sections on 'guidance' ('based on an authoritarian relationship established between therapist and patient'), 'environmental manipulation,' and 'externalization of interests' (p. 56).

Werman (1984), in his book on supportive psychotherapy, also avoids a definition. While acknowledging that terms such as 'supportive psychotherapy' and 'insight-oriented psychotherapy' are popularly used, he points out that the names attached to the modalities 'are neither very accurate nor sharply descriptive' (p. ix).

Conte (1994) states that supportive psychotherapy 'is probably the most common form of psychotherapy used for patients in acute crisis situations,' but 'there still remains some confusion over what supportive psychotherapy is and is not' (p. 496).

Pinsker (1994) states: 'supportive psychotherapy is characterized by a very limited approach that entails ventilation, the "holding environment," abreaction, reassurance, reality-testing, clarification, suggestion, advice and limit-setting' (p. 531).

WORKING DEFINITION

Supportive psychotherapy focuses on aspects of the psychotherapeutic encounter which promote a decrease in psychopathology without the primary goal of enhancing self-understanding. Novalis, Rojcewicz, and Pelle (1993) describe the following aims: (a) to promote a supportive therapist–patient relationship; (b) to enhance the patient's strengths, coping skills, and capacity to use environmental supports; (c) to reduce the patient's subjective distress and behavioural dysfunction; (d) to achieve for the patient the greatest practical degree of independence from his or her psychiatric illness; and (e) to foster the greater degree of autonomy in treatment decisions for the patient. Supportive psychotherapy is technically eclectic in that it does not presuppose a particular theory of psychopathology.

Importance of Education

Since supportive psychotherapy is not based on any one particular theory of mental disorder, mental functioning, or personality development, it is often thought of as therapy by default, or as a type of treatment to be relegated to residents or non-psychiatric therapists (Werman, 1984). However, the viewpoint that improvement in patients receiving psychotherapy depends less on the theoretical orientation of the therapist than it does on certain personal characteristics of the therapist and features of the therapy process underscores the importance of general and supportive factors in all kinds of psychotherapy and indicates that more attention should be directed to the instruction of trainees in supportive techniques (Marmor, 1975; Luborsky, Singer, & Luborsky, 1975; Strupp, 1978b; Karasu, 1986, Frank & Frank, 1991; Grunebaum, 1983; Pinsker, 1994). Research has found high intercorrelations among a set of patients' expressions in psychotherapy that were evidence of patients' experiences of a helping alliance with the therapist, and these expressions significantly predicted the outcome of psychotherapy (Luborsky, 1984). Strupp (1978a) believes that, although native ability is an asset in the therapist, some of the attributes of the good therapist can be taught.

The Doctor–Patient Relationship and Supportive Psychotherapy

In many ways, supportive psychotherapy develops as a natural continuation of the doctor–patient relationship that begins in the initial assessment meeting. Indeed, this relationship may begin even before the first meeting, because of patient expectation. The referring physician's comments about the psychiatrist, what the patient may have heard about the psychiatrist's reputation, ideas the patient may have about psychiatrists from films and magazine cartoons, all contribute. Once the patient has arrived for assessment, there are several factors which may influence the development of the relationship and of which the psychiatrist and trainee must be aware. These include: age and gender of the therapist; his or her dress and grooming; location of the office (in a hospital or in a private office building); decor of the office (Grunebaum, 1983); and attitude of the reception staff. Those coming for help are vulnerable and likely to be sensitive to *perceived* coldness, abruptness, or lack of consideration. Once regular psychotherapy sessions begin, one non-specific supportive aspect is the predictability of the therapist. That is, the assurance the patient obtains from knowing that the psychiatrist is always, or almost always, available for scheduled appointments; and that, regardless of most exigencies of his or her personal life, the psychiatrist will be interested, accepting, and supportive. In other words, he or she is a reliable ally. Unreliability may be viewed by the patient as harmful (Grunebaum, 1986).

The traditional doctor–patient relationship on which patients' expectations are based can best be described as the purchase of specialized services from an identified expert by someone in need of such services. Changes in this model over the last twenty to thirty years have altered patients' expectations, possibly vitiating the effectiveness of the psychiatrist's efforts in doing supportive psychotherapy. First, the widespread dissemination of information and misinformation in the news media and lay publications, and the proliferation of self-help articles and books, may affect patients' expectations about the value of the knowledge and skill of psychiatrists. Expectations the patient has about the psychiatrist and about the treatment are important ingredients in supportive psychotherapy, but the efficacy of supportive psychotherapy is not based solely on patients' expectations. That is, it is not placebo treatment (Patterson, 1985). Second, the spate of publicity about the sexual abuse of patients by psychiatrists and other therapists may weaken patients' trust in psychiatrists, particularly male psychiatrists. Last, it is common now for the patient not to pay directly for such expert services, payment coming instead from an insuring agent. Third-party payment could affect the accountability of both patient and physician, and influence the doctor–patient relationship.

Patient evaluation, including comprehensive history and mental-status examination, leading to a formulation and diagnosis, provides the psychiatrist an opportunity to demonstrate many of the desirable personal characteristics of a psychotherapist. These include: interest in the patient as a unique person, tact and sensitivity in obtaining information, and empathic understanding. Although, for teaching purposes, interviewing skills are distinguished from psychotherapy, supportive psychotherapy can begin with a sensitive interview and examination.

Conceptual Framework for Supportive Psychotherapy

Although supportive psychotherapy does not emanate from any one specific theory of psychopathology or mental functioning, it would be a mistake to conclude that there is no underlying rationale. The rationale derives from the following clinical observations and ethical principles. First, troubled people have always talked to others for the purpose of obtaining relief and bringing about some change in behaviour (Katz, 1986). Second, each person coming for help has value and deserves help. Third, each person, in the role of patient, is a unique individual who has had unique experiences during the developmental years as well as in adult life. Even though such a person may have a diagnosable disorder, a diagnosis conveys a limited amount of information about that person and his or her problems. Fourth, research suggests that there are certain elements common to all effective psychotherapies (Marmor, 1975) and using these elements will help patients, regardless of the source of the problems. These include a patient–therapist relationship based on trust and rapport; release of tension through ventilation; understanding of the basis of the patient's symptoms and problems; operant reconditioning by means of the therapist's subtle signs of approval/disapproval; suggestion and persuasion; identification with the therapist; reality-testing (practising of new adaptive techniques); and emotional support from the therapist. Fifth, the patient possesses the ability to benefit from these elements operating in a human relationship with a specially trained person, the psychiatrist, as a nurturing, parent-like figure (Strupp, 1978a).

PSYCHOANALYTIC PERSPECTIVES

Psychoanalytically oriented therapists (Werman, 1984) generally believe that a dynamic understanding of the patient is essential for the therapist. Most psychiatrists practising supportive psychotherapy accept the importance of such dynamic factors as unconscious motivation; the influence of past experience in the understanding of patients' problems; and the significance of transference feelings in some supportive therapies. However, the acceptance of all aspects of psychoanalytic metapsychology is not necessary in order to practise effective supportive psychotherapy.

In 1951, Gill stated, 'While the two poles of either strengthening the defenses, or of analyzing them as first steps toward reintegrating the damaged ego, stand as gross opposites of two theoretical modes of approach, the psychotherapy of any specific case will show intricate admixtures of both' (p. 63). In Gill's conceptualizing, the concept of strengthening the defences provides the organizing framework for all the supportive approaches. He specified two ways in which defences can be strengthened:

1 Praise, or, in general, give narcissistic support for, those ego activities in which defence is combined with adaptive gratification, and discourage by subtle or direct techniques those activities which provide maladaptive gratification.
2 Take care not to attack unwittingly an important defence which is critically stabilizing personality organization; for example, leave unexamined the denial of dependency wishes in the treatment of a middle-adolescent patient.

Wallerstein, in 1986, suggested that the establishment of a positive dependent transference attachment is a basic feature of all supportive psychotherapy approaches. It is a basic element in the operation of the so-called transference cure. This concept is used to indicate the willingness and desire of the patient to reach certain goals and achieve certain changes as things being done 'for the therapist,' in gratitude for the gratification of needs within the attachment relationship. To the extent that some aspects of transference remain unanalysed in all supportive psychotherapies, in all psychodynamic therapies, and in most, if not all, analyses, it can be said that this factor is an important element of all psychotherapeutic work. As Wallerstein reported, the findings of the Psychotherapy Research Project indicate that, in the therapies characterized by a high degree of unanalysed positive dependent transference attachment, positive changes that do take place have surprising endurance. In the research project, it was concluded that half of the patients studied showed clear-cut evidence of the important operation of this mechanism.

Several varieties of the positive dependent transference attachment are described by Wallerstein. These include the 'Transfer of the Transference' and the 'Displacement of the Neurosis into the Transference.'

In the mechanism described as the 'Transfer of the Transference,' the patient finds a way to displace the positive dependent feelings, thoughts, and fantasies from the person of the therapist onto an available and suitable person in the immediate environment, usually family members, but sometimes other external helping professionals. This transfer carries enough valence and durability that the manifest tie within and to the therapist in the therapy itself can be relinquished.

In the mechanism described as the 'Displacement of the Neurosis into the Transference,' the patient comes to feel that, since he or she can experience positive dependent transference gratification within the treatment, he or she can then relinquish dependent and passive attitudes and behaviours towards others in the external world. The patient comes to feel that the therapist requires that he or she make changes in his or her everyday life as the price of the continuing therapeutic relationship. Although the mechanism of enacting the conflicts within the transference are the same as those operative within the transference neurosis, the difference is that, in this case, the patient does not do so with the aim and intention of understanding and resolving the core conflicts, but does so in the unanalysed service of being used to enforce new behaviour expectations.

Another supportive mechanism is the corrective emotional experience, as described by Gill (1954). This concept implies the provision of a steadfastly concerned therapeutic stance, equidistant from the conflicting intrapsychic forces within the patient, and corrective in precisely the sense of not being drawn to respond in counteraction to the patient's transference expectations and pulls. Using this technique the therapist is able to help the patient untangle distortions in object representations, and subsequently develop more satisfying relationships, even with little appreciation of the maladaptive patterns involved or understanding of the underlying neurotic conflict.

Indications for Supportive Psychotherapy

There is no consensus on the indications for supportive psychotherapy, and, indeed, an opinion about indications is likely to be strongly influenced by the theoretical orientation of the person providing the opinion. For example, Werman (1984) acknowledges that supportive psychotherapy is indicated for 'a vast number of individuals,' but assumes that supportive psychotherapy is chosen when 'the patient's psychological equipment is fundamentally inadequate' (p. 3). Dewald (1994), in contrast, believes that the vast majority of patients coming for treatment are seeking the prompt symptomatic relief that supportive psychotherapy can provide. Given that research results fail to favour one type of psychotherapy over any other in heterogeneous populations (Luborsky et al, 1975), and that personal and therapeutic relationship factors are crucial ingredients in effective psychotherapy, including the more technical therapies (Grunebaum, 1983; Bergin & Lambert, 1978; Luborsky, McClellan, Wood, O'Brien, & Auerbach, 1985), it is appropriate to view supportive psychotherapy as the treatment of choice for many patients.

Supportive Psychotherapy as Treatment of Choice

Supportive psychotherapy is the treatment of choice for the following patients:

1 patients experiencing adjustment disorders without histories of chronic severely maladaptive behaviour;
2 patients with some maladaptive personality characteristics who seek treatment for an acute crisis;
3 patients with severe personality disorders who are not suitable for other kinds of psychotherapy;
4 patients with major mental disorders receiving pharmacotherapy;
5 patients who have responded badly to an acute severe, or chronic disabling, medical disorder.

Supportive psychotherapy does not exclude the development of insight concerning preconscious and rational material (Dewald, 1994), and at times incorporates techniques from other approaches, such as psychoanalytically oriented, behavioural, and cognitive therapies.

Goals of Supportive Psychotherapy

The goals of supportive psychotherapy depend on the type of patient and the severity of the psychopathology. Ideally, the major goal is to reduce symptoms, improve the patient's morale and confidence, increase autonomy (Pinsker, 1994), and help the patient develop some understanding of the symptoms and their origin. However, at times, goals may be very restricted: for example, to keep the patient functioning well enough to remain in the community instead of being admitted to hospital (Dewald, 1994).

Limits and Therapeutic Boundaries of Supportive Psychotherapy

Although supportive psychotherapy can be considered eclectic, there are limits to its practice. Such therapy does not focus on unconscious conflict, transference, and resistance; nor does it consistently use the didactic techniques and advice commonly found in cognitive and behavioural therapies.

Since there is no set prescription for the behaviour of psychiatrists doing supportive psychotherapy, as there is in psychoanalytically oriented psychotherapy, and since the supportive therapist is expected to be openly friendly, there is perhaps a greater potential risk for supportive psychotherapists to violate professional boundaries. When do warmth and friendliness become undue familiarity? When practising supportive therapy, psychiatrists must monitor their behaviour carefully and be guided by their knowledge of the patient's strengths and vulnerabilities obtained through comprehensive assessment and continuing treatment sessions. They must also keep in mind the fiduciary nature of the relationship and be aware of early stages of weakening boundaries (Simon, 1995).

Techniques of Supportive Psychotherapy

During the course of any psychotherapeutic treatment, the therapist must continuously assess for the level of personality strength. Patients with lower-level personality organization who employ immature defences, and have difficulty with object constancy and affect regulation and containment, require increased supportive intervention. Patients with higher levels of personality organization may derive sufficient support from the standard frame of the treatment process and from the mutual work of developing insights which lead to new adaptations and coping strategies. For these patients the experience of empathically attuned and insightfully correct understanding may contain sufficient support to allow the work to progress effectively.

The following is a partial list of techniques commonly used in supportive psychotherapy (Conte, 1994; Pinsker, 1994; Wolberg, 1967; Strupp, 1978a; Luborsky, 1984).

1 *Communication:* The communication through words and manner of an acceptance and understanding of the patient in his or her distress, and an acceptance of the patient's desire to change.

2 *Information:* Information about the mental disorder, including its prevalence, etiological factors, prognosis, and effective treatment, can be reassuring. When emotional turmoil interferes with the patient's ability to assimilate such information, it is often helpful to provide the patient with written information for future reference.

3 *Reassurance:* This has many aspects. A patient may be reassured by finding out that the psychiatrist is a reliable ally. Telling the patient about experience with other patients with similar symptoms or problems, a form of limited self-disclosure, is also reassuring. Patients also need to be told that they are not 'insane' and there is hope for improvement. The psychiatrist's exploration of the patient's effectiveness in coping with past life problems, together with a discussion of techniques that might be helpful for current problems, is also reassuring.

4 *Acknowledgment:* The therapist acknowledges the strengths and assets of the patient in dealing with personal problems (Grunebaum, 1983), and helps the patient maintain areas of competence and adaptive defences (Luborsky, 1984). It is also important to acknowledge and commend the patient's progress towards achieving goals of therapy.

5 *Hope:* The psychiatrist, during interactions with the patient, generates hopeful but reasonable expectations about improvement (Luborsky, 1984).

6 *Suggestion and advice:* In order to foster patient autonomy, suggestions are best formulated as questions (e.g., 'Have you thought of talking to your husband about his drinking?'). Another useful method is to explore options by the use of hypothetical questions (e.g., 'What do you think your husband would say if you talked to him about his drinking?'). Direct advice should be reserved for situa-

tions where it is essential to prevent harm to the patient, but otherwise should be avoided, if possible. Supportive psychotherapy is not counselling.

7 *Expression of thoughts and feelings:* Ventilation is frequently useful (together with appropriate empathic statements from the psychiatrist), but it should not continue to the point where the patient uses it in place of *doing* something to solve problems. Some patients need encouragement to express themselves openly to the psychiatrist, especially about personal and private concerns. Others need support and encouragement to express themselves openly in their personal and social relationships.

8 *Reinforcement:* Encouragement and the verbal or non-verbal rewarding of mature adaptive behaviour are useful techniques.

9 *Clarifications and confrontations:* These are useful to help the patient focus on behaviours that have not been adaptive, and possibly on patterns of maladaptive behaviour.

10 *Reinforcing the alliance:* The therapeutic alliance is reinforced by the psychiatrist's referring to experiences in therapy that he or she and the patient have been through together. The alliance is also strengthened by the psychiatrist's conveying to the patient that, together, they are engaging in a search for an understanding of the patient's symptoms and for measures that will bring relief.

11 *Modulating anxiety:* Conflict between various agencies within the personality or with reality leads to anxiety, which is modulated by defence mechanisms. If anxiety becomes excessive, the patient can experience intense feelings of helplessness, of being overwhelmed, of being disorganized or impotent. Anxiety, within normal limits, is viewed as a primary affect which alerts a patient to danger but also acts as a motivator to stimulate appropriate defences and adaptive behaviour. Within psychotherapy the therapist pays continual attention to the level of anxiety. Too much or too little impedes the progress of treatment. In general, supportive techniques decrease the level of anxiety while expressive techniques increase it.

Some forms of treatment may challenge the psychiatrist's ability to utilize supportive techniques. For example, a psychiatrist working in a subspecialty clinic (e.g., a mood-disorders clinic) may have such a narrowly defined task that other aspects of the patient's distress are not dealt with. It is a challenge for psychoanalysts concerned with the proper use of expressive techniques (Dewald, 1994), especially therapeutic abstinence as a technical manoeuvre (Pinsker, 1994; Werman 1984), to be optimally spontaneous and forthcoming in supportive psychotherapy. Behaviour therapists and cognitive therapists may seem too didactic to be supportive to patients.

Training Recommendations

Residents should be taught about the elements that are believed to be effective in all psychotherapies. Supportive psychotherapy should not be depicted as a second choice, used only when patients are not suitable for some more specific kind of psychotherapy. Rather, it is a treatment of choice for some patients. In fact, it comprises a useful and effective set of strategies and techniques that can be employed, beginning in the initial assessment interview and examination. Training should include opportunities for residents to observe their teachers doing supportive psychotherapy, and for teachers to observe residents' sessions with patients.

References

Bergin, A.E., & Lambert, M.J. (1978). The evaluation of therapeutic outcomes, in S.L. Garfield & A.E. Bergin (Eds.), *Handbook of psychotherapy and behaviour change: An empirical analysis* (2d ed.). New York: Wiley.

Conte, H.R. (1994). Review of research in supportive psychotherapy: An update. *American Journal of Psychotherapy, 48,* 494–504.

Dewald, P.A. (1994). Principles of supportive psychotherapy. *American Journal of Psychotherapy, 48,* 505–518.

Frank, J.D., & Frank, J.B. (1991). *Persuasion and Healing: A comparative study of psychotherapy.* (3d ed.). Baltimore: Johns Hopkins University Press.

Gill, M.M. (1951). Ego psychology and psychotherapy. *Psychoanalytic Quarterly, 20,* 62–71.

Gill, M.M. (1954). Psychoanalysis and exploratory psychotherapy. *Journal of the American Psychoanalytic Association, 2,* 771–797.

Grunebaum, H. (1983). A study of therapists' choice of a therapist. *American Journal of Psychiatry, 140,* 1336–1339.

Grunebaum, J. (1986). Harmful psychotherapy experience. *American Journal of Psychotherapy, 40,* 165–176.

Karasu, T. (1986). The specificity versus the nonspecificity dilemma: Toward identifying therapeutic change agents. *American Journal of Psychiatry, 143,* 687–695.

Katz, P. (1986). The role of the psychotherapies in the practice of psychiatry: The position of the Canadian Psychiatric Association. *Canadian Journal of Psychiatry, 31*, 458–465.

Luborsky, L. (1984) *Principles of psychoanalytic psychotherapy: A manual for supportive–expressive treatment.* New York: Basic.

Luborsky, L., McClellan, A.T., Wood, G.E., O'Brien, C.P. & Auerbach, A. (1985). Therapist success and its determinants. *Archives of General Psychiatry, 42*, 602–611.

Luborsky, L., Singer, B., & Luborsky, L. (1975). Comparative studies of psychotherapies. *Archives of General Psychiatry, 32*, 995–1008.

Marmor, J. (1975). The nature of the psychotherapeutic process revisited. *Canadian Psychiatric Association Journal, 20*, 557–565.

Novalis, P.M., Rojcewicz, S.J. Jr, & Pelle, R. (1993). *Clinical manual of supportive psychotherapy.* Washington, DC: American Psychiatric Press.

Patterson, C.H. (1985). What is the placebo in psychotherapy? *Psychotherapy, 22*, 163–169.

Pinsker, H. (1994). The role of theory in teaching supportive psychotherapy. *American Journal of Psychotherapy, 48*, 530–541.

Simon, R. (1995). The natural history of therapist sexual misconduct: Identification and prevention. *Psychiatric Annals, 25*, 88–89.

Strupp, H. (1978a). The nature of the therapeutic influence and its basic ingredients. In A. Burton (Ed.) *What makes behaviour change possible?* New York: Brunner/Mazel.

Strupp, H. (1978b). The therapist's theoretical orientation: An overrated variable. *Psychotherapy: Theory, Research and Practice, 15*, 314–317.

Wallerstein, R.S. (1986). *Forty-two lives in treatment: A study in psychoanalysis and psychotherapy.* New York: Guilford.

Werman, D.S. (1984). *The practice of supportive psychotherapy.* New York: Brunner/Mazel.

Wolberg, L.R. (1967). *The Technique of psychotherapy* (2d ed.). New York: Grune & Stratton.

10. Guidelines for the Practice of Psychotherapy with Children and Adolescents

Marshall Korenblum

Why is it important for clinicians of varied backgrounds to have access to practice guidelines in the area of child and adolescent psychotherapy (hereinafter referred to as 'child therapy,' and encompassing individual, family, and group formats unless otherwise specified)? On a practical note, there are simply too few subspecialists to meet the need of the child-psychiatric population (Offord, Boyle, & Racine, 1989; Heseltine, 1983; Cleghorn, Miller, & Humphrey, 1982). Mental health professionals who are not child psychiatrists can therefore expect to (and already do) treat a significant number of young people (Looney, Ellis, & Benedek, 1985; Parker, 1992). Often, however, these clinicians feel inadequately trained (Looney, 1980).

Guidelines also offer heuristic value. Familiarity with child therapy can enhance one's understanding of the origins of adult psychopathology (e.g., the role of temperament and trauma in the genesis of personality disorders); a greater appreciation of how phenomenology changes over time (e.g., depressive symptoms across the lifespan) can be gleaned; the clinician is better prepared for working with difficult adult populations.

Forensic patients, for instance, like some children, frequently use denial or are pressured to attend therapy by others. Borderline patients, like some children, tend to express primitive affects, may act out, and elicit intense transference and countertransference phenomena. Geriatric patients, like some children, often require observational and non-verbal techniques to assist in diagnosis and treatment, and involve collateral informants or systemic interventions because of cognitive limitations which impair communication. Indeed, some have suggested that 'child' cases are actually the most challenging adult cases that general mental health practitioners will ever see (Kendziora & O'Leary, 1993).

For the clinician who actually chooses to *do* child therapy, acting as an agent of prevention and being able to observe large changes over reasonably short periods of time can be extremely rewarding.

Practice guidelines are useful for parents, as well as for professionals. In this era of increased accountability, parents have a right to publicly accessible, evidence-based indications as to 'best practices' for the treatment of their children's emotional problems. The therapeutic endeavour almost always represents a partnership between clinician and parent (or primary caregiver). An educated partnership strengthens this alliance.

The importance of developing a shared collaborative relationship with parents cannot be overemphasized (Sanders & Dadds, 1993; Sanders & Lawton, 1993). Especially with younger children, parental resistance can be a major cause of premature drop-out from therapy and poor treatment outcome, whether the focus is on the child or the parents.

Some authors have even called for a 'Copernican revolution' in which parenting is no longer the Sun orbiting the Earth (the child), but the centre about which the child revolves (Kendziora & O'Leary, 1993). According to this model, dysfunctional parenting would become a disorder in its own right, with a spectrum of interventions ranging from brief written instructions, with no therapist contact; to specific advice, plus active training via video-modelling, rehearsal, and feedback; to intensive behavioural family intervention involving sophisticated behavioural management techniques which simultaneously focus on parent–child interactions, marital stress, anger control, and extrafamilial tensions (Sanders, 1996). In fact, *DSM-IV* (American Psychiatric Association, 1994) has a V-Code category called 'Parent–Child Relational Problem,' thus lending credibility to the importance of this area as a focus of attention.

Modern conceptualizations of childhood psychopathology acknowledge the bidirectionality of parent–child influences, viewing aberrant development as arising from 'misattunements' or poor 'fit' between temperament (of both child and parent) and child (or parent)-rearing.

It certainly behooves the therapist of any child, especially the preadolescent, to engage the parents in a contracting process in which they accept the relationship between their actions and their child's behaviour, and achieve consensus about the nature of the problem. The reverse is also true – that it is important to obtain an alliance with the child, especially with adolescents, if the parents are being counselled.

While all of the psychotherapies described elsewhere in this volume have been used with the child population, and share many underlying principles, there are sufficient differences to warrant distinct guidelines. For child therapy, these differences include: (1) different effects and frame requirements, depending on the patient's developmental stage; (2) a systemic perspective because of the degree to which children are dependent upon context (e.g., family and school). These contexts may have tremendous impact on the outcome of psychotherapy, and there-fore need to considered in any treatment plan; (3) a multidisciplinary perspective because of the frequent need for collaboration with other professionals; (4) unique emphasis on non-verbal (e.g., play) techniques because of linguistic and cognitive limitations; (5) the sensitivity of chil-dren to separation; (6) special considerations with respect to consent, capacity, confidentiality, and research; (7) intense countertransference, especially with abused children, and intense transference (e.g., erotic and aggressive), especially with adolescents; (8) greater need to set lim-its on 'acting in' and 'acting out'; (9) unique legal and ethical obligations when a disclosure of abuse occurs during the course of psychotherapy.

Historical Overview

The antecedents of contemporary child therapy can be traced to religious and philosophical beliefs about the nature of childhood. In the Middle Ages, for instance, baptism and exorcism were common approaches to childhood behavioural problems. These practices were predicated on assumptions of 'evil' or original sin.

In the seventeenth and eighteenth centuries, Locke and Rousseau advocated deconditioning for childhood fears. In the nineteenth century, Itard's work with the 'wild boy of Aveyron' began to approximate today's comprehensive inclusion of cognitive, affective, behavioural, social, and educational components.

Modern psychodynamic psychotherapy is generally thought to have begun with Freud's 1909 report of treating Little Hans via his father, and the adolescent 'Dora' (Freud, 1905/1953, 1909/1955). Anna Freud (1963), Melanie Klein (1932), and Hermine von Hug-Hellmuth (1921) subsequently systematized the use of play as a central metaphor and change agent in the therapy of children, equating it with free association in the analysis of adults.

Levy (1939), Alpert (1959), and Mahler and Furer (1982) introduced modifications of psychoanalytic play therapy for use with more disturbed populations (e.g., specific traumas and pervasive developmental disorders), which included parents.

In the 1950s and 1960s treatments based on learning theory led to behaviour modification for various 'habit disturbances'; group therapy incorporating activity was used for passive, constricted children (Slavson, 1955); family therapy for relational and communication problems came into its own (Haley, 1963; Satir, 1967); and brief, time-limited therapy began to be defined for this age group (Proskauer, 1969).

The therapeutic armamentarium has continued to expand, with parent management programs for conduct-disordered youth (Dumas, 1989), and exciting new applications of data from infant psychiatry based on attachment theory (Muir, 1992; Lojkasek, Cohen, & Muir, 1994), which address the parent–infant dyad as the unit of treatment.

In summary, there is no unified, integrated conceptual model of child therapy (Carek, 1972). Neither is there such a model for adult psychotherapy. While many of its principles and techniques have been 'borrowed' from adult psychiatry, child therapy continues to evolve, and, as it does, its own unique stamp will probably be further refined.

Empirical and Research Foundations

Evaluating the efficacy of child therapy is complicated by many factors. Techniques, and therefore outcome, can vary, depending on who is seen (child, parents, or family), the mode of treatment (talk, play, or activity), the central focus (affects, cognitions, behaviours, or social skills), and the setting (office, home, school, or other).

In trying to establish diagnostically homogeneous groups, one is confronted by the reality of co-morbidity, which may run as high as 50 per cent (Bird et al, 1988), and both *DSM-IV* and ICD-10 assume that a single individual has a disorder. With children, one is frequently dealing with interpersonal dysfunction as the presenting and most important problem.

Developmental factors are probably the most serious impediments to evaluation. Because children are often unreliable informants, it is necessary to use several different sources of information for purposes of measuring symptom change. Unfortunately, parents and teachers (the commonest sources) often disagree (Offord et al, 1989).

In longitudinal studies, measurement tools may have to change according to a child's age. Researchers are then left to wonder whether differences over time are real, or a function of differences in the instruments used.

Base rates of certain behaviours wax and wane at different ages, and so outcome has to be assessed against developmental norms. Treatment effects have maturational processes as strong competitors for explaining observed changes. Unfortunately, many studies combine children of diverse ages, thus obscuring possibly meaningful processes, or use age instead of developmental stage as a marker.

Age alone is a very poor construct because it fails to elucidate underlying change mechanisms and again can mask important patterns. In the ten-to-thirteen age range, for instance, it is well known that pubertal status can vary widely. This factor, however, is rarely assessed in therapy studies.

The impact of context varies with stage. For younger children, parent and family functioning can influence who drops out of treatment, the degree of change among those who remain, and maintenance of gains over time (Kazdin, 1990). As a corollary, parent-training methods are more likely to be optimally effective in this age group. For adolescents, peer relations become particularly important, as does the need for privacy. As a result, group and individual therapies have greater relevance.

Long-term effects of treatment are important to evaluate. Yet, outcome is usually assessed immediately after treatment has ended, or at most perhaps one year later. Greater validity would be established if gains could be shown to persist into adulthood, and change mechanisms would be better understood if longitudinal patterns – for example, 'sleeper effects' – could be identified.

A truly developmental perspective requires a complex paradigm which accounts for changes in the child over time, both symptomatically and adaptively (i.e., global functioning), as they relate to and interact with changes in the interpersonal environment. A static model will not suffice.

Practical impediments to appraising psychotherapy exist because of age. Ethical constraints are often greater than in adult research because of the need to demonstrate informed consent. Parents may be less cooperative both because they may *not* be the target of a study and because they *are*. Even simple blood tests must be justified by clear clinical benefit when the subjects are under sixteen (Steinhauer, Bradley, & Gauthier, 1992).

Despite these problems, a number of methodological improvements have occurred over the past fifteen years. For one, assessment tools have become much more standardized. Diagnostic interviews for children (Edelbrock & Costello, 1988; Puig-Antich & Ryan, 1986), and symptom rating scales for depression, anxiety, tics, eating disorders, obsessions and compulsions, and hyperactivity are now available. They are all compatible with *DSM-IV*, demonstrate excellent reliability and validity, and can be used to establish baselines against which therapeutic responses can be determined.

Of course, such inventories do not provide the comprehensive assessment of feelings, personality style, coping mechanisms, or strengths that the clinical interview does (Kestenbaum, 1991; Lewis, 1991), but they certainly facilitate researchable studies. Even the documentation of development with respect to various realms of adaptive functioning can be done in a standardized fashion (John, Gammon, Prusoff, & Warner, 1987; Sparrow, Balla, & Cicchette, 1984).

As well, the assessment of non-clinical youth has advanced significantly (Achenbach & Edelbrock, 1981), thus establishing a firm base upon which to detect therapeutic change.

Finally, treatment approaches for children have been operationalized. Therapy manuals exist for psychoanalytically oriented treatments (Kernberg & Chazan, 1991), family therapy (Alexander & Parsons, 1982), cognitve therapy (Horne & Sayger, 1990), parent training (Forehand & McMahon, 1981), social-skills training (Michelson, Sugai, Wood, & Kazdin, 1983), mother–infant interventions (Muir, 1992), and brief psychotherapy of varied modalities (Dulcan, 1984), to name but a few.

Psychotherapy Outcome and Efficacy

METHODOLOGICAL ISSUES

Unfortunately, pharmacotherapy for children has not been uniformly effective, and outcome studies of drug treatments have been disappointing (Jensen, Ryan, & Prien, 1992). Consequently, research into psychosocial interventions is vital.

In evaluating the effectiveness of child therapy, one must begin with certain caveats. Behaviour modification and cognitive/behavioural techniques account for about half of all treatment studies over the past twenty years (Kazdin, Bass, Ayers, & Rodgers, 1990). Other, more traditional therapies in child psychiatry, such as family therapy, play therapy, or combined approaches, have been only infrequently examined. Very few studies using controlled clinical trials have looked at psychodynamic psychotherapy (Fonagy & Moran, 1990).

Unfortunately, the very modalities which have been least studied are the ones which are used most frequently in clinical practice (Silver & Silver, 1983), often in combination. This gap between how treatment is studied and how it is practised is apparent in other ways.

Route of referral, duration of treatment, types of dysfunctions, settings, and involvement of parents or teachers as reported in the literature often differ from what is done in 'real life' (Kazdin et al, 1990; Weisz, Donenberg, Han, & Weiss, 1995; Seligman, 1995). The impact of these differences on the ability to assess the efficacy of child therapy is not small. In most studies, children are recruited for treatment and are not actual clinical cases. Selection bias is thus significant. It has been shown, for instance, that mothers who respond to advertisements on behalf of their children are likely to be motivated by their own psychopathology, or the fact that they have poor access to health care and social supports (Harth & Thong, 1990).

Studies choose subjects with only one or two focal problems, to enhance homogeneity. Therapists receive concentrated pre-therapy training, and therapies are usually highly structured, being guided by a manual, monitored for adherence to the protocol, and defined by a fixed end point. Patients are randomly assigned to treatment or rigorous control conditions.

In the real world, therapy is (usually) not of fixed duration. It keeps going until the patient is better, or he or she drops out. Therapy usually consists of trial-and-error, self-adjusting eclectic combinations of modalities or orientations. If one approach doesn't work, another is tried. Patients usually enter therapy after actively searching for the clinician and type of treatment which they prefer. Real patients and families usually have multiple, interacting problems, and therapy is geared to addressing those problems so that the outcome is one of improved general functioning, not just symptomatic relief. In fact, research studies tend to have better outcomes than clinic-based studies because clinic cases are more seriously disturbed, and research studies over-represent behavioural approaches (Weisz, Weiss, Han, Granger, & Morton, 1995).

Recent attempts to use more realistic, less 'laboratory-oriented' models of outcome, and which include lesser-studied modalities such as long-term and psychoanalytic therapy, are yielding some interesting results. Fonagy and Target (1996) undertook a retrospective chart review of more than 750 cases of child psychoanalysis and psychotherapy at the Anna Freud Centre. They used pre- versus post-treatment changes as the outcome measure, and incorporated acceptable criteria such as

DSM-III-R (APA, 1987) diagnoses (reliably rated), and the Hampstead Child Adaptation Measure, which was modelled on Luborsky's Health–Sickness Rating Scale (Luborsky, 1984) and the Children's Global Adaptation Scale (Shaffer, Gould, & Brasic, 1983).

The authors found that long-term (greater than six months), intensive (four to five times/week) therapy was significantly more effective than short-term (less than six months), non-intensive (one to three times/week) therapy for pre-adolescent patients, while the reverse was true for teenagers. Children with internalizing disorders did better than externalizers, but the difference disappeared when intensity and duration of treatment were controlled for. Intensive treatment was especially beneficial when the disorder was severe. When the disorder was less severe, there was no difference between intensive and non-intensive therapy. Groups who did poorly and dropped out prematurely fell into the categories of pervasive developmental disorder, attention deficit/hyperactivity disorder, mental retardation, and conduct disorder, especially if they were adolescents.

Interestingly, the influence of parental pathology on outcome varied according to developmental level. Severe maternal psychopathology predicted poorer outcome in children under six years, but positive outcome in those aged six to twelve years. The authors speculate on the greater damage done by earlier trauma, and the greater degree of exposure in pre-schoolers as opposed to latency-aged children.

The study is limited by its retrospective nature and lack of control groups. It is, nevertheless, the first large-scale attempt to measure outcome of a long-term, insight-oriented therapy with children, and it has the advantages of analysing a cohort in their naturalistic (therapeutic) context. Some of the results support findings from other controlled studies (e.g., the lack of difference between externalizers and internalizers), as well as other naturalistic studies.

Seligman (1995), for instance, analysed the results of a *Consumer Reports* survey (1995) of mental health utilization. While this survey did not include children, it did show that long-term therapy (lasting more than two years) produced more improvement than short-term therapy, in a direct, dose–response curve fashion. Furthermore, as in Fonagy and Target's study (1996), symptomatic improvement was correlated with global improvement (work, social, and personal domains), and the most improvement occurred when treatment lasted longer than six months.

Seligman praises the survey as a reliable, valid self-report measure of *effectiveness*, as opposed to *efficacy*, of psychotherapy. 'Imagine what a decent efficacy study of long-term dynamic therapy would require: control groups receiving no treatment for several years; a credible comparison treatment of the same duration ... but [one that] is inert; a step-by-step manual covering hundreds of sessions; and random assignment of patients. The ethical and scientific problems of such research are daunting ... The efficacy study is the wrong method for empirically validating psychotherapy as it is actually done because it omits too many crucial elements' (Seligman, 1995, p. 966).

Shirk and Russell (1992) examined 29 non-behavioural controlled treatments (taken from a meta-analysis of 108 studies). They found that studies with more serious methodological problems (which occurred in 62 per cent of their sample) yielded smaller treatment effects than those without such flaws. The best studies reported effect sizes that were more than twice as big as those reported in the worst studies. Estimates of effectiveness were not independent of the therapeutic allegiance of the researcher. Substantially smaller effects were reported by behaviourally oriented investigators.

Furthermore, the sample did not reflect how child therapy is actually practised. Compared with surveys of clinicians (Silver & Silver, 1983; Koocher & Pedulla, 1977), client-centred, group, and brief therapies were overrepresented. The average effect size for group treatments was significantly smaller than that for individual treatments. Over 20 per cent of the studies had ten or fewer sessions, and many of the contacts lasted less than forty-five minutes. In this sense, the 'dose' or 'strength' of the treatments were 'weaker' than those reported in practice surveys.

Almost 25 per cent of the treatments took place in correctional facilities, which was used as the sole inclusion criterion. Such populations are known to be extremely heterogeneous and often do poorly in therapy because they are forced into it, and, in actual practice, much less than 25 per cent of child therapy occurs in that context. Thus, subjects used in research studies may not represent patients treated in the community.

Play therapy was not included in the authors' meta-analysis. Behavioural researchers don't have the same investment in play as they do in behavioural interventions. At the same time, psychodynamic researchers have not developed a satisfactory play measure (Kernberg, 1992). Yet, this form of therapy is widely used, and play is considered a central mechanism of change in the dynamic treatment of young children.

In summary, findings from research may not generalize to clinical practice, and comments about certain types of therapy being ineffective, especially long-term individual psychodynamic therapy, cannot be regarded as robust because of confounding variables which reduce the size of reported treatment effects.

Does child therapy work? If one takes a broad-based meta-analytic approach, then the answer is 'Yes.' Studies including age ranges from two to eighteen years, cutting across modalities and types of problem, and as recent as 1995, show mean effect sizes ranging from .71 to .84 (Brown, 1987; Casey & Berman 1985; Weisz et al, 1987; Weisz & Weiss, 1989; Weisz, Weiss, et al, 1995), which is similar to outcomes in meta-analytic studies of adult psychotherapy. The average child after treatment functioned better than 78 per cent of control-group children.

Nevertheless, a specific treatment is likely to vary in effectiveness as a function of child, parent, family, community, therapist, therapy, and temporal/developmental factors. For a given intervention, one would want to know: the impact of treatment relative to no and other treatment; the necessary and sufficient components of treatment that effect change; parameters that could be systematically varied to improve outcome; the relative effectiveness of various combinations of treatment; and the role of process as it effects outcome (e.g., therapeutic alliance).

Until such research is conducted, clinicians will have to combine their knowledge of the literature with their own experience (and those of their peers, through study groups or supervision) in order to arrive at informed decisions as to the best match of treatment/child/problem.

TREATMENT SELECTION

Can we be more specific? Do we know which treatments work with which children? According to Weisz, Weiss, et al (1995), behavioural interventions are more effective than non-behavioural ones, but the latter are seriously underrepresented in the studies examined; both externalizing and internalizing problems respond equally well to therapy; outcomes are better for adolescents than children, but only for girls – there is no gender difference in pre-teens; qualified mental health professionals are more effective than either students or paraprofessionals (parents or teachers who are trained for specific therapies) when dealing with internalizing (depression, anxiety) problems, but the reverse is true for externalizing problems – teachers and parents are actually more effective than professionals or students, who show no differences; therapy effects are specific, that is, have the greatest impact on targeted symptoms, but the perception of improvement depends very much on the source of evaluation and the type of problem. Positive treatment effects for externalizing problems (aggression, delinquency) are most likely to be reported by teachers, parents, and other observers. Positive effects for internalizing problems are most likely to be reported by peers or the children themselves.

Aggressive and antisocial behaviour (conduct disorder) is one of the most extensively studied problem domains. Patterson, Reid, and Dishion (1992) have demonstrated improved behaviour at home and school using a developmental, programmatic approach which surpassed results from family therapy alone, placebo discussion groups, and no treatment. Significant symptomatic improvement has also been shown at home, at school, and in the community, using parent management training, cognitive therapy, and variations of family therapy (Dumas, 1989; Kazdin, Siegel, & Bass, 1992).

Cognitive behavioural therapy for depressed children and adolescents has resulted in significant reductions in functional impairment and depressive symptomatology compared with placebo discussion groups, waiting list only, and no treatment (Lewinsohn, Clarke, Hops, & Andrews, 1990; Reynolds & Coats, 1986; Stark, Reynolds, & Kaslow, 1987). Single-case designs have shown that gains can be maintained for as long as five years following a major depressive episode, without medication (Asarnow & Carlson, 1988).

Results of brief, focused individual and family treatments have been mixed, or difficult to evaluate because of methodological flaws (Dulcan, 1984). Isolated case reports using adaptations of adult forms of brief dynamic therapy with adolescents (e.g., Luborsky's CCRT method) suggest great promise (Golombek & Korenblum, 1995), but await proper trials incorporating randomized controlled protocols.

FAMILY THERAPY

Meta-analytic studies of family therapy show effect sizes ranging from .45 (Hazelrigg, Cooper, & Borduin, 1987) to .70 (Markus, Lange, & Pettigrew, 1990). Diagnostically, the greatest successes have appeared in families with: a schizophrenic child, in which psychoeducation to reduce 'expressed emotion' reduces the probability of relapse (Goldstein et al, 1978) and rehospitalization (Leff, Kuipers, Berkowitz, Eberlein-Vries, & Sturgeon, 1982); anorexia nervosa and bulimia, in which weight gain and normal menstrual functioning are better maintained than with individual therapy (Russell, Szmukler, Dare, & Eisler, 1987); and conduct disorder, where parent management training (Eisenstadt, Eyberg, McNeil,

Newcomb, & Funderburk, 1993; McMahon, 1994), functional family therapy (Alexander, 1988), and multisystemic family therapy (Henggeler, Borduin, Melton, Mann, & Smith, 1991) have all resulted in lower recidivism rates among delinquents and improved family functioning.

Unfortunately, externalizing disorders are overrepresented in most studies of family therapy. Furthermore, reliable, valid, and treatment-sensitive assessment tools are lacking, as are measures of adherence to a manualized approach. Family-based process research is just in its infancy, and investigators have relied on small, heterogeneous samples which lack control groups or define certain constructs idiosyncratically (Diamond & Dickey, 1993).

INFANT PSYCHIATRY

Studies of interventions to help disturbed mother–infant relationships are emerging from the new field of infant psychiatry. This is the one area where outcome studies of combined psychotherapeutic treatments, especially ones which clearly delineate the decision processes behind the choice of combination, have been conducted.

Infants are increasingly referred to clinics because of relationship problems with their caregivers (Sameroff & Emde, 1989). Their problems manifest as functional disturbances of feeding, sleeping, and behavioural regulation (e.g., 'tantrums'), or are identified in association with parental abuse and neglect, with and without parental mental illness.

Four models of intervention have been described: support and maternal psychotherapy, which aim to change the quality of the relationship indirectly; and guidance and infant-led therapy, which address the dyad directly (Lojkasek et al, 1994).

In support, the mother is helped to access community resources such as housing, work, child care, or self-help groups. It is almost always combined with guidance, and has therefore been essentially impossible to evaluate on its own. While its rationale makes sense (lower maternal stress allows greater maternal availability and responsivity), its effects are only indirect.

Guidance falls into two subcategories: developmental and relational. The former aims to increase maternal knowledge of developmental milestones and is generic and psychoeducational. The latter has its roots in infant-stimulation programs and involves a therapist who guides the mother to attend and respond to selected cues of her own infant.

Studies of guidance have shown significant improvements in the quality of the dyadic relationship (Cramer et al, 1990; Landy, Schubert, Cleland, & Montgomery, 1984), cognitive improvements (Metzl, 1980), positive changes in maternal perception of the infant and improved parenting skills (Nurcombe et al, 1984), and normalized developmental expectations and childrearing attitudes (Field, Widmayer, Stringer, & Ignatoff, 1980). In one study, group differences in cognitive functioning did not appear until two years after the intervention, suggesting a 'sleeper effect' (Rauh, Achenbach, Nurcombe, Howell, & Teti, 1988), and were maintained after seven years (Achenbach, Phares, Howell, Rauh, & Nurcombe, 1990).

Maternal psychotherapy which focuses on parenting has been evaluated in a controlled fashion for help with anxiously attached infants (Lieberman, Weston, Pawl, 1991). After one year, significant improvement in the quality of the dyadic relationship was noted. In a comparative evaluation, Cramer et al (1990) assessed brief psychodynamic therapy of the mother versus relational guidance. Both groups improved significantly on measures of presenting symptoms; the dyadic relationship; and mother's representations. of self, infant, and her mother. The only differences were that the maternal-psychotherapy mothers had higher self-esteem, while the relational-guidance mothers were less intrusive and controlling when with their infants.

Infant-led psychotherapy is a two-step intervention in which regular time is set aside for the mother to observe the free play of her infant with the therapist present, and then she discusses her observations and experiences with the therapist (Johnson, Dowling, & Wesner, 1980; Muir, 1992). The mother is specifically instructed to follow her baby's lead and not initiate activity. It aims to enhance mutual responsiveness and sensitivity. The therapist does not instruct or give advice, but tries to enhance the mother's understanding of her relationship with the infant, via an examination of transference and the mother's own internal working models (Bowlby, 1988b; Fonagy et al, 1991).

Unfortunately, few outcome studies evaluating this modality have been published. Ostrov, Dowling, Wesner, and Johnson (1982) noted improved sensorimotor and language skills in the baby, along with improved marital relationship, more cooperative play with siblings, and increased attachment to fathers. Johnson et al (1980) reported improved dyadic relationships for the majority of more than 100 mother–infant pairs. Neither study was controlled.

Practice Guidelines

ASSESSMENT FOR PSYCHOTHERAPY

To use Frances, Clarkin, and Perry's (1984) terminology, many of the principles for choosing the setting, format, orientation, duration, and frequency of adult psychotherapy can be usefully applied to children. A complete review of the indications and contraindications for all psycho-therapies is therefore redundant.

There are, however, certain unique features of working with this age group which are worth delineating. First, some general tenets (which cut across all modalities) will be outlined, and then more format-specific issues will be covered.

In many cases, children's abnormalities consist of a failure to progress in the expected fashion along one or more dimensions of development, rather than specific symptoms *per se*. The assessment must therefore look at functioning relative to that expected for the child's developmental stage.

The social context of the referral must be taken into account. Who is concerned about the child, and why? Because children's ability to con-ceptualize and verbalize experiences differs from that of adults, tech-niques for history-taking and conducting a mental-status exam need to be adapted to ensure stage-appropriateness, and almost always need to be supplemented with other sources of information, such as parents and/or teachers.

Unfortunately, different informants do not always agree – with each other and with the child. These discrepancies may arise for a number of reasons: informants may differ in their access to emotional/behavioural data, especially if the symptoms are situation-specific (e.g., only at home or only at school); informants differ in how they evaluate the behaviours they do observe; and informants may differ in their willingness to report various thoughts or feelings.

It is known, for instance, that parents are more likely to report exter-nalizing behaviours and are more accurate with factual information (Kashani, Orvaschel, Burk, & Reid, 1985; Orvaschel, Weissman, Padian, & Lowe, 1981). Children, on the other hand, are more likely to report internalizing symptoms (e.g., anxiety or depression) and may be the only source of attitudes or some shameful events such as sexual abuse.

Despite possible parent–child incongruities, involving parents is important. If individual therapy is selected, their support will be needed to maintain the alliance and drive them to appointments. If supportive therapy is selected, access to pertinent information from the child's real life may be quite valuable, since young children are often unreliable in conveying the interface between intrapsychic and interpersonal worlds. If parent counselling or family therapy is selected, then, obviously, the parents will play a central role in implementation.

When tired, sick, or fearful, children may regress, and in those under the age of ten, symptoms may be labile (Edelbrock, Costello, Dulcan, Kalas, & Conover, 1985). It is therefore advisable to see the child more than once to get a sense of the consistency or reactivity of symptoms. At times, home or school visits may be valuable adjuncts since they permit observation *in vivo*. If this is not practical, home videos can be used to assist in diagnosis and recommendations, especially if they are available both pre- and post-morbidly (Korenblum, 1996).

Children's symptoms often cluster into certain groupings. These can then be used to assist choice of format or orientation. For example, eating, sleeping, bowel/bladder, speech, or motor symptoms suggest a disturbance of bodily function which may indicate a more somatically oriented treatment. Symptoms related to memory, perception, and academic failure suggest higher cognitive dysfunction (such as learning disability), which would indicate a need for educational remediation. Anxiety and depression are affect disturbances which could be treated with cognitive or dynamic individual psychotherapies. Antisocial, oppositional, or aggressive behaviour usually call for family or group therapy, supplemented by environmental manipulation.

The overall goal of the assessment and formulation is not merely to obtain a description of the problematic behaviours, thoughts, or feelings, but to understand their meaning and function in relation to the child and his or her environment (Cox & Rutter, 1985).

Informed treatment decisions with children should be tailored to their cognitive, linguistic, and social level. Often, interactive play and/or projective techniques can assist in the decision. Such techniques are a means of surmounting limitations in children's ability or willingness to introspect or to report their feelings and concerns. They also introduce an element of fun, which places both the child and the interviewer at ease.

Examples include role play with puppets, animals, or other small figures. Via displacement, the child's concerns, perceptions, and characteristic modes of relating can be identified. With older children, board games can serve the same function. Both the content and form of play should be considered.

Drawing a picture is a very useful visuomotor tool which provides a less-filtered window into the child's internal world and can be used to assess various non-verbal functions. Usually one asks the child to sketch a person, the child's family, or inanimate objects such as a house or tree. Scoring systems exist to help evaluate such productions (Koppitz, 1968; Naglieri, 1988). As with play, the manner in which the child responds to and implements the request is as informative as the content itself (e.g., extreme reluctance or oppositional behaviour might suggest non-dynamic or other-than-individual types of interventions).

Interactive verbal and non-verbal techniques include Winnicott's 'squiggle' drawing game (1971), Gardner's Mutual Story-Telling game (1985), and completion of the Despert fables (1937), which are a series of short stories designed to evoke certain standardized affective themes. Through use of an interactional assessment tool, further data are gleaned with respect to the capacity to engage in a psychotherapeutic modality (be it individual, family, or group) which requires a relationship to be built.

Generally, all of these play and projective methods are most relevant with children under ten years of age, although drawings can be useful through to adulthood. Once a child enters the pre-teen and adolescent years, a more traditional (i.e., direct verbal) approach to mental status and assessing for treatment suitability can be used.

TREATMENT SELECTION

Sharp distinctions between intrapsychic and interpersonal therapies are probably not valuable with adults. With children, it is even more important to consider psychological, familial, and social interventions in a mutually inclusive, dynamically fluid, complementary fashion because of the degree to which children are dependent and constantly changing.

The question of how to select a treatment modality therefore becomes one of deciding which blocks to development need to be addressed, and in what order, and which systems are most amenable to change at a given time.

Individual Psychotherapy

In *relative* terms, then, individual therapy is most appropriate when: a child displays ego-dystonic symptoms such as anxiety or depression; the problem is so shameful that the child requests privacy (e.g., sexual abuse); there is sufficient observing ego (given the developmental stage) to keep acting out to a manageable minimum; the environment supports the therapy. Most important is the support of the parents, but the school and peer subsystems must also be able to accommodate both the process and the outcome of therapy.

Relative contraindications include: legal entanglements which involve secondary gain for the child or family (e.g., custody/access disputes, or to 'look good in court' for a delinquent adolescent); serious substance abuse in the identified patient; acute psychosis; or perpetuation of the individual pathology by severe family dysfunction such as scapegoating.

Family Therapy

Family therapy is most clearly indicated when there is consensus that the presenting problem is primarily interactional, involving distortions of communication, socialization, role definition, boundaries, and structure. Individual pathology is either minor or ego-syntonic. The problem often manifests in behavioural rather than affective or cognitive dimensions. As with individual therapy, the family should be 'in pain' (i.e., view the behaviour as 'family-dystonic),' and the various subsystems need to be adaptive enough to accommodate and support change in individual members and in the family as a whole.

Group Therapy

Since the indications for group therapy with children are essentially the same as with adults, they are not reviewed here in any detail. This modality can be particularly useful for adolescents because of their need for peer acceptance, and their greater trust in peers than adults for help with personal problems. With younger children, the emphasis is often on activity rather than talk, and shared focus on a common task can be used to build social skills as a 'by-product.'

Any psychiatric illness which interferes with social cognition or behaviour, from depression to learning disorder, can form the basis of an appropriate referral for group therapy. Children tend to enjoy the here-and-now, problem-solving approach which is frequently used.

Other Interventions

Although some consider 'environmental manipulation' a dirty word

(Carek, 1972), a true generalist will always consider the impact of social factors on psychotherapy, no matter what the modality. This impact is often greater with children.

Therapists are sometimes asked to become directly involved in the patient's world. At other times, the therapist him- or herself may initiate such contact. The primary indications for actively relating to the 'outside' environment (usually the school, but also social agencies, courts, camps, etc.) are: to ensure the continued viability of the therapy; to enhance necessary structure in the child's life; to assist outside institutions in correctly understanding the child's needs (within the bounds of confidentiality); to obtain feedback on the impact of therapy on the child's environment; to make sure that everyone is 'on the same wavelength' with respect to therapeutic goals and implementation of treatment strategies.

On rare occasions, direct advocacy with a view to having the child placed in a different environment is required. If the environment poses a clear and present danger to the child, there is certainty that other responsible adults cannot or will not act, and a safer alternative actually exists, then the therapist is obliged ethically – and in circumstances to be outlined later, legally – to act on behalf of the child (Cooper & Wanerman, 1977).

Fortunately, such extreme instances are not that frequent. However, degrees of chaos, depreciation, and danger are all too common. In these instances, the therapist must use his or her clinical judgment as to when it is time to act. Comparing progress (or regress) against developmental norms often provides the clearest guideline.

There are, of course, limitations to extratherapeutic involvements. Perhaps the greatest is encouraging dependency in the child/family (Steinhauer, 1985). The therapist may unwittingly confirm the child's/family's sense of helplessness by doing something which they are quite capable of handling themselves. Even worse, the therapist may provide secondary gain for regressive behaviour by, for instance, acceding to a request to excuse the child from certain responsibilities (e.g., school exams, court appearances).

Outside agencies may idealize the therapist as the person with all the 'answers,' or as a magician who can 'cure' the child. Expectations need to be tempered with reality. The therapist should present him- or herself as someone who can facilitate communication among all those who have an interest in the child, and who may be able to foster supportive attitudes based on an accurate understanding of the child's needs.

Conversely, the therapist sometimes idealizes the outside agency, and imagines that the school, for instance, will be able to mobilize all sorts of resources to provide intensive support for the child. These expectations may be equally unrealistic. A balanced appreciation of the interaction between and limitations of both therapy and the 'real world' is usually the most helpful.

COMBINING TREATMENTS

When a child is in individual therapy, how should the parents be involved? When should one combine individual and family therapy, and in what manner?

The more a family lacks the ability to accommodate change at one level with adaptation at another, the more likely one will need multi-modal therapy (Steinhauer, 1985). Furthermore, combining therapies allows internal, external, and transferential realities to be dealt with simultaneously. The effects are often synergistic, with the gains made in one therapy fuelling progress in the other. In particular, the role and boundary definition provided by family therapy helps to clarify 'whose pathology belongs to whom,' thus suggesting the most effective level at which to intervene.

One or Two Therapists?

Should the same person provide both therapies? In underserviced geographic locations, the answer may be pragmatically determined. There may *be* no one 'else' to provide the 'other' therapy, and so the modalities will be concurrent and combined, of necessity. In larger urban centres, however, the option of collaboration may exist.

If a clinician is therapeutically 'bilingual' enough to shift easily between intrapsychic and interpersonal domains, the experience can be very enriching. As mentioned above, the material which emerges from one therapy can be used to inform and guide the other. Splitting by the family, and competition between therapists, are avoided.

In infant psychiatry, psychotherapy with the parent alone prevents the observation and working-through of the relational problem which may constitute the presenting complaint, and may take too long for the infant's well-being (Lojkasek et al, 1994). It is understandable that infants have been excluded from most interventions for this age group. 'A baby has none of the conventional attributes of a psychiatric patient. He can't talk about his problems. He can't form a therapeutic alliance. He has no capacity for insight. Such patients are usually labelled 'not suitable for treatment' (Fraiberg, Shapiro, & Chemiss, 1983, p. 56). However, only 'combined,' that is, infant-led, therapy considers maternal perceptions, thoughts, and feelings in a manner which allows linkage to a corrective emotional experience in the here-and-now.

Nevertheless, when one person 'does it all,' the therapist's ego boundaries can be severely tested. While integration would presumably occur with the consent of all parties (when the child is older than infancy), it can sometimes feel like a conflict of interest. Protecting the confidentiality of the child in individual therapy usually poses the biggest challenge. With adolescents, in particular, consent would rarely be granted willingly, and proceeding in the face of such a gross breach of trust or of respect for autonomy would be the 'kiss of death' for the individual therapy. Similarly, if the parental dyad has been seen as part of a flexible family therapy, then remembering what the couple wanted to be kept private can become difficult. Sometimes, the child or family resent having to 'share' the therapist.

For these reasons, collaboration between two clinicians is often preferred. Several advantages accrue. The case is treated from two vantage points simultaneously, thus stimulating both patients and therapists to be aware of alternative, complementary strategies. The burden of responsibility can be shared. Structure and a 'holding environment' can be more easily created. Scapegoating can be rapidly identified and dealt with.

The two therapists must respect each other, avoid competition, and communicate sufficiently to limit splitting. The frequency of communication and parameters of confidentiality should be discussed with the child and parents in advance, as part of the contracting. Under these conditions, concurrent but separate individual and family therapy can work quite well.

In general, the younger the child, the more 'externalized' the pathology, and the more behavioural the individual therapy, the greater the indication for a combined and integrated (i.e., single therapist) approach. The older the child (especially if adolescent), the more 'internalized' the pathology, and the more psychodynamic the individual therapy, the greater the indication for a concurrent but separate (i.e., two therapists) approach (Weiner, 1970).

Parental Involvement

Even when family therapy is not formally part of the treatment plan, and a child is being seen in individual therapy, it is wise to involve the parents in some fashion. Maintaining an alliance to support the therapy, obtaining periodic information about the child's real-life activities, and modifying the home environment to support therapeutic goals are just some of the reasons for which liaison with parents is important (Cooper & Wanerman, 1977).

Parents can be engaged in several different ways. For some parents, the assessment of their child represents an opportunity for reporting marital concerns. Referral to a separate marital therapist is then indicated. At other times, parental concerns are child-focused and are expressed as confusion over the child's behaviour or diagnosis.

In this case, informational books or reading material can be provided; referral to a self-help organization or psychoeducational parents' group can be made; support groups for advice on discipline (therapist- or parent-led) can be helpful; or formal parent counselling by a collaborative therapist can occur.

The question of whether the child's therapist him- or herself should fulfil any of these functions requires flexibility. The guidelines suggested above for whether one or two therapists is appropriate can be applied here as well. In therapy lasting one school year or longer, a meeting with parents, child, and individual therapist to have a mutual 'progress report' and consolidate therapeutic goals should take place at times such as Christmas and June. These occasions provide an opportunity for 'fine-tuning' the therapy, revising formulations, and evaluating the need for further treatment.

CONSENT AND CONFIDENTIALITY

Informed Consent

(See chapter 18, 'Consent Issues in Psychotherapy.')

Medical psychotherapy as defined in this volume is a form of treatment for psychological problems. As such, it is subject to certain laws. As an illustration, the current consent legislation in the province of Ontario is used as an example. In the jurisdiction of Ontario, the Advocacy, Consent, and Substitute Decisions Statute Law Amendment Act (Bill 19) came into effect in 1996. Part of this legislative package is the Health Care Consent Act.

The Health Care Consent Act has very clear definitions of consent, capacity, and guidelines for establishing informed consent (College of

Physicians and Surgeons of Ontario, 1996). With respect to children and child therapy, the act presumes that *all* persons, regardless of age, are capable of making decisions about treatment, provided that they understand information relevant to the decision and can appreciate the consequences of making or not making a decision. In fact, one may not assume that a patient lacks capacity just because of age.

This guideline is consistent with the parameters of Bill 77, An Act Respecting the Protection and Well-Being of Children and Their Families (otherwise known as the Child and Family Services Act, or CFSA), which has been in effect in Ontario since 1984, and is specifically designed to meet the social and psychological needs of children under the age of eighteen.

Under section 4(5) of this act, it is stated that 'a person's consent ... is not invalid by reason only that the person is less than 18 years old.' Furthermore, 'a service provider may provide counselling to a child twelve years of age or older, and no other person's consent is required' (section 28). Hence, twelve-year-olds are legally allowed to seek and obtain therapy confidentially. In fact, parents cannot have access to their child's (over the age of twelve) therapy records unless the child gives written permission (section 167[2]).

Obviously, procedures for obtaining informed consent are important. They protect children from harm, recognize autonomy, and honour the dignity of an individual (Cooke, 1977). This is perhaps even more critical when requesting participation in research. In the United States, for instance, the National Commission for the Protection of Human Subjects (1977) recommended that investigators honour the dissent of minors. No lower age limit was specified.

The problem, however, is that legislation defines *age* and not *stage*. It does not account for variations in development. It doesn't consider contextual variables such as family dysfunction or parental needs. And it assumes that 'capacity' is primarily an autonomous cognitive function.

Clinicians understand that cognitive capacities are often affected by emotions, unconscious factors such as ambivalence, and external stresses. With children, in particular, temporary regression is extremely common, as is vulnerability to fatigue, fright, and other external stressors. When consent is allowed to be 'express or implied,' relevant to some treatments but not others, and valid at some times but not at others (Section 15 [1 & 2]), there is even greater latitude for uncertainty. How does one reconcile contradictions between verbal and non-verbal behaviour, for instance? Such phenomena are widespread in children, whose linguistic capacities may not be sophisticated.

Empirical evidence suggests cause for concern when assuming that children *a priori* possess full capacity, undifferentiated from standards which are used for adults. Lewis (1981), for example, examined the degree to which 108 adolescents used formal operations when making decisions.

Teenagers ranging from twelve to eighteen years of age were presented with several dilemmas which required them to give advice to a hypothetical peer. These included whether to trust a researcher about whom conflicting reports had been received, and how to decide on a surgical procedure about which two doctors disagreed.

The results showed that children as old as fifteen had difficulty imagining risks and future consequences, identifying the need for inde- pendent opinions, and recognizing the potential vested interests of professionals who were giving them advice. Compared with eighteen-year-olds, they lacked fundamental decision-making skills.

Children also tend to focus on what they are most familiar with and their immediate environment, instead of new or potentially helpful experiences. Schwartz (1972) studied thirty-six children who had been hospitalized for participation in a research protocol dealing with short stature. Despite extensive interviewing and preparation, none of the subjects under age eleven showed any awareness that they had been admitted to a research unit for research purposes. Of the nineteen children older than eleven, only six were even partially aware, and the two who had the clearest understanding eventually decided to drop out.

Schwartz speculated that, besides cognitive limitations, unconscious wishes to be 'cured' may have interfered with the children's ability to perceive reality accurately.

While physicians are advised to determine each patient's capacity to consent, and may therefore come to the conclusion that a child is not capable after interviewing him or her, it is the presumption of capacity which is being challenged here.

Confidentiality

With regard to content issues and confidentiality, *some* rules are very clear, but there is a much larger 'grey zone' of uncertainty. If, during the course of psychotherapy (or assessment), a physician 'has reasonable grounds to suspect that a child is or may be or may have suffered abuse,' then the clinician *must* report the suspicion and the information upon which it is based to a Children's Aid Society (section 68[3] of the CFSA).

Under the act, 'child' is defined as anyone under the age of sixteen, and therefore does not apply to older adolescents. Also, the act is meant to apply to perpetrators who 'have charge of the child' (section 37[2]), not strangers who have no relationship to the child.

While the law is obvious with respect to physical and sexual abuse, the duty to disclose suicidal or homicidal intent, or illegal activities, is not at all clear. If a parent or other adult who has charge of the child fails to seek or allow *treatment* for self-destructive or dangerous, aggressive behaviour, then it is reportable.

In and of itself, however, suicidal, homicidal, and illegal behaviour is subject only to the clinician's judgment in terms of designating the child to be in need of protection and reporting to authorities. Of course, Criminal Code considerations such as aiding and abetting suicide would apply. In Ontario, there is currently no precedent like the Tarasoff case in the United States, that is, a duty to warn a potential victim of impending harm, but the College of Physicians and Surgeons is actively considering and supporting such a proposal (Carlisle, 1996).

Whether one shares psychotherapeutic material voluntarily or by mandate, ethical conflicts of interest almost always arise. With young patients, 'the best interests of the child' is a theoretically useful guide, but one that is not always easy to implement practically. Determining the child's best interests is not a value-free task, and the interests of various stakeholders often compete.

Although the ultimate decision as to a finding of abuse is not the physician's, the initiation of the process would stem from his or her disclosure to authorities. At times, the consequences can be dramatically disruptive to both the therapy and the child's life.

Clinical experience suggests that, in contracting for psychotherapy, the parameters of confidentiality be established at the outset. The identified patient should be told that his or her physical and psychological safety and well-being will be of paramount concern to the therapist. If, during the course of therapy, the clinician has reason to be concerned, the patient should be told of this and informed that other parties may need to be involved (usually the parents). Thus, the therapist promises not to 'go behind the child's back.'

Together, child, parents, and therapist should establish a hierarchy of people to contact in a situation where safety is an issue *before* therapy begins. In this way, the potential for confusion and crisis is minimized, and agreement is obtained from everyone.

After a disclosure, every attempt should be made to 'heal' what may be perceived to be a breach of trust. The patient should be reminded (in a non-critical fashion) of the agreed-upon contract, and a therapeutic alliance with the healthy aspects of the ego should be consolidated.

In general, a decision about when to share material should be guided by the therapeutic goals, along with the orientation and format of therapy. If the patient has weak ego functions, especially judgment, impulse control, and frustration tolerance; significant superego deficits; the therapy is behaviourally oriented and supportive; concurrent family therapy or parent counselling is occurring; and the behaviour is largely determined by interpersonal dynamics such as scapegoating, inconsistent discipline, or inadvertent reinforcement by parents (Weiner, 1970), then disclosure of potentially harmful or antisocial acts is more easily accomplished and relevant to the task of assisting psychological structuralization, and converting ego-syntonic to ego-dystonic behaviour.

If, on the other hand, the child suffers from more internalized conflicts, the therapy is psychodynamic and insight-oriented, individual therapy alone is the existent modality, and the behaviour serves neurotic purposes such as a need to be punished or narcissistic functions such as a need for recognition, then working through within the framework of the relationship may be more effectively accomplished by respecting confidentiality (and holding one's breath, hoping that serious risk does not ensue).

THE THERAPEUTIC FUNCTIONS OF PLAY

The central role of play in child therapy has been compared to hypnosis, free association, and fantasy in adult psychiatry (Hug-Hellmuth, 1921; Erikson, 1950). According to Ekstein and Friedman (1957), the 'royal road to the child's unconscious' is play. For a child, 'playing it out' is equivalent to an adult's 'talking it out.'

Play serves at least four functions: discharge of energy, mastery of anxiety, experimentation and development of new skills through practice, and identification via role modelling. Through play, the child engages in pleasurable activity, turns passive into active, and 'rearranges reality' such that overwhelming events can be 'broken up' into more psychologically 'digestible' ones, allowing traumas to be worked through (Waelder, 1933).

Play is both self- and other-directed. The pure discharge of motoric energy is the clearest example of play as self-expression. Role playing involving another person illustrates the communicative aspect of play. Both facets – intrapsychic and interpersonal – must be attended to in child therapy. While one may predominate over the other at any given moment, the emphasis is relative only. Each interacts with the other in a fluid dynamic.

Knowledge of the functions of play is important because it helps guide one's selection and use of play materials, which, in turn, should be determined by the goals of therapy. If the goal is abreaction, catharsis, and regression, as might be indicated for the severely inhibited, obsessional, or traumatized child, then the setting needs to accommodate this.

In general, for the child under five years of age, a separate playroom is desirable. Designed for regression and motoric discharge, such a room allows both therapist and child to 'relax' in terms of worrying about damage to property, thus minimizing the need for frequent limit-setting. Typical materials would include sand, water, clay, and finger-paints.

For the older child (five to ten years), or one with whom the goal is communication or self-expression as a means to resolve conflict, it may be better to incorporate toys into one's usual office setting, so that talk and play can be combined. In this instance, typical materials would include paper and crayons, puppets and dolls, cars, trucks, or animals, and a doll's house. In addition, the older latency child is often struggling with conflicts related to skill acquisition and competition. For him or her, cards and board games are valuable tools.

Types of Play Therapy

Actual interventions fall into directive-structured or non-directive categories (Carek, 1972). The former are used in supportive, focal, or time-limited therapies, in which relationship-building with a 'real' therapist and a corrective emotional experience are the central mechanisms of change (Hambidge, 1955).

The therapist is a participant in the play, with varying degrees of activity. He or she may simply comply and follow the child's 'script'; he may play the assigned role but add his own ideas; he may take the initiative and (for example) 'phone' the child, or assign the puppet roles, thus explicitly modelling and giving permission to engage in 'make-believe'; he may play a competitive game. Greater activity is called for when the child is inhibited by anxiety and a harsh, punitive superego.

If games are used, it is best to avoid choices such as Monopoly or chess. They require too much time, concentration, and skill to foster a free-flowing atmosphere of communication or self-expression. Instead, games of chance (e.g., cards) are preferred. The therapist should play reasonably well, since 'throwing' a game is often detected as dishonesty, and many children have as much anxiety about winning as they do about losing. Instead, the child can be given a 'handicap' to even out any skill disparity, and then the rules can be observed.

Non-directive interventions are more appropriate for exploratory, 'insight-oriented,' psychoanalytic approaches. The therapist is a non-participant/observer whose main role is interpretive, and to whom the child relates as a transference figure. Interpretation can take place via displacement, that is, in the play, or in reality. Where possible, it is better to stay in the realm of make-believe, as reality-based interpretations are often intellectualized (from the child's point of view), dampen the spontaneous expression of affect, and may be less easily assimilated. They sometimes feel like a 'frontal assault' on the child's defences.

Limit-Setting and Boundaries

Limit- and boundary-setting is often a difficult technical issue. Play is useful and constructive in so far as it maintains a therapeutic alliance and fosters self-awareness. Motoric or affective discharge for discharge's sake alone, or if it threatens the safety of the therapist, child, or integrity of the office, is not constructive and must be limited.

Strong countertransference can be mobilized when a child is out of control. The therapist must confront his or her own conflicts around control, aggression, passivity, and narcissism in order to handle primitive displays of impulsivity in children. Overidentification with an abused child (for instance), or a strong need to be liked, can lead to paralysing permissiveness. An inability to tolerate spontaneity or 'messy' outbursts of affect can lead to premature, punitive interventions.

While clarification, confrontation, and interpretation are the therapist's main tools, on rare occasions non-verbal acts such as physical restraint are called for. Restraint should be a choice of last resort. It is indicated when harm to person or property is imminent (or has occurred), to assist self-control, to defuse a power struggle, and to re-establish an atmosphere in which it is safe to talk.

It should always be accompanied by an explicit statement of intention: 'I'm not trying to hurt you. I am making sure that neither one of us gets hurt, and I will hold you until you can control yourself.' 'It is usually more effective and less complicated with a younger, smaller child. Restraint should not be used with a child over the age of nine or ten, except in the most extreme circumstances. If a child of that age or older cannot control him- or herself, then the therapist should end the session.

Restraint has many drawbacks. It can literally or symbolically involve sexual stimulation; it feeds masochistic wishes of the child; it is a gross deviation from the neutrality of a supposed transference object; it places the therapist at risk of being accused of assault; in the absence of a therapeutic alliance, it may actually reinforce fantasies of omnipotence in the child, which can be quite frightening ('See, not even *you* can contain me!').

Perhaps the wisest comment about restraint is that an ounce of prevention is worth a pound of cure. Recognition of early warning signs of loss of impulse control should be the goal of both child and therapist. During assessment, the clinician should screen for minimal levels of affect and behaviour regulation. If these are absent, then treatment modalities other than individual psychotherapy should be considered, or consultation around adjunctive approaches, such as pharmacotherapy, should be obtained.

Similar warnings apply to physical expressions of affection or attempts to calm a child. Although well-meaning, affectionate touching can emphasize inequality between therapist and patient and may be interpreted as inappropriate sexualization of the relationship. Prior discussion with the parents as to what methods are used to soothe their highly anxious or frightened child can usually lead to creative alternatives (e.g., allowing the child to enter the session with a favourite blanket or pacifier). On the other hand, a handshake at the end of a session can be an expression of mutual respect and a non-verbal way of the child saying 'Thanks.'

Goals of Play Therapy

Play therapy (or play as part of therapy) operates as a positive force for change in a number of ways. The relationship itself fosters growth through new identifications, reworking of transference distortions, and corrective emotional experiences which are part of the safe, nonjudgmental context. Ventilation, abreaction, and catharsis allow discharge of affect which may have been repressed.

Insight is enhanced. The role of insight with children is somewhat controversial (Shapiro & Esman, 1985). 'The development of awareness should not be viewed as a panacea, but as an aid for the child to cope more effectively' (Carek, 1972, p. 27). With adults, insight has come to signify a cognitive and affective appreciation of the 'why' of behaviour.

With children, whose reality-testing and capacity for self-reflection ('observing ego') are developmentally determined, a more realistic goal may be an enhanced awareness of the 'what' of behaviour. Certainly connecting thoughts, feelings, and behaviour is a valid aim of child therapy as is helping the child to appreciate his own contribution to each. But, as Whyte (1960) has noted, 'self-awareness is basically self-eliminating. Consciousness is like a fever which hastens curative processes by eliminating its source' (p. 28).

The ultimate goal of child therapy, and the means by which it is 'curative,' is the removal of blocks to development. Awareness sufficient to attenuate distortions of adaptation, be they consciously or unconsciously derived, intra- or interpersonally maintained, is both the means and the end of the therapeutic endeavour with children.

TERMINATION

'Leaving this treatment is not like dying, because you can see the person again, but it is like having someone close die, because you are really on your own' (Schmukler, 1990, p. 473). This was a sixteen-year-old boy's comment on termination, and it poignantly captures the bittersweet ambivalence of ending a close therapeutic relationship.

While much has been written about termination of therapy with adults, there are comparatively fewer guidelines for when and how to end with children. There is a rich literature within child analysis, but it consists primarily of case descriptions. Even in that domain, controversy exists about whether one can truly speak of termination, given the debate over whether or not children can develop a transference neurosis (Schmukler, 1991).

This dearth is rather surprising in view of the gains which have been made over the last thirty years in understanding the importance of attachment, separation, and loss in children (Bowlby, 1969, 1973, 1980, 1988a). Nevertheless, the application of this knowledge to psychotherapeutic technique for children older than three years has lagged (Rutter, 1995).

Gillman (1991) has suggested that therapists are guilty of 'childism' – the tendency to avoid acknowledging the significance which a clinician may have to a child. This, in turn, may arise out of ignorance of development, countertransference separation anxiety, or simply generalizations based on children's limited ability to verbalize their feelings.

Whatever the sources of this relative neglect, or 'blind spot,' it is clear that the usual criteria of termination for adults cannot be applied to children. 'Mature' object relations, genital primacy of libido, and the ability to work are all irrelevant or developmentally impossible for pre-teens, and only partially achievable even by the end of adolescence.

Vulnerability to separation, dependency on adults, and incomplete personality development require a different approach. Furthermore, the *parents'* relationship to the child's therapist also needs to be taken into account, because parents will frequently prolong or shorten the child's treatment for their own needs.

Deciding when and how to end depends on the goals established at the beginning of therapy, the duration and severity of presenting symptoms, the orientation of the therapist, and a past history of separations. A shorter course of therapy will be indicated for cases in which the symptoms are of recent onset or milder severity, the goals of therapy are more supportive or synthetic, the orientation is more cognitive or behavioural, and there is no past history of insecure attachment or traumatic separation. Longer treatment is usually indicated for chronic or severe symptoms; when conflict resolution and psychodynamic insight are the goals; in children who have demonstrated problems in engaging or detaching from significant others owing to experiences of early loss; or multiple disruptions of caretaking.

Criteria for determining when the child is ready to stop should encompass his or her adjustment both in and out of therapy. In the 'real world,' there should be evidence of resumed progressive development in terms of peer relationships, academic achievement (the child's equivalent of work), hobbies or extra-curricular activities, and family relationships. Knowledge of these areas may have to come directly from the sources – usually parents and teachers – if the child is very young. Progress should be clear not just because of avoidance of conflict or constriction of risk. Instead, active engagement in the stage-appropriate tasks of development should be reported.

Within the therapy, a number of factors can signal preparation for termination (Weiner, 1970; Carek, 1972; Kernberg, 1991). These include: reacting to therapist absences (due to vacation, illness, or even just weekends) with little anxiety and good tolerance in the context of a strong therapeutic alliance; statements about the therapist which indicate 'object constancy' (i.e., the ability to preserve a stable representation of the therapist in the face of strong negative affect) and 'object permanence' (the ability to remember the therapist despite long absences); realistic ambivalence; identification with the therapist and his or her function (i.e., an introspective attitude); less investment in therapy and more in reality, along with a sense of the passage of time in the therapy, (i.e., a shared history and a possible future, if necessary); higher-level defences such as humour and sublimation, as well as increased flexibility, range, and adaptiveness of defences, especially modulation of affect and impulse control, as shown by improved frustration tolerance, ability to delay gratification, and expressions of relief and gratitude in connection with termination alongside sadness; symptom reduction, decreased acting out, and a strengthened observing ego as shown by the ability to laugh at one's self and empathize with others; play activity and/or reports of dreams which are more pleasurable.

One should expect a certain degree of symptom reoccurrence as a 'protest' against the impending separation, and perhaps the child's way of preserving the memory of the relationship, in effect saying, 'Remember how we started and where we came from, Doc?' These symptoms, however, should subside with interpretation and limit-setting, and should call for a re-evaluation of the decision to terminate if they are dangerous and persistent. As Kernberg has noted (1991), one should be able to answer the question 'If the child were being seen for the first time *now*, would you recommend therapy?' with a confident 'No.'

Countertransference reactions can be particularly strong when working with children. The commonest is perhaps guilt over abandonment (O'Reilly, 1987), and can lead to unnecessary prolongation of treatment. Patient and therapist may unconsciously engage in a 'dance,' trying to decide who is leaving whom. For this reason, self-analysis or peer supervision, especially for the less experienced clinician, is advisable to assist with implementing plans for termination.

The actual method of ending depends again on the goals, format, and orientation of the therapy, and differences of opinion exist. The timing of the decision, for instance, carries both risks and benefits. Too long a 'lead time' may engender a defensive weakening of the alliance. On the other hand, in a child who is severely disturbed, or who has a history of multiple, traumatic losses, more time will be needed to work through the issues associated with ending.

If the therapy has been psychoanalytically oriented, then the frequency of sessions should not be decreased. Fewer sessions will deprive both patient and therapist of opportunities to explore the meaning of ending and may confuse the child in terms of altered process. Qualitative, not quantitative, change is the harbinger of true conflict resolution. Kernberg (1991) goes as far as advising that termination *not* coincide with vacations or school endings, because then it's not a 'true' test of how the child would cope in real life. Similarly, she cautions clinicians not to become more of a 'real' object as the end nears. If the child decides to re-enter therapy at a future date, such deviations from the agreed-upon *modus operandi* could interfere with the development of a transference neurosis.

On the other hand, if the therapy is more synthetic, supportive, or relationship-oriented (as opposed to exploratory or insight-oriented), then decreasing the frequency of sessions is advised in order to lessen the impact of perceived abandonment, 'wean' the child off of therapy, and reassure the patient that he or she will be all right and 'can do it' (Weiner, 1970).

It is wise to involve the parents in the termination process in some fashion. One can anticipate 'symptom reoccurrence' or 'acting out' on their part, as mentioned above, as *they* become anxious over 'getting their child back' without the support of the therapist. If they have been in concurrent family therapy or parent counselling, this may be less necessary, since the issues would presumably be dealt with in that forum. If, however, individual child therapy is the only modality, then the child's therapist should meet with the parents at least a few times to ensure their support for the termination.

WORK WITH ADOLESCENTS

Psychotherapy with disturbed adolescents – whether individual, family, or group – is certainly challenging. Many clinicians avoid treating adolescents because of the latter's tendencies to act out and drop out (of therapy). Therapists as distinguished as Anna Freud have described the treatment of teenagers as 'a hazardous venture from beginning to end' (Freud, 1958, p. 256), while Josselyn (1957) considers it to be among 'the most frustrating, baffling, anxiety-arousing experiences a psychiatrist can have' (p. 14).

While adolescents generally turn to their parents or friends when seeking help for psychological problems (Offer, Howard, Shonert, & Ostrov, 1991), that fact may reflect the lack of accessibility and poor quality of professional help, more than adolescent 'resistance' *per se*

(Kellam, Branch, Brown, & Russell, 1981). Adolescents are said to be 'poor candidates' for psychotherapy. Empirical research shows that this attitude is unwarranted. In most adult outpatient clinics, only 50 per cent of patients return for their first agreed-upon therapy appointment, and 70 per cent have left treatment (unilaterally) by the fifth session (Phillips, 1988). By comparison, only 20 per cent of teenagers terminate therapy unilaterally, and when open-ended contracts are considered separately from time-limited (up to six months) ones, only 7 per cent drop out of the latter modality (Suzuki, 1989).

In fact, Balser (1966) reports that about 80 per cent of disturbances that develop during adolescence respond well to short-term therapy, and more recent case reports support this finding (Golombek & Korenblum, 1995). 'Adolescents usually respond with gratifying ease and speed to proper treatment because of their flexibility and resilience' (Gallagher & Harris, 1964, p. 64). As Seiffge-Krende (1989) notes, 'Adolescence is a period when we can detect early signs of potentially serious trouble, offering a unique opportunity to intervene' (p. 473).

The Subphases of Adolescence

As a guideline, it is important to recognize that adolescence is not a homogeneous process. Early, middle, and late adolescents differ from each other in characteristic ways (Blos, 1962) which dictate different therapeutic approaches (Golombek, 1983; Esman, 1985).

Early teenagers (roughly twelve to fourteen years old) are predominantly 'oral.' Their major preoccupation is with dependency, and their conflict is around trust. Still in the throes of pubertal changes, they tend to be action-oriented and less reflective. They characteristically demand, 'I want, I need, I have to have.' Therapists working with this age group often feel like they are being sucked dry or used as a gas station, just to fill their patients up. Techniques used should approximate those used with younger children, often incorporating activity or 'play' accessories such as board games. Concurrent family or group therapy is often appropriate, and individual therapy should be highly supportive.

Middle adolescents (fourteen to sixteen years old) are more 'anal.' Like the two- or three-year-old who is out to prove his or her autonomy, this teenager declares 'I can do everything myself.' Omnipotent grandiosity, narcissism, and splitting are common, making verbal sparring the order of the day. Therapists need to be able to tolerate this kind of interaction in order to facilitate self–other differentiation and help the teenager feel safe (i.e., contained) with respect to aggressive urges. It is as if the patient is trying to define him- or herself by opposing the therapist, and discovering what he or she is *not*, in order to clarify what he or she *is*. This calls for an active stance in the context of non-judgmental empathy.

Concurrent parent counselling (by another therapist) may be useful to provide structure for the 'affective storms,' but family therapy is likely to be strongly resisted. A flexible mixture of support and insight in individual therapy is usually helpful. Despite their 'phobia' of dependence, middle adolescents are actually easier to engage than early teenagers because of their greater cognitive (Piagetian) capacities, and their natural inclination to begin philosophically grappling with issues of existence, morality, and mortality.

Late adolescents (seventeen to nineteen) present saying, 'I want to be understood; I want to love and be loved by another separate person.' They are much more capable of ambivalent, 'whole–object' relationships, and have the cognitive capacity for self-reflection. The difference from adults is the degree to which these gains are tenuous. Under stress, regression can appear, and therapists can feel frustrated or confused unless they are prepared for this fluidity. Individual therapy alone demonstrates respect for autonomy, and exploratory (insight-oriented) approaches are more feasible in view of enhanced ego strengths.

Countertransference with Adolescents

When a clinician is working with adolescents, his or her conceptual beliefs and personality of the clinician are of crucial importance (Sanchez,1986; Korenblum, 1993). If the therapist holds the mistaken view that adolescent turmoil is inevitable and universal (as many mental health professionals do), then he or she may underdiagnose serious psychopathology (Offer et al, 1991). If the clinician has unresolved residual conflicts from his or her own adolescence, then there may be a neurotic tendency to over- or counteridentify with the patient. Anthony (1969) has convincingly described how adults tend to stereotype adolescents to defend against their own narcissistic, sexual, and aggressive anxieties.

Teenagers are masters at pointing out our flaws. It is part of their developmental need to de-idealize parental figures. As a result, our needs to be flattered, to be caretakers, to be sexually desirable, to have control, and to be correct can feel as if they are being assaulted. Neurotic fears of criticism, engulfment, being seduced, passivity, or being wrong may be exposed, similar to countertransference reactions when working with borderline adults (Kroll, 1988).

Personal beliefs about abortion, sexual activity, drug use, religion, and politics may clash with those of the patient, and we may be tempted to diagnose non-existing pathology just to protect our self-esteem.

When teenagers devalue their therapists, it is important to understand the underlying dynamics. Their rage may represent: a defence against wishes for nurturance, which are particularly threatening for middle and late adolescents, who are trying to deny dependence; a defence against envy of the therapist; projection of low self-esteem; or a manifestation of transference.

Therapeutic Alliance

To achieve engagement, the therapist must allow the teenager to be comfortable, but still involve him or her beyond the level of the superficial (Weiner, 1970). This requires a delicate titration of anxiety. The patient can't feel so relaxed that appointments become 'bull-sessions.' But, if the teenager is paralysed by irrational anxieties about what a psychiatrist can or cannot do to him or her (for instance), then obviously communication will be hindered.

One must also help the patient to acknowledge his or her own role in determining the course of treatment. Whether the therapy is short-term or open-ended, clearly defined goals or foci should be chosen, mutually agreed upon, and adhered to. This process models boundary-setting, negotiation, and persistence. Requiring consensus between therapist and patient on the choice of goals conveys respect for the teenager's decision-making wishes and capacities, and reinforces ownership of the process and outcome.

A *therapeutic* alliance is characterized by strengthened ego functions: reality testing, object relations, judgment, regulation of impulses and affects, mastery, and synthesis, along with a general attitude of curiosity, introspection, and shared confrontation of painful affects.

The key to maintaining a therapeutic alliance usually lies in the careful and systematic attention to affective states as they present in the 'here and now' of the treatment process. Whether one is conducting interpersonal, cognitive, behavioural, or psychodynamic therapy, the primary task is usually to connect thoughts, feelings, and behaviours in ways which the teenager has heretofore not recognized.

At times, teenagers defensively try to distort the therapeutic process by seducing the therapist into 'unholy alliances' with superego or id (Meeks, 1986). In the former, the clinician is put in the position of the judgmental, punitive policeman-parent – 'Why can't I smoke in your office?' In the latter, one is set up to collude with or derive vicarious gratification from the patient's sexual or aggressive urges – 'Do you want to hear more about my hot date with Nancy last night, Doc?' Less commonly, an unholy alliance with pathological ego defences is sought, via prolonged philosophical discussions which consist of nothing more than intellectualization, for instance.

Practical guidance as to what one should actually *do* to facilitate an alliance is offered by Church (1989). She compared novice with experienced therapists by coding audiotapes of therapy sessions with middle-adolescent patients (blind as to therapist status). The patient's responses to various interventions were categorized: ignoring, changing the subject, disagreement, simple agreement (factual statements), and agreement followed by new information about their thoughts and feelings (complex agreement). She found very significant differences in the responses to experienced versus novice therapists. The teenagers agreed with 92 per cent of the experienced therapists' interventions – 60 per cent in a complex fashion and 32 per cent in simple fashion. By contrast, the patients either ignored (8 per cent), actively disagreed with (18 per cent), or changed the subject (28 per cent) in response to novices' interventions, for a total 'rejection' rate of 54 per cent.

While the goal of therapy is not to simply persuade the patient to agree with the therapist, it is clear that the experienced clinicians were able to elicit new information about their teenagers' thoughts and feelings to a much greater degree than were the novices, and fostered a more positive alliance. Why?

Church found that novices attempted to control the discussion by being too directive, asking closed-ended questions, and making interpretations which were theory-driven instead of relating to actual process in the session. If the patient initiated discussion about therapy or the therapeutic relationship, the novices tend to ignore the comments or change the topic. They devoted much more time to less threatening issues such as scheduling, or the patient's behaviour outside the office.

Experienced therapists, on the other hand, responded neutrally and empathically to patient-led comments about therapy, and focused much more on affect, as opposed to behaviour. They readily acknowledged when they had made an error, even apologizing when some aspect of the contract had been transgressed. The alliance subsequently became stronger. Their interventions were experience-near, based on 'here and now' phenomena of the session. While active, in the sense of immediately responding to important leads, they were less controlling, and framed their interventions as hypotheses to be jointly examined, rather than pronouncements from 'on high.'

Church concludes that adolescents will most easily discuss their feelings and thoughts about therapy when therapists respond promptly to explicit and implicit references to the relationship; a focus on affect and cognition engenders greater openness than a focus on behaviour *per se*; directive comments, in which advice or opinions are offered (especially when unsolicited), seem counter-productive; apologizing for mistakes strengthens the relationship; interventions should be based on material from the sessions, not experience-distant theory.

Transference Interpretations

With regard to transference interpretations, a number of guidelines should be followed (Swift & Wonderlich, 1990): emphasize the 'here and now' aspects, rather than the genetic roots; be slow to interpret positive transference, since a certain degree of idealization is necessary to cement the therapeutic alliance, but be quick to interpret negative transference; always work from the 'top down' (i.e., conscious to unconscious, defence to anxiety), and rarely, if ever, make direct impulse or id interpretations; interpret more actively with late and less actively with early adolescents because of the latter's fragile self-esteem and diminished introspective tendency; be judicious in the use of interpretation – many non-dynamic interventions (such as education, humour, advice, limit-setting) may be equally useful, depending on the goals of therapy.

Self-Disclosure

Is self-disclosure helpful to the adolescent patient? Weiner and King (1977) offer some useful guidelines, noting that the context of disclosure is more important than the content *per se*. The risks include: changing the focus of therapy from patient to therapist; leaving the therapist open to both transferential and reality-based manipulation ('I'll tell you something if you tell me something'); and abandonment of neutrality, creating the opportunity for the 'unholy alliances' mentioned above. On occasion, however, certain properly-timed disclosures can facilitate reality testing, and that is the main benefit. With very disturbed patients, whose ego is becoming overwhelmed, as evidenced by preoccupation with primary process, or poor self–other boundaries, clear statements about who the therapist is (and is not) can be useful. Self-disclosure is therefore indicated if it helps distract the patient from unconscious impulses, emphasizes the reality and separateness of the therapist from the patient and his or her parents, offers a model of identification for handling painful affects (e.g., acute grief), and distinguishes between fantasy and action.

Disclosure for the sake of honesty alone, or to become the patient's 'friend,' is not useful. It tends to undermine the professionalism and expertise which the patient expects and needs to make therapy a safe place. On the other hand, a request for information about how to handle a certain situation, especially if the patient is experientially deprived, intellectually limited, or socially and emotionally detached, can be evaluated and responded to if the orientation is primarily supportive and a therapeutic relationship has already been established.

Confidentiality and Contact with Parents

The previously mentioned parameters of confidentiality apply to this age group as well. Generally, the older and higher-functioning the teenager, the more confidentiality should be respected. When the clinician feels compelled to share certain information, he or she can emphasize that the teenager will be told first, and that, even if certain behaviours are communicated to others, the thoughts and feelings of the patient will remain private.

In liaising with parents, the phone line should remain open to receiving material *from* them, even if the direction of information is limited the other way. Too often, parents feel (and are) shut out of the therapeutic process. They should be told that the therapist reserves the right to let the teenager know of their call, so that the therapist is not put in the position of keeping secrets. However, data from the family can be extremely useful, especially with an 'externalizing' teenager who tends to deny, or a severely depressed teen who is relatively mute.

Parents can be reassured that their input is valued and will play a role in the course of their son or daughter's therapy, as long as the purpose is to help the clinician understand their child better. Attempts to coerce either the patient or the therapist to behave (or not behave) in a certain manner, would, of course, be unacceptable. But just knowing that they *can* call if need be often has a beneficial effect on the alliance with the family.

Paradoxical Techniques and Other Parameters

On occasion, certain adolescents and their families are highly 'resistant.' They seem to defeat themselves and therapists when the usual psychotherapeutic interventions are offered. In these instances, consideration may be given to so-called paradoxical techniques (Rohrbaugh, Tennen, Press, & White, 1981; Fisher, Anderson, & Jones, 1981). However, these manoeuvres carry significant risks, and should only be tried after a thorough evaluation of the patient or family's dynamics, and preferably by clinicians familiar with their use. They work best with individuals or families who are overly structured and rigid. They are contraindicated in situations where structure and boundaries are lacking and/or the potential for dangerous acting out is high.

Indeed, certain situations call for extraordinary parameters such as placement in a hospital inpatient unit or residential treatment centre. The use of psychotherapy with the pregnant, runaway, violent, or drug- abusing adolescent is best left to a specialist in adolescent psychiatry. A review of these circumstances is beyond the scope of this chapter, but texts by Holmes (1964), Meeks (1986), and Wexler (1991) cover such topics.

Termination with Adolescents

Regarding termination, the stage-appropriate developmental tasks of adolescents should serve as markers for determining when therapy has been successful, and therefore when it is time to end. Has the teenager come to terms with his or her body image and sexual orientation? Has the patient begun to separate and individuate from parents, relinquishing incestuous ties and gradually de-idealizing them in the process? Has he or she begun to formulate a moral/ethical belief system? Is there an indication of assuming responsibility for making a choice of vocation or postsecondary education? Is there a capacity for ambivalent, whole–object relationships, as demonstrated by seeing both the good and bad qualities of the therapist, parents, and significant others? Are the ego functions of reality testing and affect regulation sufficiently strong and flexible to permit continued growth? Is the sense of identity more cohesive and stable?

If the answers to these questions are 'Yes,' then it is time to consider ending therapy. The family should support the decision, especially if the teenager is still living at home. Parents, after all, may be going through a 'middlescence' of their own, struggling with parallel developmental tasks but from the perspective of middle age: separating from parents (the teenager's grandparents) via illness or death; adjusting to waning sexuality (the so-called menopause–menarche syndrome); re-evaluating ethics, values, and perhaps job definition.

The exact *modus operandi* of terminating will depend on the goals of therapy, as described in the previous section. However, in view of most teenagers' profound ambivalence over dependency, flexibility is crucial. Experimentation with decreased frequency of sessions, or even allowing the patient to leave therapy briefly and then return, is appropriate in terms of giving him or her a sense of control over the process. More disturbed teens may need a transitional object, a so-called teddy bear of adolescence (Ekstein, 1983), to help them through the ending. A simple appointment card may suffice, if explicitly designated as such.

Provided that the therapist can confront conflicting countertransference feelings (usually trouble letting go versus a wish to 'kick out'), and the family is flexible enough to have their changed teenager 'back' (i.e., out of therapy), then it is probably time to heed Meeks's dictum (1986, p. 266): 'Individuation is best served by assisting the adolescent towards a workable character synthesis and then quickly moving aside so that the adolescent's strengths propel him towards real and available objects outside of the therapy office.'

Cost-Effectiveness

While cost is certainly an important consideration, the purpose of practice guidelines is to assist clinical decision making, not resource allocation. To evaluate cost-effectiveness, there would need to be agreement on whose costs – the child's, the parent's, the school's, the insurance company's – and which costs – direct treatment costs or indirect expenses, such as time lost from work (McIntyre & Zarin, 1996)?

The personal cost of pain, suffering, and inconvenience cannot easily be assigned a dollar value. What is the cost of impaired peer relations to a five-year-old as compared with a fifteen-year old? These judgments are arbitrary, and thus reliable cost data are sorely lacking (Rush, 1996). Furthermore, cost issues are not necessarily germane to what is best for the patient. Empirical evidence may, for example, suggest a treatment that simply cannot be delivered because of lack of providers, inaccessibility, or expense (Merriam & Karasu, 1996).

Instead, quantitative and qualitative, and experimental–laboratory and naturalistic-clinical, paradigms should complement each other.

Practice guidelines such as those described in this chapter should be applied with an attitude of critical enquiry, in the spirit of 'clinician-scientist.'

Let us hope that we have moved beyond the split conveyed in the old saying 'Researchers know everything about nothing. Clinicians know nothing about everything.'

References

Achenbach, T.M., & Edelbrock, C.S. (1981). Behavioral problems and competencies reported by parents of normal and disturbed children aged 4 through 16. *Monographs of the Society for Research in Child Development, 46* (1, No. 188). Chicago: Society for Research in Child Development.

Achenbach, T.M., Phares, V., Howell, C.T., Rauh, V.A., & Nurcombe, B. (1990). Seven-year outcome of the Vermont Intervention Program for low-birthweight infants. *Child Development, 61,* 1672–1681.

Alexander, J.F. (1988). Phases of family therapy process: A framework for clinicians and researchers. In L.C. Wynne (Ed.), *The state of the Art in family therapy research*. New York: Family Process.

Alexander, J.F., & Parsons, B.V. (1982). *Functional family therapy.* Monterey, CA: Brooks/Cole.

Alpert, A. (1959). Reversibility of pathological fixations associated with maternal deprivation in infancy. *Psychoanalytic Study of the Child, 14,* 169–185.

American Psychiatric Association (APA). (1987). *Diagnostic and statistical manual of mental disorders* (3d ed., revised). Washington, DC: Author.

American Psychiatric Association (APA). (1994). *Diagnostic and statistical manual of mental disorders* (4th ed.). Washington, DC: Author.

An Act Respecting the Protection and Well-Being of Children and Their Families (Bill 77). (1984). Toronto: Queen's Printer for Ontario.

Anthony, E.J. (1975). The reactions of adults to adolescents and their behavior. In A.H. Esman (Ed.), *The psychology of adolescence: Essential readings*. New York: International Universities Press.

Asarnow, J.R., & Carlson, G.A. (1988). Childhood depression: Five-year outcome following combined cognitive–behavior therapy and pharmacotherapy. *American Journal of Psychotherapy, 42,* 456–464.

Balser, B.H. (1966). A new recognition of adolescence. *American Journal of Psychiatry, 122,* 1281–1282.

Bird, H.R., Canino, G., Rubio-Stipec, M., Gould, M.S., Ribera, J., Sesman, M., Woodbury, M., Huertas-Goldman, S., Pagan, A., Sanchez-Lacay, A., &

Moscoso, M. (1988). Estimates of the prevalence of childhood maladjustment in a community survey of Puerto Rico: The use of combined measures. *Archives of General Psychiatry, 45*, 1120–1126.

Blos, P. (1962). *On adolescence: A psychoanalytic interpretation.* New York: The Free Press.

Bowlby, J. (1969). *Attachment and loss. Vol. 1 Attachment.* New York: Basic.

Bowlby, J. (1973). *Attachment and loss. Vol. 2. Separation, anxiety, and anger.* London: Hogarth Press.

Bowlby, J. (1980). *Attachment and loss. Vol. 3. Loss, sadness, and depression.* London: Hogarth Press.

Bowlby, J. (1988a). *A secure base: Clinical implications of attachment theory.* London: Routledge & Kegan Paul.

Bowlby, J. (1988b). *A secure base: Parent–child attachment and healthy human attachment.* New York: Basic.

Brown, J. (1987). A review of meta-analyses conducted on psychotherapy outcome research. *Clinical Psychology Review, 7*, 1–23.

Carek, D.J. (1972). *Principles of child psychotherapy.* Springfield, IL: Charles C. Thomas.

Carlisle, J. (1996). Duty to warn: Report from Council. College of Physicians and Surgeons of Ontario (CPSO), *Members' Dialogue, 4*, 21–22.

Casey, R.J., & Berman, J.S. (1985). The outcome of psychotherapy with children. *Psychology Bulletins, 98*, 388–400.

Church, E. (1989). Facilitating the therapeutic relationship in adolescent psychotherapy. Paper presented at the Annual Meeting of the American Orthopsychiatry Association, New York City.

Cleghorn, J.M., Miller, G.H., & Humphrey, B.C. (1982). Psychiatric manpower in Ontario. Part I: A survey and recommendations. *Canadian Journal of Psychiatry, 27*, 617–628.

College of Physicians and Surgeons of Ontario (CPSO). (1996). *A guide to the Health Care Consent Act.* Toronto: Author.

Consumer Reports (1995, November). Mental health: Does therapy help? Pp. 734–739.

Cooke, R.E. (1977). An ethical and procedural basis for research on children. *Journal of Pediatrics, 90*, 681–682.

Cooper, S., & Wanerman, L. (1977). *Children in treatment: A primer for beginning psychotherapists.* New York: Brunner/Mazel.

Cox, A., & Rutter, M. (1985). Diagnostic appraisal and interviewing. In M. Rutter & L. Hersov (Eds.), *Child and adolescent psychiatry: Modern approaches* (2d ed.). Oxford: Blackwell Scientific.

Cramer, B., Robert-Tissot, C., Stern, D.W., Serpa-Rusconi, S., De Muralt, M.,

Besson, G., Palacio-Espasa, F., Bachmann, J., Knauer, D., Berney, C., & D'Arcis, U. (1990). Outcome evaluation in brief mother–infant psychotherapy: A preliminary report. *Infant Mental Health Journal, 11,* 278–300.

Despert, J.L. (1937). Technical approaches used in the study and treatment of emotional problems in children, V: The playroom. *Psychiatry Quarterly, 11,* 677–690.

Diamond, G., & Dickey, M.S. (1993). Process research: Its history, intent, and findings. *Family Psychology, 9,* 23–25.

Dulcan, M.K. (1984). Brief psychotherapy with children and their families: The state of the art. *Journal of Amererican Academy of Child Psychiatry, 23,* 544–551.

Dumas, J.E. (1989). Treating antisocial behavior in children: Child and family approaches. *Clinical Psychology Review, 9,* 197–222.

Edelbrock, C., & Costello, A.J. (1988). Structured psychiatric interviews for children. In M. Rutter, A.H. Tuma, & I.S. Lann (Eds.), *Assessment and diagnosis in child psychopathology.* New York: Guilford.

Edelbrock, C., Costello, A.J., Dulcan, M.K., Kalas, R., & Conover, N.C. (1985). Age differences in the reliability of the psychiatric interview of the child. *Child Development, 56,* 265–275.

Eisenstadt, T.H., Eyberg, S., McNeil, C.B., Newcomb, K., & Funderburk, B. (1993). Parent–child interaction therapy with behavior problem children: Relative effectiveness of two stages and overall treatment outcome. *Journal of Clinical Child Psychology, 22,* 42–51.

Ekstein, R. (1983). The adolescent self during the process of termination of treatment: Termination, interruption, or intermission? In S.C. Feinstein &   P. Giovacchini (Eds.), *Adolescent psychiatry* (Vol. 11, pp. 125–146). Chicago: University of Chicago Press.

Ekstein, R., & Friedman, S.W. (1957). The function of acting out, play action, and play acting in the psychotherapeutic process. *Journal of American Psychoanalytic Association, 5,* 581–600.

Erikson, E.H. (1950). *Childhood and society.* New York: Norton.

Esman, A.H. (1985). A developmental approach to the psychotherapy of adolescents. In S.C. Feinstein & P. Giovacchini (Eds.), *Adolescent psychiatry* (Vol. 12, pp. 119–133). Chicago: University of Chicago Press.

Field, T.M., Widmayer, S.M., Stringer, S., & Ignatoff, E. (1980). Teenage, lower-class, black mothers and their preterm infants: An intervention and developmental follow-up. *Child Development, 51,* 426–436.

Fisher, L., Anderson, A., & Jones, J.J. (1981). Types of paradoxical intervention and indications/contraindications for use in clinical practice. *Family Process, 20,* 25–35.

Fonagy, P. & Moran, G.S. (1990). Studies on the efficacy of child psychoanalysis. *Journal of Consulting and Clinical Psychology, 58,* 684–695.

Fonagy, P., & Target, M. (1996). Predictors of outcome in child psychoanalysis: A retrospective study of 763 cases at the Anna Freud Centre. *Journal of the American Psychoanalytic Association, 44,* 27–77.

Fonagy, P., Steele, H., & Steele, M. (1991). Maternal representations of attachment during pregnancy predict the organization of infant–mother attachment at one year of age. *Child Development, 62,* 891–905.

Forehand, R., & McMahon, R.J. (1981). *Helping the noncompliant child: A clinician's guide to parent training.* New York: Guilford.

Fraiberg, S., Shapiro, V., & Cherniss, D. (1983). Treatment modalities. In J.D. Call, E. Galenson, & R.L. Tyson (Eds.), *Frontiers of infant psychiatry* (Vol. 6). New York: Basic.

Frances, A., Clarkin, J., & Perry, S. (1984). *Differential therapeutics in psychiatry: The art and science of treatment selection.* New York: Brunner/Mazel.

Freud, A. (1958). Adolescence. *Psychoanalytic Study of the Child, 13,* 255–278.

Freud, A. (1963). The concept of developmental lines. *Psychoanalytic Study of the Child, 18,* 245–265.

Freud, S. (1953). Fragment of an analysis of a case of hysteria. In J. Strachey (Ed. and Trans.), *The standard edition of the complete psychological works of Sigmund Freud* (Vol. 7, pp. 7–122). London: Hogarth Press. (Original work published 1905)

Freud, S. (1955). Analysis of a phobia in a five-year-old boy. In J. Strachey (Ed. and Trans.), *The standard edition of the complete psychological works of Sigmund Freud* (Vol. 10, pp. 5–149). London: Hogarth Press. (Original work published 1909)

Gallagher, J.R., & Harris, H.I. (1964). *Emotional problems of adolescents.* New York: Oxford University Press.

Gardner, R. (1985). The initial clinical evaluation of the child. In D. Shaffer, A.A. Ehrhardt, & L.L. Greenhill (Eds.), *The clinical guide to child psychiatry.* New York: Free Press.

Gillman, R.D. (1991). Termination in psychotherapy with children and adolescents. In A.G. Schmukler (Ed.), *Saying goodbye.* Hillsdale, NJ: Analytic Press.

Goldstein, M.J., Rodnick, E.H., Evans, J.R., Philip, R.A., May, R.A., & Steinberg, M.R. (1978). Drug and family therapy in the aftercare of acute schizophrenics. *Archives of General Psychiatry, 35,* 1169–1177.

Golombek, H. (1983). Personality development during adolescence: Implications for treatment. In H. Golombek & B. Garfinkel (Eds.), *The adolescent and mood disturbance.* New York: International Universities Press.

Golombek, H., & Korenblum, M.S. (1995). Brief psychoanalytic psychotherapy with adolescents. In R.C. Marohn & S.C. Feinstein (Eds.), *Adolescent psychiatry* (Vol. 20). Hillsdale, NJ: Analytic Press.

Haley, J. (1963). *Strategies of psychotherapy.* New York: Grune & Stratton.

Hambidge, G. (1955). Structured play therapy. *American Journal of Orthopsychiatry, 25,* 601–610.

Harth, S.C., & Thong, Y.H. (1990). Sociodemographic and motivational characteristics of parents who volunteer their children for clinical research: A controlled study. *British Medical Journal, 300,* 1375–1376.

Hazelrigg, M.D., Cooper, H.M., & Borduin, C.M. (1987). Evaluating the effectiveness of family therapies: An integrative review and analysis. *Psychology Bulletin, 101,* 4228–4442.

Henggeler, S.W., Borduin, C.M., Melton, G.B., Mann, B.J., & Smith, L.A. (1991). Effects of multisystemic therapy on drug use and abuse in serious juvenile offenders: A progress report from two outcome studies. *Family Dynamics in Addictions Quarterly, 1,* 40–51.

Heseltine, G.F. (1983). *Towards a blueprint for change: A mental health policy and program perspective.* Toronto: Ontario Ministry of Health.

Holmes, D.J. (1964). *The adolescent in psychotherapy.* Boston: Little, Brown.

Horne, A.M., & Sayger, T.V. (1990). *Treating conduct and oppositional disorders in children.* Elmsford, NY: Pergamon.

Hug-Hellmuth, H. (1921). On the technique of child analysis. *International Journal of Psycho-Analysis, 2,* 287–305.

Jensen, P.S., Ryan, N.D., & Prien, R. (1992). Psychopharmacology of child and adolescent major depression: Present status and future directions. *Journal of Child and Adolescent Psychopharmacology, 2,* 31–45.

John, K., Gammon, G.D., Prusoff, B.A., & Warner, V. (1987). The social adjustment inventory for children and adolescents (SAICA): Testing of a new semistructured interview. *Journal of the American Academy of Child and Adolescent Psychiatry, 26,* 898–911.

Johnson, F.K., Dowling, J., & Wesner, D. (1980). Notes on infant psychotherapy. *Infant Mental Health Journal, 1,* 19–33.

Josselyn, I.M. (1957). Psychotherapy of adolescents at the level of private practice. In B.H. Balser (Ed.). *Psychotherapy of the adolescent.* New York: International Universities Press.

Kashani, J.H., Orvaschel, H., Burk, J.P., & Reid, J.C. (1985). Informant variance: The issue of parent–child disagreement. *Journal of the American Academy of Child Psychiatry, 24,* 437–441.

Kazdin, A.E. (1990). Premature termination from treatment among children referred for antisocial behavior. *Journal of Child Psychology and Psychiatry, 31,* 415–425.

Kazdin, A.E., Bass, D., Ayers, W.A., & Rodgers, A. (1990). Empirical and clinical focus of child and adolescent psychotherapy research. *Journal of Consulting and Clinical Psychology, 58*, 729–740.

Kazdin, A.E., Siegel, T., & Bass, D. (1992). Cognitive problem-solving skills training and parent management training in the treatment of antisocial behavior in children. *Journal of Consulting and Clinical Psychology, 60*, 733–747.

Kellam, S.G., Branch, J.D., Brown, C.H. & Russell, G. (1981). Why teenagers come for treatment. *Journal of the American Academy of Child Psychiatry, 20*, 477–495.

Kendziora, K.T., & O'Leary, S.G. (1993). Dysfunctional parenting as a focus for prevention and treatment of child behavior problems. In T.H. Ollendick & J. Prinz (Eds.), *Advances in clinical child psychology* (Vol. 15). New York: Plenum.

Kernberg, P.F. (1991). Termination in child psychoanalysis: Criteria from within the sessions. In A.G. Schmukler (Ed.), *Saying goodbye*. Hillsdale, NJ: Analytic Press.

Kernberg, P.F. (1992). Discussion of 'A re-evaluation of estimates of child therapy effectiveness.' *Journal of the American Academy of Child and Adolescent Psychiatry, 31*, 710.

Kernberg, P.F., & Chazan, S.E. (1991). *Children with conduct disorders: A psychotherapy manual*. New York: Basic.

Kestenbaum, C.J. (1991). The clinical interview of the child. In J.M. Wiener (Ed.), *Textbook of child and adolescent psychiatry*. Washington, DC: American Psychiatric Press.

Klein, M. (1932). *The psychoanalysis of children*. London: Hogarth Press.

Koocher, G.P., & Pedulla, B.M. (1977). Current practices in child psychotherapy. *Professional Psychology, 8*, 275–287.

Koppitz, E.M. (1968). *Psychological evaluation of children's human figure drawings*. New York: Grune & Stratton.

Korenblum, M.S. (1993). Diagnostic difficulties in adolescent psychiatry: Where have we been, and where are we going? In S.C. Feinstein (Ed.), *Adolescent psychiatry* (Vol. 19). Chicago: University of Chicago Press.

Korenblum, M. (1996). Through the looking-glass: The home video as diagnostic aid. Grand Rounds presentation to the Department of Psychiatry, Sunnybrook Health Science Centre, Toronto, ON, April.

Kroll, J. (1988). *The challenge of the borderline patient*. New York: Norton.

Landy, S., Schubert, J., Cleland, J.F., & Montgomery, J.S. (1984). The effect of research with teenage mothers on the development of their infants. *Journal of Applied Social Psychology, 14*, 461–468.

Leff, J., Kuipers, L., Berkowitz, R., Eberlein-Vries, R., & Sturgeon, D. (1982). A controlled trial of social intervention in the families of schizophrenia patients. *British Journal of Psychiatry, 141*, 121–134.

Levy, D. (1939). Release therapy. *American Journal of Orthopsychiatry, 9*, 13–36.

Lewinsohn, P.M., Clarke, G.N., Hops, H., & Andrews, J. (1990). Cognitive–behavioral treatment for depressed adolescents. *Behavior Therapy, 21*, 385–401.

Lewis, C.C. (1981). How adolescents approach decisions: Changes over grades seven to twelve and policy implications. *Child Development, 52*, 538–544.

Lewis, M. (1991). Psychiatric assessment of infants, children, and adolescents. In M. Lewis (Ed.), *Child and adolescent psychiatry: A comprehensive textbook.* Baltimore: Williams & Wilkins.

Lieberman, A.F., Weston, D.R., & Pawl, J.H. (1991). Preventive intervention and outcome with anxiously attached dyads. *Child Development, 62*, 199–209.

Lojkasek, M., Cohen, N.J., & Muir, E. (1994). Where is the infant in infant intervention? A review of the literature on changing troubled mother–infant relationships. *Psychotherapy, 31*, 208–220.

Looney, J. (1980). Psychiatrists' transition from training to career: Stress and mastery. *American Journal of Psychiatry, 137*, 32–36.

Looney, J., Ellis, W., & Benedek E. (1985). Training in adolescent psychiatry for general psychiatry residents: Elements of a model curriculum. In S.C. Feinstein & P. Giovacchini (Eds.), *Adolescent psychiatry* (Vol. 12). Chicago: University of Chicago Press.

Luborsky, L. (1984). *Principles of psychoanalytic psychotherapy: A manual for supportive–expressive treatment.* New York: Basic.

Mahler, M., & Furer, M. (1982). Child psychosis: A theoretical statement and its implications. *Journal of Autism & Child Schizophrenia, 2*, 213–218.

Markus, E., Lange, A., & Pettigrew, T.F. (1990). Effectiveness of family therapy: A meta-analysis. *Journal of Family Therapy, 12*, 205–221.

McIntyre, J.S. & Zarin, D.A. (1996). The role of psychotherapy in the treatment of depression: Review of two practice guidelines. *Archives of General Psychiatry, 53*, 291–293.

McMahon, R. (1994). Diagnosis, assessment, and treatment of externalizing problems in children: The role of longitudinal data. *Journal of Consulting and Clinical Psychology, 62*, 901–917.

Meeks, J.E. (1986). *The fragile alliance: An orientation to the psychiatric treatment of the adolescent.* Malabar, FL: Robert E. Krieger.

Merriam, A.E., & Karasu, T.B. (1996). The role of psychotherapy in the treatment of depression: Review of two practice guidelines. *Archives of General Psychiatry, 53*, 301–302.

Metzl, M.M. (1980). Teaching parents a strategy for enhancing infant development. *Child Development, 51*, 583–586.

Michelson, L., Sugai, D.P., Wood, R.P., & Kazdin, A.E. (1983). *Social skills assessment and training with children.* New York: Plenum.

Muir, E. (1992). Watching, waiting, and wondering: Applying psychoanalytic principles to mother–infant intervention. *Infant Mental Health Journal, 13,* 319–328.

Naglieri, J.A. (1988). *Draw a person: A quantitative scoring system manual.* San Antonio, TX: Psychological Corporation/Harcourt, Brace, Jovanovich.

National Committee for the Protection of Human Subjects of Biomedical and Behavioral Research. (1977). *Report and Recommendations: Research involving children.* Washington, DC: DHEW Publication No. OS 77–0004.

Nurcombe, B., Howell, D.C., Ruah, V.A., Teti, D.M., Ruoff, P., Murphy, B., & Brennan, J. (1984). An intervention program for mothers of low-birthweight infants: Preliminary results. *Journal of the American Academy of Child Psychiatry, 23,* 319–325.

Offer, D., Ostrov, E., & Howard, K.I. (1984). *Patterns of adolescent self-image.* San Francisco: Jossey-Bass.

Offer, D., Howard, K.I., Shonert, K.A., & Ostrov, E. (1991). To whom do adolescents turn for help? Differences between disturbed and nondisturbed adolescents. *Journal of the American Academy of Child and Adolescent Psychiatry, 30,* 623–630.

Offord, D.R., Boyle, M.H., & Racine, Y.A. (1989). *Ontario Child Health Study: Children at risk.* Toronto: Ontario Ministry of Community and Social Services.

O'Reilly, R. (1987). The transfer syndrome. *Canadian Journal of Psychiatry, 32,* 674–678.

Orvaschel, H., Weissman, M.M., Padian, N., & Lowe, T.L. (1981). Assessing psychopathology in children of psychiatrically disturbed parents: A pilot study. *Journal of American Academy of Child Psychiatry, 20,* 112–122.

Ostrov, K., Dowling, J., Wesner, D.O., & Johnson, F.K. (1982). Maternal styles in infant psychotherapy: Treatment and research implications. *Infant Mental Health Journal, 3,* 162–173.

Parker, Z. (1992, May). Do all psychiatrists see children and adolescents? Implications for graduate training. *Bulletin of the Canadian Academy of Child Psychiatry, 2,* 28.

Patterson, G.R., Reid, J.B., & Dishion, T.J. (1992). *Antisocial boys.* Eugene, OR: Castalia.

Phillips, E.L. (1988). *Patient compliance.* New York: Hogrefe & Huber.

Proskauer, S. (1969). Some technical issues in time-limited psychotherapy with children. *Journal of the American Academy of Child Psychiatry, 18,* 154–169.

Puig-Antich, J., & Ryan, N. (1986). *The schedule for affective disorders and schizophrenia for school-aged children (Kiddie-SADS)* (4th ed.). Pittsburgh: Western Psychiatric Institute and Clinic.

Rauh, V.A., Achenbach, T.M., Nurcombe, B., Howell, C.T., & Teti, D.M. (1988).

Minimizing adverse effects of low birthweight: Four-year results at an early intervention program. *Child Development, 59*, 544–553.

Reynolds, W.M., & Coats, K.I. (1986). A comparison of cognitive–behavioral therapy and relaxation training for the treatment of depression in adolescents. *Journal of Consulting and Clinical Psychology, 54*, 653–660.

Rohrbaugh, M., Tennen, H., Press, S., & White, L. (1981). Compliance, defiance, and therapeutic paradox: Guidelines for strategic use of paradoxical interventions. *American Journal of Orthopsychiatry, 51*, 454–467.

Rush, J.A. (1996). The role of psychotherapy in the treatment of depression: Review of two practice guidelines. *Archives of General Psychiatry, 53*, 298–300.

Russell, G.F.M., Szmukler, G., Dare, C., & Eisler, I. (1987). An evaluation of family therapy in anorexia nervosa and bulimia nervosa. *Archives of General Psychiatry, 44*, 1047–1056.

Rutter, M. (1995). Clinical implications of attachment concepts: Retrospect and prospect. *Journal of Child Psychology & Psychiatry, 36*, 549–571.

Sameroff, A.J., & Emde, R.N. (1989). *Relationship disturbances in early childhood.* New York: Basic.

Sanchez, E. (1986). Factors complicating psychiatric diagnosis of adolescents. In S.C. Feinstein & P. Giovacchini (Eds.), *Adolescent psychiatry* (Vol. 13). Chicago: University of Chicago Press.

Sanders, M.R. (1996). New directions in behavioral family intervention with children. In T.H. Ollendick & J. Prinz (Eds.), *Advances in clinical child psychology* (Vol. 18, pp. 283–330). New York: Plenum Press.

Sanders, M.R., & Dadds, M.R. (1993). *Behavioural family intervention.* Needham Heights, MA: Allyn & Bacon.

Sanders, M.R., & Lawton, J.M. (1993). Discussing assessment findings with families: A guided participation model for information transfer. *Child and Family Behaviour Therapy, 15,* 5–35.

Satir, V. (1967). *Conjoint family therapy.* Palo Alto, CA: Science and Behavior Books.

Schmukler, A.G. (1990). Termination in mid-adolescence. *Psychoanalytic Study of the Child, 45*, 459–474.

Schmukler, A.G. (Ed.) (1991). *Saying goodbye: A casebook of termination in child and adolescent analysis and therapy.* Hillsdale, NJ: Analytic Press.

Schwartz, A.H. (1972). Children's concepts of research hospitalization. *New England Journal of Medicine, 287*, 588–592.

Seiffge-Krenke, I. (1989). Problem intensity and the disposition of adolescents to take therapeutic advice. In M. Brambring, F. Losel, & H. Skowronek (Eds.). *Children at risk: Assessment, longitudinal research and intervention.* New York: Walter de Gruyter.

Seligman, M.E.P. (1995). The effectivess of psychotherapy: The *Consumer Reports* study. *American Psychologist, 50,* 965–974.

Shaffer, D., Gould, M.S., & Brasic, J. (1983). A children's global assessment scale (CGAS). *Archives of General Psychiatry, 40,* 1228–1231.

Shapiro, T., & Esman, A.H. (1985). Psychotherapy with children and adolescents: Still relevant in the 1980's? *Psychiatric Clinics of North America, 8,* 909–921.

Shirk, S.R., & Russell, R.L. (1992). A re-evaluation of estimates of child therapy effectiveness. *Journal of the American Academy of Child and Adolescent Psychiatry, 31,* 703–709.

Silver, L.B., & Silver, B.J. (1983). Clinical practice of child psychiatry: A survey. *Journal of the American Academy of Child Psychiatry, 22,* 573–579.

Slavson, S. (1955). *Fields of group psychotherapy.* New York: International Universities Press.

Sparrow, S.S., Balla, D.A., & Cicchette, D.V. (1984). *The Vineland Adaptive Behavior Scales: Interview editions, survey form.* Circle Pines, MN: American Guidance Service.

Stark, K.D., Reynolds, W.M., & Kaslow, N. (1987). A comparison of the relative efficacy of self-control therapy and a behavioral problem-solving therapy for depression in children. *Journal of Abnormal Child Psychology, 15,* 91–113.

Steinhauer, P.D. (1985). Beyond family therapy: Toward a systemic and integrated view. *Psyciatric Clinics of North America, 8,* 923–945.

Steinhauer, P.D., Bradley, S.J., & Gauthier, Y. (1992). Child and adult psychiatry: Comparison and contrast. *Canadian Journal of Psychiatry, 37,* 440–449.

Suzuki, R. (1989). Adolescents' dropout from individual psychotherapy – is it true? *Journal of Adolescence, 12,* 197–205.

Swift, W.J., & Wonderlich, S.A. (1990). Interpretation of transference in the psychotherapy of adolescents and young adults. *Journal of the American Academy of Child and Adolescent Psychiatry, 29,* 929–935.

The Advocacy, Consent, and Substitute Decisions Statute Law Amendment Act (Bill 19). (1996). Toronto: Queen's Printer for Ontario.

Waelder, R. (1933). The psychoanalytic theory of play. *Psychoanalytic Quarterly, 2,* 208–220.

Weiner, M.F., & King, J.W. (1977). Self-disclosure by the therapist to the adolescent patient. In S.C. Feinstein & P. Giovacchini (Eds.), *Adolescent Psychiatry.* (Vol. 5). Chicago: University of Chicago Press.

Weiner, I.B. (1970). *Psychological disturbance in adolescence.* New York: Wiley-Interscience.

Weisz, J.R., Donenberg, G.R., Han, S.S., & Weiss, B. (1995). Bridging the gap between laboratory and clinic in child and adolescent psychotherapy. *Journal of Consulting and Clinical Psychology, 63,* 688–701.

Weisz, J.R. & Weiss, B. (1989). Assessing the effects of clinic-based psycho-therapy with children and adolescents. *Journal of Consulting and Clinical Psychology, 57,* 741–746.

Weisz, J.R., Weiss, B., Alicke, M.D., & Klotz, M.L. (1987). Effectiveness of psycho-therapy with children and adolescents: Meta-analytic findings for clinicians. *Journal of Consulting and Clinical Psychology, 55,* 542–549.

Weisz, J.R., Weiss, B., Han, S.S., Granger, D.A., & Morton, T. (1995). Effects of psychotherapy with children and adolescents revisited: A metanalysis of treatment outcome studies. *Psychological Bulletin, 117,* 450–468.

Wexler, D.B. (1991). *The adolescent self: Strategies for self-management, self-soothing, and self-esteem in adolescents.* New York: Norton.

Whyte, L.L. (1960). *The unconscious before Freud.* New York: Basic.

Winnicott, D.W. (1971). *Therapeutic consultations in child psychiatry.* London: Hogarth Press.

11. Guidelines for Combining Pharmacotherapy with Psychotherapy

David M. Magder, Zindel V. Segal, Barry Gilbert, and Sidney H. Kennedy

The inclusion of a chapter on the combined use of pharmacotherapy and psychotherapy in a book on the guidelines for psychotherapy reflects the general acceptance of an integrated treatment approach in most psychiatric disorders. Despite combined treatment being 'time-honored' (Gabbard, 1990, p. 146) in the clinical practice of psychiatry, until recently there was significant polarization within psychiatry (Frances, Clarkin, & Perry, 1984; Klerman, 1991; Paykel, 1995). Those who viewed themselves as biologically oriented often ignored psychotherapy. Many of those practising and promoting psychotherapy as the treatment of choice in a broad range of psychiatric disorders were sceptical about the efficacy of medications and untrained in their use. While that latter view has shifted, some therapists continue to express concerns that drug therapy may be unnecessarily toxic, especially where psychotherapy could be used instead (Hollon & Fawcett, 1995; Munoz, Hollon, McGrath, Rehm, & VandenBos, 1994) or that the introduction of medications into an established therapy might skew the therapeutic relationship (Klerman, 1991).

One of the strongest incentives for psychotherapists to consider using drugs is economic. The recent trend of third-party insurers as well as individual patients to scrutinize treatment has put pressure on psychiatry to deliver not only treatments that have been proven effective, but also ones that will consume the minimum amount of time and cost, including the psychological cost to the patient. This development has influenced primary-care physicians and non-medical therapists as well as psychiatrists (Lazarus, 1994; Schreter, 1993).

As well as a general encouragement to use combined therapies (Frances et al, 1984), several investigators have focused on the evaluation of combined psychotherapy and medication (Beitman & Klerman, 1991; Manning & Frances, 1990a). There is evidence that, in practice, psychiatrists do endorse the use of combined therapy (Donovan & Roose, 1995) and that ideological boundaries are more flexible than is often realized (Sullivan, Verhurst, Russo, & Roy-Byrne, 1993). Increasingly, psychiatrists with a psychodynamic background have viewed combined treatment as a natural approach to clinical management with mutually enhancing results (Frances et al, 1984; Basch, 1988; Gabbard, 1990). Division of opinion exists. A concern for the possible negative effects of introducing medications into psychotherapy remains even while some who promote insight-oriented psychotherapy acknowledge that certain symptoms can be relieved only by pharmacological agents (Hollender & Ford, 1990).

Improvements in side-effect and safety profiles, as well as ease of dosing for new medications used to treat a spectrum of mood, anxiety, and eating disorders, have been encouraging developments for both patients and therapists. Increased training, experience, and comfort among psychiatrists in the use of medications also contributes. For some nonmedical psychotherapists (Lazarus, 1994) as well as psychodynamically oriented psychiatrists (Basch, 1988; Gabbard, 1990; Hollender & Ford, 1990), the issue is not whether to use combined therapy, but how it should be approached. Methods of applying combined treatment are discussed later in the chapter.

The literature on combined therapy suggests four converging trends. One is that attention to psychotherapeutic principles will enhance compliance in the administration of medications (Burgess, 1993; Gabbard, 1990; Karasu, 1990; Paykel, 1995) as well as addressing aspects of the patient's problems which are not responsive to medications (Basch, 1988). Another emerges from the comparative controlled trials involving cognitive behavioural therapy or interpersonal therapy with pharmacotherapy (Hollon & Fawcett, 1995; Hollon, Shelton, & Loosen, 1991a). The third appears to have originated in the theoretical and clinical discussions on integrating psychotherapy (Beitman, Hall, & Woodward, 1992; Karasu, 1990) and integrating psychiatric treatments in general (Beitman & Klerman, 1991). Finally, as a clinical reflection of the last point, psychotherapists are recognizing that the prescription of medication within a primarily psychotherapeutic treatment can enhance the response to psychotherapy (Basch, 1988; Gabbard, 1990; Hollender & Ford, 1990).

The trend towards integration highlights the debate on the mind–body dichotomy. Attitudes influence clinical practices (Karasu, 1990). Even though the argument is far from resolved, these authors take the position that the question of mind–body separation is misleading. With increasing evidence in favour of mutually interacting biological and psychological subsystems (Andreasen, 1995; Beitman et al, 1992; Gabbard, 1995a), we consider integration of psychological mechanisms and neuroscience as a given in the combined use of medications and psychological interventions.

In this regard, it is important to emphasize that the prescribing of pharmacotherapy does not occur within a relationship vacuum. Non-specific psychotherapeutic factors within the therapist, including warmth, empathy, and genuineness (Truax & Carkhuff, 1967), therapeutic optimism, the instillation of hope, as well as patient education, the expectations of both therapist and patient (Frank, 1973; Gabbard, 1990; Strupp, 1970), and the symbolic nature of the act of prescribing medications (Hollender & Ford, 1990) may all influence compliance and outcome. The placebo effect in research on pharmacotherapy reflects this process (Beitman et al, 1992). The biological psychiatrist intentionally or unintentionally operates within a framework of such non-specific psychotherapeutic factors. However, a casual approach to the prescription of medications without the role of non-specific influences clearly in mind will likely disappear as psychiatrists become more sophisticated and those who develop clinical research protocols increasingly demand awareness of such factors (e.g., Fawcett, Epstein, Fiester, Elkin, & Autry, 1987). In the following discussion, the operation of non-specific psychotherapeutic factors will be assumed to be implicit in all forms of therapy, including drug therapy. However, one cannot assume that all therapists are equally sophisticated in managing these factors (Munoz et al, 1994), and both research and day-to-day clinical results may vary accordingly.

Empirical Review of Combined Treatment

Although individual case reports suggest a potentially rich role for integrating psychotherapy with pharmacotherapy (Beitman, 1991), the results of research to confirm these impressions have been less than conclusive (Hollon & Fawcett, 1995). This results in part from the fact that larger numbers of patients in each comparison group are required to show a difference among active treatments (Hollon, Shelton, & Loosen, 1991b). The most substantial research directed at combined treatment has been with three diagnoses: mood disorders, schizophrenia, and anxiety disorders (Beitman et al, 1992).

The literature is further hampered by the emphasis on studying populations with one 'pure' disorder, rather than populations with mixed disorders (both Axis I and Axis II) that are more typical of populations seen in treatment by psychiatrists. As well, the limited outcome measures from most studies are not well correlated with quality-of-life issues that clinicians in practice constantly face (Hollon & Fawcett, 1995).

Combined treatment may be more valuable when there is significant co-morbidity, such as with substance-abuse or Axis II disorders. Here the target symptoms for each treatment modality may be distinct, and treatment may be carried on concurrently (Rush & Kupfer, 1995). Patients with a history of chronic illness are more likely to need concurrent psychotherapy. Patients with prior history of treatment may be approached, in the absence of clear indications for psychotherapy, with combined medication and management. After some symptom resolution, a later decision regarding ongoing psychotherapy may be made based on the degree of symptom response and on the ability of the person to function generally.

Co-morbidity in the psychiatric population is greater than was earlier believed (National Comorbidity Survey; Kessler et al, 1995). For example, 51 per cent of people with a dysthymic disorder and 42 per cent of people with major depression have an Axis II disorder (Marin, Koesis, Frances, & Klerman, 1993). There are no randomized trials that provide data that would help practitioners make treatment decisions with this sizeable population. This group tends to have more chronic illness (Sotsky et al, 1991) and probably needs longer-term treatments.

There is little research to establish guidelines for treatment over the longer term, despite the fact that many psychiatric disorders (including many mood, anxiety, and personality disorders) are chronic. In the area of chronic disorders, clinicians must draw on the accumulated clinical experience in the literature. Especially with Axis II disorders, most of the clinical experience reported uses long-term dynamic psychotherapy, often combined with medication. Here, medication may provide symptom relief and mood stability that allow progression of the deeper psychotherapeutic work which may be necessary for patients' improved quality of life (Ostow, 1979). More research is needed to evaluate efficacy of combined therapy modalities in treating co-morbidity and chronic illness.

In the next section of this chapter, focusing on methods of providing combined therapy, the treatment of unipolar depression is used as a prototype for discussing combining treatment modalities. The psychotherapy modalities chosen are cognitive behavioural therapy, and interpersonal therapy, since the majority of combined-therapy research has been done on these modalities.

Psychodynamic psychotherapy is the modal form of intervention among psychiatrists and the type of psychotherapy most likely to be practised in combination with pharmacotherapy. Regrettably, this type of psychotherapy has been underevaluated in combined-therapy research, and even in direct comparisons with medication, for example, in the treatment of depression (Persons, Thase, & Crits-Christoph, 1996). More of the research has focused on cognitive behavioural therapy and interpersonal therapy. One recent study does compare brief dynamic psychotherapy combined with a medication favourably in relation to the medication alone in the treatment of panic disorder (Wiborg & Dahl, 1996).

Since evidence from randomized controlled studies of psychodynamic psychotherapy is sparse, the best alternative is to extrapolate the data which exist regarding other forms of psychotherapy for the purposes of discussing combined treatment, especially since a meta-analysis of the efficacy of brief dynamic psychotherapy has found it to be as effective as other forms of psychotherapy in the disorders studied (Crits-Christoph, 1992). Of course, we must await further data on psychodynamic therapies in combination with medication in order to address this question more directly.

MOOD DISORDERS

In relation to major depression, specific psychotherapies such as cognitive behavioural therapy (CBT) and interpersonal therapy (IPT) have been shown to be as effective as drug therapy in the acute treatment of non-psychotic mild to moderate forms of the illness (American Psychiatric Association, 1993). In a number of situations, psychotherapy may even be preferable (Munoz et al, 1994). There is some indication that medications influence somatic symptoms, while psychotherapy may foster improvement in social functioning (Manning & Frances, 1990b).

Surprisingly, in several influential studies, combination treatments did not achieve statistical significance in showing an advantage over each individual therapy. However, neither treatment approach appears to interfere with the effectiveness of the other (Manning & Frances, 1990b). Potential benefits of combined pharmacotherapy and psychotherapy include a greater breadth and depth of response to treatment, enhanced quality of life, reduced relapse and recurrence rates, and facilitation of the use of lower doses of medication (American Psychiatric Association, 1993; Hollon & Fawcett, 1995; Munoz et al, 1994). As standards of training and expertise in administration of both kinds of treatments improve, these effects could become clearer (Munoz et al, 1994).

These potential benefits have significance when considering treatment beyond the acute stage, and for previously 'treatment-resistant' patients. Significant numbers of patients, 25–50 per cent, fail to respond to antidepressant medication, respond incompletely, or are vulnerable to relapse (Rosenbaum, Fava, Nierenberg, & Sachs, 1995). This large group of patients may prove in the long run to benefit most from an integrated approach. All of these possible advantages have to be weighed against drawbacks such as cost and the potential for side-effects when two treatments are used instead of one (Manning & Frances, 1990b).

Dysthymia has not been studied to the same extent as major depressive disorder. Few studies comparing pharmacotherapy in the treatment of dysthymia have been undertaken, and those that exist involved small groups of patients and with no controls. Combined treatment has not been investigated to any significant extent (Markowitz, 1994).

Mood-stabilizing medications and/or electroconvulsive therapy (ECT) are the cornerstones of treatment in bipolar disorder, although a variety of psychological interventions may be an important adjunct (American Psychiatric Association, 1994). Psychotherapy helps patients with bipolar disorder to come to terms with the significance of their illness and improves compliance (Jamison, 1991). Cognitive-therapy interventions have been shown to be useful in improving lithium compliance and reducing the necessity for hospitalization (Cochran, 1984).

Zaretsky and Segal (1994), in a survey of the literature, found that psychosocial interventions combined with medication improved the outcome, compared with medications alone. They suggested that a variety of mechanisms provide the active ingredients, including closer monitoring of affective symptomatology, earlier environmental modification, enhanced compliance with medication, enhanced social support, improved familial adjustment, regulation of daily routines and enhancement of coping strategies. Zaretsky and Segal suggest that the role of psychotherapeutic involvement in the depressed phases of the patients' illness may be to reduce the necessary dosage of antidepressant medication, which may consequently reduce the risk of these medications triggering hypomania or rapid cycling.

ANXIETY DISORDERS

In the treatment of agoraphobia, there is evidence that medication and psychological treatments are mutually potentiating (Mavissakalian, 1991). Exposure treatment is aided by the use of medication (imipramine). The response to imipramine is helped by instructions concerning exposure. The long-term results suggest that improvement is best maintained by patients whose initial response, was most significant. Combining medication with psychological treatment may not only maximize this initial response, but also help to reduce relapse (Mavissakalian, 1991). In panic disorder, the addition of brief dynamic psychotherapy to treatment with clomipramine has been shown to significantly reduce the relapse rate at the nine-month follow-up (Wiborg & Dahl, 1996).

Studies of combined treatment are not as fully developed in obsessive–compulsive disorder (Jenike, 1991), social phobia (Uhde & Tancer, 1991), or generalized anxiety disorder (Beaudry, 1991). In most instances the effects of psychotherapy in combination with medication are compared with those of psychotherapy with a placebo. As might be expected, the results favoured the active medication condition, but, without including, as a minimum, 'medication only' control groups, little can be said about the value of combined treatment. The addition of a pharmacological agent certainly did not interfere with the psychotherapies reviewed in these more limited studies. Most of the authors believed that a combined approach improved compliance.

SCHIZOPHRENIA

As with bipolar disorder, medications remain the necessary cornerstone of treatment in schizophrenia, but a variety of psychotherapeutic approaches, including individual, group, and family therapy, and social-skills learning, enhance the outcome (Fenton & Cole, 1995; Goldstein, 1991; Marder, Johnston-Cronk, Wirshing, & Eckman, 1991). They are aimed at helping the patient and family deal with the initial crisis of the illness and subsequent relapses, identifying stress and developing coping mechanisms, improving medication compliance, and possibly providing a basis for eventual reduction of medication (see chapter 12,

'Guidelines for Psychotherapy with Patients Suffering from Severe and Persistent Mental Illness').

EATING DISORDERS

Two studies have compared combined pharmacotherapy and psychotherapy in the treatment of bulimia nervosa. Imipramine combined with structured intensive group therapy did not prove to be superior to the group therapy alone for the eating disorder. However, the addition of the medication helped by reducing anxiety and depression (Mitchell et al, 1990). Agras et al (1992) demonstrated that the combination of desipramine and CBT produced better results than either treatment alone, but only when continued for twenty-four weeks. In reviewing the literature on the psychopharmacological treatment of eating disorders, Kennedy and Goldbloom (1995) concluded that the psychotherapeutic approaches should also be included. The value of family therapy (Russell, Szmukler, Dare, & Eisler, 1987) must be considered, as well as individual psychotherapy.

Clinical Indications for Combined Treatment

THE GENERAL APPROACH TO TREATMENT

Combined therapy can begin at the very outset of treatment, or follow a period of initial treatment with either modality. Thus, medication can be added to deal with symptoms that do not respond to psychotherapy; psychotherapy may be added when initial symptom resolution by medication is incomplete or if further problems in functioning are uncovered after initial symptom improvement. The decision to use combined therapy depends on diagnosis, co-morbidity, and, in the absence of clear guidelines from empirical studies, patient preferences.

In any psychiatric treatment, whether psychological or biological, most therapists implicitly follow the same overall approach: (1) introduce a specific treatment and, over a given course of time, evaluate progress; (2) if the results are positive, continue in the initial course; (3) if the results do not seem to be either sufficient or beneficial, or produce unacceptable side-effects, consider some form of modification of the original therapy, either altering, expanding, or switching to a new approach.

In dynamic psychotherapy the process described in the preceding paragraph has been recognized in the formal analysis of resistance, but the term has been applied more broadly to include not only psychoanalytic therapy, but also behaviour therapy (Wachtel, 1982). In an even wider sense, defined as the diagnosis and dismantling of 'blocks' in therapy, this concept has been applied as an integrating principle for psychotherapy of all kinds (Pinsof, 1983). Similarly, from the biological perspective, psychopharmacologists continually monitor patient responses and toxic reactions, reducing or increasing dosage, augmenting with additional medications or stopping one drug and changing to another as indicated, in effect diagnosing and overcoming 'blocks' in the treatment.

COMBINED TREATMENT IN DEPRESSION

The same general approach of starting a treatment, evaluating its efficacy, and either continuing it, adding to it, or changing it applies to the implementation of combined treatment. On the basis of the authors' involvement in mood disorders and the extensive research on depression, major depression is used as the prototype here. As discussed in the introduction to the previous section, on empirical research, while the current data mainly support the use of CBT or IPT, brief psychodynamic therapy (BPT) will also be considered in the choice of psychotherapy. Table 11.1 lists psychotherapeutic approaches, and table 11.2 pharmacological options, which could be considered, and figure 11.1 gives a flow chart for treatment based on these options.

If the depression is mild to moderate, either psychotherapy or medications could be used alone as the first step in treatment. If the depression is severe but the patient shows no psychotic features and there is no imminent risk of suicide, adjunctive psychotherapy could still be considered, although current practice guidelines would indicate that antidepressants are the preferred treatment (American Psychiatric Association, 1993). Treatment response in previous episodes, if any, should be taken into account. Psychotherapy may be the treatment of choice in certain specific situations, for example, with pregnant women, or in the presence of some co-morbid physical illnesses (Gabbard, 1995a; Rush & Kupfer, 1995). However, there is a substantial data base to support the continuation of tricyclic or SSRI antidepressants throughout pregnancy.

When a patient has psychotic features or poses a significant risk for suicide, antidepressants, with or without hospitalization, are necessary. ECT should also be considered. If the patient responds to the initial

Table 11.1: Psychotherapeutic Approaches in the Treatment of
Major Depression

1 Empirically Validated in Direct Comparison with
   Antidepressant Medication
   a. Cognitive Behavioural Treatment
   b. Interpersonal Therapy

2 Useful Adjunctive Treatments
   a. Family/Marital Therapy and/or Support
   b. Brief Psychodynamic Therapy
   c. Group Therapy

Table 11.2: Pharmacological Agents in the Treatment of Depression

1 *First-Line Agents*
   a. *Serotonin Reuptake Inhibitors and Modified Reuptake Inhibitors*

Fluoxetine	Sertraline
Fluvoxamine	Venlafaxine
Paroxetine	Nefazadone

   b. *Cyclic Agents*

Nortriptyline	Doxepin
Desipramine	Clomipramine
Protriptyline	Trimipramine
Amitriptyline	Maprotiline
Imipramine	

   c. *Monoamine Oxidase Inhibitors*

| Phenelzine | Tranylcypromine |

   d. *Other*

| Moclobemide | Trazodone |
| Buproprion | |

2 *Augmenting Agents*
   a. Lithium
   b. T3
   c. L-tryptophan
   d. Buspirone

Source: Kennedy, 1995

treatment, usually within six to twenty weeks, depending on the treatment and the need for minor adjustments, the therapy is continued in maintenance or terminated. Termination is more appropriate with a focused, time-limited psychotherapy than in a drug therapy.

Figure 11.1: Flow Chart for the Combined Treatment[1] of Major Depression[2]

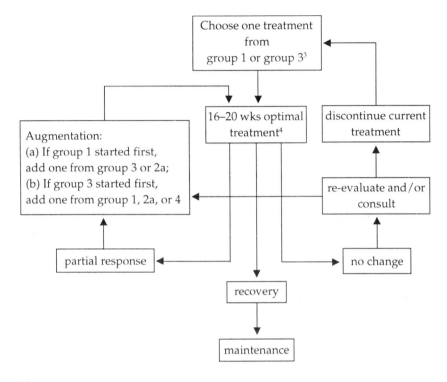

Notes:
1 According to this flow chart, combined pharmacotherapy and psychotherapy would occur when either treatment is augmented by the addition of the other.
2 Most relevant for the initial three or four cycles of this decision process.
3 In severe depression start with group 3. If there are contraindications to medication, start with group 1.
4 For medication dosages see Kennedy, 1995.

When a patient experiences non-response, partial response, or major side-effects, the next stage becomes more critical from the point of view of combined treatment. Although changes in the modality or frequency of psychotherapy might be considered, the psychotherapist might also prescribe medication, most likely within the context of the particular psychotherapy. The therapist who has started with medication usually will either adjust dosage; add an augmentation agent such as lithium, T3, buspirone, or tryptophan; or switch to a new antidepressant within the same family or from a new family. The psychopharmacologist would seldom consider introducing psychotherapy at this point, before trying at least two different medications. However, in our clinic, we are exploring, in a randomized controlled trial, the effects of CBT with antidepressant medication for twelve weeks compared with lithium augmentation for patients who have partial antidepressant response after eight weeks of pharmacotherapy. The patients will be followed up to evaluate the relative effects of these two approaches in preventing relapse or recurrence.

In all cases where there has been no response to the initial sequence of treatment, and in some cases of partial response, the patient should receive a detailed symptom review to establish primary and possible comorbid diagnoses. Consultation could be considered. The physician who primarily uses pharmacological approaches may consider the possibility that lack of response reflects the influence of psychological factors on compliance or comfort with the medication. Some of the clinical vignettes presented later in this chapter illustrate how the prescription of medications may help a stalled psychotherapy as well as the value of psychological management in smoothing medication compliance and/or response.

In the treatment of depression, as one moves from the acute treatment phase to the continuation and maintenance phases (Kupfer, 1991), almost any combination of treatment may prove useful in confronting treatment resistance. In fact, psychotherapists who are not constrained by the need to adhere to strict research protocols may have a great deal in common with psychopharmacologists who persistently prescribe multiple combinations of drugs in an effort to optimize or maximize treatment. It is likely that these psychotherapists shift back and forth through a mixture of therapeutic approaches which would include dynamic, interpersonal, cognitive, educational, and supportive features, with some including marital or family therapy, depending on the appearance of blocks in the treatment (Pinsof, 1983). It would seem reasonable to expect that combined drug and psychological treatment would be a natural extension of this approach reflected in clinical practice (Manning & Frances, 1990b; Sullivan et al, 1993). It is important to emphasize that, if no robust statistical benefit can be ascribed to combined therapy, the prescription of medications, at a minimum, does not interfere with psychotherapy. At the very least, psychotherapy combined with medication has shown a trend towards increasing the probability, magnitude, and breadth of response, as well as encouraging the acceptability of either (Hollon & Fawcett, 1995).

METHODS OF PROVIDING COMBINED TREATMENT

Combined therapy can be administered by one individual, and in psychiatric practice this is probably the most common and perhaps the most appropriate approach. An external view or intervention can be useful even for experienced and sophisticated therapists. The guidelines in this chapter and the flow chart (figure 11.1) are primarily based on the assumption of a therapist working alone, but may apply as well to two clinicians working together. Combined therapy could be the result of teamwork between a physician, not necessarily a psychiatrist, and a non-medical therapist, or between two physician-therapists. Table 11.3 provides guidelines for two clinicians working together (Kelly, 1992).

When one therapist administers both, success is enhanced by a theoretical position of integration, in which medications and psychological interventions are considered interchangeable. Such integration recognizes the 'fundamental compatibility of biology and psychodynamics' (Gabbard, 1990, p. 148). However, the already large and growing amount of information about both new and old medications, as well as about new psychotherapeutic approaches, for example, manual-driven therapies, and variations of more established methods, can make integration difficult (Chiles, Carlin, Benjamin, & Beitman, 1991).

When more than one therapist is involved, comfort with each other as well as the opportunity for easy and open communication are essential (Busch & Gould, 1993; Chiles et al, 1991; Kelly, 1992).

TRANSFERENCE AND COUNTERTRANSFERENCE

A number of common transference and countertransference situations can occur when medication is prescribed within an already established psychotherapy or when pharmacotherapy is the main approach (Gabbard, 1990). Gabbard suggests that empathically exploring the transference issues triggered by introducing the prescription of medication into an established psychotherapy may advance the psychotherapy and/or improve compliance with medications. Some of the clinical examples in the next section illustrate this point as well.

According to Gabbard (1990), patients may see the prescription of medications as an empathic failure on the part of the psychiatrist. Others will interpret it as a threat of domination by a powerful parental figure, or, conversely, as an indication that they no longer need to take responsibility for any aspect of their illness. For some patients it may

Table 11.3: Guidelines for the Pharmacotherapist and the Psychotherapist Working Together

---

1 Guidelines for the Pharmacotherapist
  a. Accept referrals for medication consultation only from psychotherapists whose skills you know and trust.
  b. Consider the non-medical psychotherapist a responsible professional and a reliable informant, but not a medical colleague, supervisee, or competitor.
  c. Make it clear to the psychotherapist that you are not a drug dispenser who automatically recommends medication. You are a consultant who appreciates the opportunity to advise the psychotherapist and the patient about potential benefits and risks of medication for this person with this disorder at this time.
  d. Adopt the stance of a physician and use a medical model.
  e. Emphasize what may be useful to the patient, not what the patient absolutely needs. This distinction will reduce patients' expectation that you view them as weak and disabled.
  f. View the request for consultation as a sign of progress in treatment, not as evidence of failed psychotherapy.
  g. Consider resistance to medication and the psychological meaning of taking it as interesting issues to be discussed with the psychotherapist, but refrain from suggesting interpretations.

2 Guidelines for the Psychotherapist
  a. Use a psychiatrist who will not just prescribe medications appropriately, but also appreciate the complexities of psychotherapy and of parallel treatment.
  b. Consider the psychiatrist a source of information about some aspects of the patient's life and psychopathology, but not a co-therapist, back-up, or competitor.
  c. Refrain from offering the patient any advice about medications, doses, or side-effects; instead, refer all such questions to the pharmacotherapist. If the questions persist, consider exploring the patient's attempt to distort your role.
  d. Realize that the mutual decision to seek a medication consultation is a sign of progress in the treatment and not an indication of failure.
  e. Psychological reactions to needing drugs, taking drugs, and benefiting from drugs are all grist for the psychotherapeutic mill. The psychological meaning of the experience, as well as transference reactions to the consultant, should be seen as an opportunity for exploration and understanding.

Source: Adapted from Kelly, 1992

provide yet another opportunity to defeat a treatment intervention. A positive transference to a medication may lead to a rapid and mostly placebo response, or act as a transitional object in the absence of the therapist. This kind of powerful transference could lead to refusal to discontinue the medication when recommended. Paranoid patients may disguise their delusional fears of a medication by referring to side-effects as a reason for discontinuing. Still other patients will experience the prescription of medication as a supportive and containing act that strengthens the therapeutic alliance.

Gabbard (1990) also describes a number of countertransference possibilities. The psychiatrist may take an overly authoritarian stance or become punitively angry when prescribing medication. Overprescription of medications may signify despair on the part of the physician. The psychiatrist may use medications to suppress intense transference feelings, in particular, hostility, rather than exploring and resolving them. As Gabbard points out, some psychiatrists may induce guilt as a way of insuring compliance. Others may fail to prescribe needed medication because of narcissistic injury. They may 'believe that doing so would be tantamount to conceding that their psychotherapeutic skills have been ineffective' (p. 142).

Clinical Considerations

In this section a number of case reports are used to demonstrate some of the clinical situations where combined therapy, occasionally occurring in unusual ways, was beneficial. As well, they are meant to illustrate the value for the psychiatrist in thinking in a manner which integrates both biological and psychological principles.

UNPLANNED OR INADVERTENT COMBINED THERAPY

Other physicians or therapists may be invaluable allies of the psychotherapist by introducing or assisting in the introduction of medications into an ongoing psychotherapeutic treatment. In some cases the alliance may be unplanned and inadvertent.

Case Report A: A family physician independently prescribed an antidepressant medication for a man in long-term psychotherapy. The psychotherapist was comfortable with the use of medications, but in the course of a long therapy had overlooked the fact that significant external events had precipitated severe depression in the patient. Amitriptyline significantly enhanced the progress of psychotherapy and the patient's comfort.

Case Report B: A man in his twenties with a history of illicit drug use in his teens and severe anxiety was being seen in psychotherapy and treated with imipramine. While there was some improvement and he was subjectively benefiting from the supportive and exploratory psychotherapy, he also continued to experience significant anxiety and pre-occupation with suicide. He had been extensively evaluated for organic causes during an inpatient hospitalization which included a non-contributory EEG. One day he arrived for a regular therapy session convinced that his symptoms were identical to those of a television character with temporal-lobe epilepsy who he had seen in an episode of a popular fictional medical program. At his insistence he was referred for another neurological assessment. Photic stimulation during EEG testing precipitated a seizure. His anxiety and thoughts of suicide decreased significantly with the addition of anticonvulsant medication. He nevertheless continued in psychotherapy for assistance in dealing with significant interpersonal problems.

Comment: In the treatment of a patient, it is important to keep in mind that, even if one aspect of the individual's problem is being successfully treated, it does not mean that there may not be other aspects or diagnoses to be dealt with, possibly using a completely different modality.

CONSULTATION

Consultation could be considered a normal part of the process of therapy. Decisions made by two psychiatrists working together could be thought of as reflecting the kind of internal debate an individual psychiatrist might have with her- or himself. The two examples of consultations that follow represent the value inherent in combining psychotherapeutic and pharmacological knowledge.

Case Report C: A fifty-two-year-old woman was suffering from her second episode of major depressive disorder with significant anxiety within two years. She was experiencing a number of somatic and psychological symptoms and had been unable to work for four to five months since this second bout began. She had no previous history of any psychological difficulties and, until that time, had led a successful family and professional life. The first episode she had had been treated quickly and effectively by a psychotherapeutically oriented psychiatrist who had prescribed an appropriate antidepressant. At the same time he helped the patient cope with a significant stress in her life, the diagnosis of a breast lump. (Her mother had died from breast cancer.) In the second episode, the psychiatrist used the same treatment strategy, including the same medication. He addressed a new psychological stress, the death of her father and the liquidation of his estate, including selling the family home. However, the patient failed to respond. The patient and her husband were becoming frightened that she might never recover.

The consultant made two recommendations. The first was to switch to another, newer antidepressant, with instructions as to dosage since the referring psychiatrist was unfamiliar with this medication. The second, which was also discussed at length with the patient and her husband, was to reassure the patient that the unique and significant stress which immediately predated the onset of her symptoms was a sufficient cause of the difficulties and it was unlikely that her distress would recur once she recovered. Although no guarantee could be given, the patient felt reassured. During a brief follow-up visit, it was determined that the woman had recovered and returned to work.

Comment: It is always difficult to know what precise factor or combination of factors leads to recovery. It could be argued that the change in medication contributed to this woman's recovery, but the fact that she responded to the original medication in the first episode and not the second suggests that other factors were at work. Reassurance about the likely psychological cause of the illness appears to have been the necessary extra ingredient. The medication had to be changed, since the patient had lost confidence in the one originally prescribed.

The consultant must attend to both psychological and biological factors and have comfort in integrating both. Not all 'psychotherapeutic' interventions necessarily need to be extensive in order to work. Placebo-like ingredients may have a significant influence on the efficacy of medication. This highlights the difficulty and importance of designing research that can accurately and adequately take all of these issues into account, allowing us to tease out their influence and design a reasonable approach to therapeutics which takes all these factors into account.

Case Report D: A thirty-eight-year-old single woman was referred by her family physician with concern about the treatment of long-standing dysthymia complicated by occasional episodes of major depression. She reported a history of having been depressed as long as she could remember and of thinking of suicide when she was 'five years old.' Her mother had told her of notes she had written about wanting to die when she was nine or ten. She described being unhappy most of her adult life and had researched a method of suicide with high lethality. She was never treated with medication until two and a half months earlier, when she approached her family doctor, describing a serious occurrence of depression lasting ten months and observed by co-workers.

The patient experienced 'chaotic' early years. Her father was an alcoholic who physically abused her and embarrassed her in front of her peers. Three of his sisters suffered from depression. She worked her own way through university and graduate school, and established herself in her chosen career. She described her relationships with men as unsuccessful, stating that she tends to attract men who are in crisis in their own lives and need caretaking. Her current depression as well as a previous one were precipitated while she was in unhappy relationships. Brief psychotherapy for the previous episode helped her out of the relationship she was currently involved in, but did not give her any guidelines for building more effective ties with men. She revealed to the consultant that, at age sixteen, she was sexually abused by a non-related but dominant male in her life. Her therapist had not known about the sexual abuse, and in fact the consultant was the first person she had told.

The formulation was of a double depression with a biological predisposition and long-standing dissatisfaction, cynicism, and disappointment in her relationships with men. Her diagnosis was chronic dysthymia, occasionally aggravated by major depression, in response to the stress of a particular relationship.

The consultant recommended continuing the same medication, with a few adjustments for side-effects. The patient and her physician were given advice regarding the direction of her psychotherapy: an approach which would focus on the significance of her father's abuse and the sexual abuse at age sixteen. It was hypothesized that she was attempting to avoid further abuse by forging links with weak but ultimately unsatisfactory men.

Comment: The accuracy of a psychological formulation developed after only one patient visit will always be limited. Even the pharmacological formulation could be incomplete on the basis of one contact. However, this woman had a partial response to the medications prescribed by her family physician. Given the chronic nature of her depression, the relatively brief psychotherapy was not sufficient to help her overcome the distortions of her earlier life, especially those influenced by significant men. The fact that the consultant uncovered the history of sexual abuse, which the psychotherapist was unaware of, underscores the importance of maintaining a combined approach, not just when prescribing, but also while taking a history. Involving the patient in the formulation and giving her suggestions about what to look for in therapy instead of only describing it to the referring physician allows her to be a more informed consumer and better able to participate in the therapeutic process.

SYNERGY

Case Report E: A thirty-eight-year-old single man suffering from chronic depression with obsessive–compulsive disorder (OCD) was referred for treatment after a creative and innovative therapist had been unable to produce any change with a variety of psychotherapeutic approaches, and the patient had refused medication. The patient, who had experienced his symptoms, including repetitive obsessional ruminations, for many years, had worn out the patience of a number of psychiatrists who attempted to help him resolve his difficulties.

The new psychiatrist recommended that the patient would likely respond best to pharmacological agents, specifically SSRIs, but the patient remained adamant in his fear of medication and his refusal to take any. Individual psychotherapy was begun, as well as couple sessions with the patient's on-again, off-again girlfriend. Although the sessions were repetitious and unproductive, the therapist continued to offer, but not press, medications, exploring the patient's resistance to drugs in the process. Finally the patient agreed to try an SSRI and responded almost immediately, with the disappearance of his depression and his obsessional symptoms. He began to sleep fewer hours during the day. He made plans, and followed through with vocational retraining, which he had refrained from doing for considerable time. The length and frequency of the sessions were reduced to focus on medication monitoring.

Comment: In this particular case, the second psychiatrist had the advantage of the previous psychiatrists' frustration with the patient to guide him in not expecting easy compliance with a medical regime while, at the same time, recognizing the likely lack of success of a specific psychotherapeutic approach. The goal of achieving pharmacological treatment was established early in the therapist's mind, but the means to achieving it were broadly psychotherapeutic. Hollender and Ford (1990) cite a similar case where exploration of the psychodynamics smoothed compliance with medication.

'SEAMLESS' PHARMACOTHERAPY AND PSYCHOTHERAPY

Case Report F: Ms D., a twenty-eight-year-old married woman, was referred by her family physician for treatment of depression and suicidal thoughts. She had been prescribed an SSRI, to which she responded poorly. Diagnosis at consultation was major depressive episode, possible dysthymic disorder. While depressed, the patient became preoccupied with memories of a trauma she had experienced as a child. Although the memory was never repressed, she had told no one about the incident. She did not believe that the memories and associated feelings were connected with her depression and suicidal feelings. The psychiatrist prescribed medication and arranged follow-up visits to monitor her response and her thoughts of suicide.

Her initial positive response to treatment began to fade after eight weeks. A good therapeutic alliance and a positive transference developed gradually. Her preoccupation with the trauma intensified obsessively. The psychiatrist encouraged her to bring these memories to their sessions in an effort to contain the intensity of the process. As her mood worsened, she became concerned that her thoughts of suicide were triggered by the memories, though she could not make a clear affective connection between her suicidal periods and her memories of the traumatic incident. The suicidal urges seemed to descend upon her almost from outside herself and were probably grossly magnified by her ongoing depression. Just before a week-long break in the treatment, the patient reported she no longer felt safe alone, despite all the safeguards against suicide they had put in place. She agreed to a hospital admission.

Over the course of a three-week admission, her mood began to stabilize on a TCA, with marked diminution of her suicidal feelings. She was able to return to work and, with the help of her psychiatrist, she monitored her mood and tried to limit her tendency to demand perfection, overload herself as she had in the past, and deny her emotional needs.

At this point, she no longer required weekly monitoring visits for medication and suicide risk. Her mood was stable as she continued to take the TCA. She then asked to continue in therapy, saying she now understood the psychiatrist's comments about her being out of touch with her feelings, in the context of her sudden urges to harm herself when she was depressed. Though these experiences may have purely resulted from a biological disturbance of her mood, the process reminded her of other times in her life when she made impulsive and sudden decisions, for no apparent reason. Now she realized that she tended to flee as involvements became too intense – both at work and in her personal relationships. She now wished to understand and to change this tendency, which had deeply affected her entire life.

Comment: This young woman presented with a serious affective illness, an underlying history of a single trauma, and characterological difficulties, including problems with tolerating affects and with making perfectionistic demands of herself. Multiple disturbances like this are common in clinical practice (Kessler et al, 1994) and may be where combined treatment is most clearly indicated. Medication addressed her acute depressive symptomatology. Ms D.'s persistent thoughts of suicide in the midst of depression may reflect a biological mood state that would not necessarily respond directly to psychotherapeutic treatment (Kantor, 1993). At the same time, her difficulty in maintaining awareness of her feelings may have contributed to the lethal nature of her suicidal urges by allowing them to build to high intensity before she became aware of them. The psychiatrist's prescription of medication also facilitated the establishment of a relationship that allowed the exploration of disturbances in her affective life that were evident to him early on in the treatment. That work might make it easier for her to withstand suicidal urges in future relapses. Supportive psychotherapy was used to enhance safety and compliance with medication and to establish a therapeutic alliance that later opened the door to work on character and developmental issues, using a psychodynamic model. As treatment progressed, therapy shifted from the supportive to the psychodynamic and interpretive end of the psychodynamic spectrum (Gabbard, 1995b). The treatments complemented each other, and the clinician's ability to shift between modalities facilitated their synergy.

MEDICATION IN THE TRANSFERENCE

Case Report G: Ms R., a thirty-eight-year-old divorced woman, was referred to a psychiatrist for treatment of anxiety. Three courses of briefer therapies, as well as treatment with medication, failed to resolve her symptoms. She had experienced anxiety for most of her life, with fluctuating periods of panic and low-grade depression. Although she recently began a new relationship and completed her professional education, her symptoms severely hampered both her work and her relationships. The psychiatrist diagnosed her as suffering from generalized anxiety disorder, panic disorder (in remission), and mixed traits on Axis II.

As therapy progressed, it became apparent to Ms R. and her psychiatrist that she was deeply troubled by her father's death (which was still unmourned almost twenty years later) and her difficult relationship with her mother. The mother, who could be loving, was also harsh and had been physically punitive . Transferences based on these relationships appeared quickly and intensely in the therapy.

After a year of treatment, her symptoms worsened, and she experienced near-panic during most of her waking hours. She requested medication. Her psychiatrist agreed and prescribed an SSRI and a benzodiazepine. These provided some relief, and her near-panic and affective instability lessened to the point that she was able to work and to continue therapy. The psychiatrist's willingness to respond to her became a key event for her, indicating she could have some impact in getting her needs met. The therapeutic alliance was strengthened, and she was able to tolerate the psychiatrist's periodic shift away from empathic immersion to a review of medication and of target symptoms.

Comment: The addition of medication to a psychodynamic therapy both facilitated and deepened the therapy through the transference meanings of medication, relief, and the act of providing them. Medication, by reducing her symptoms, allowed her to do psychological work, including unfinished mourning, that she previously had been unable to do. A significant clinical literature supports the benefits of the same psychiatrist providing both psychotherapy and medication, thus containing all treatment in one relationship (Ostow, 1979).

Conclusion

The empirically proven success of pharmacotherapy in a wide range of psychiatric disorders has created a polarized debate about the relative utility of pharmacotherapy and psychotherapy in many of these disorders. Those with an integrated mind–body view of not only psychiatric disorders, but also all clinical medicine, are now challenged to respond with a clearer definition of both the specific and the non-specific factors in psychotherapy and the appropriate and efficient means for their application. As the percentage of treatment-resistant cases of depression illustrates, in spite of a significant and powerful pharmacological armamentarium, there are many gaps in our understanding of the treatment of this ubiquitous disorder. The interlocking synergy of combining psychotherapy with pharmacotherapy may help these patients, as well as non-responders with other diagnoses, to improve.

Many of the studies comparing antidepressants and psychotherapy were done with tricyclic antidepressants which have a high side-effect profile and lead to more drop-outs (Mitchell et al, 1990). With the newer medications, which seem to have fewer side-effects, the results may be different. At the same time, specific psychotherapies could become more accurate and targeted for specific diagnoses, and more effective.

The most significant finding from the research on combined therapy may be one that was not found. Adding medications to psychotherapy does not interfere with the psychotherapy. Psychotherapy researchers can, with confidence, explore the theoretical and practical value of integrating medications into their practice.

The research and individual case studies point to directions that various psychotherapeutic modalities could take. Awareness of the non-specific factors in the prescription of medication would aid compliance. Family or marital counselling could reduce the stress surrounding or maintaining a condition. In some conditions, specific psychotherapies could compete on equal footing with medication, producing broader resolution of problems than drugs alone can provide. As comparative research proceeds, more diagnoses may fall within this category. Combined therapy would enhance the value of either treatment alone.

Psychotherapists have a great deal to learn from the eclecticism of psychopharmacologists. The latter integrate clinical procedures with their basic biochemical and neurophysiological sciences. Psychotherapy could gain from a similar openness to the basic psychological sciences. The *process* of pharmacotherapeutics can be instructive. In clinical practice and research, therapists could integrate different psychotherapy modalities while treating a given patient. Lithium is used to augment fluoxetine. CBT could be used to augment IPT, or vice versa. Psychotherapists would have to become trained and comfortable in a wide variety of modalities.

Medicine in general could benefit from the contributions of psychotherapy to pharmacology in the management of treatment failure, compliance, placebo response, and the influence of psychosocial stress. Many ingredients of psychotherapy may actually decrease physical morbidity and delay mortality (Spiegel, Bloom, Kraemer, & Gottheil, 1989).

The ability to deliver sophisticated combined therapy should be a major training goal for psychiatry. As Hollender and Ford (1990) state in their introductory text to dynamic psychotherapy: 'as long as the therapist is aware of the potential complications and prescribes judiciously, the net therapeutic benefit can be great' (p. 177). The ideal clinician would be able to integrate both biologically and psychologically relevant data in assessing, prescribing, and implementing treatment. He or she would be a significant role model and teacher, not only for students in psychiatry, but also for physicians in the rest of medicine.

References

Agras, W.S., Rossiter, E.M., Arnow, B., Schneider, J.A., Telch, C.F., Raeburn, S.D., Bruce, B., Perl, M., & Koran, L. M. (1992). Pharmacological and cognitive–behavioral treatment for bulimia nervosa: A controlled comparison. *American Journal of Psychiatry, 149*, 82–87.

American Psychiatric Association (APA). (1993). Practice guideline for major depressive disorder in adults. *American Journal of Psychiatry, 150* (Suppl., 4), 1–26.

American Psychiatric Association (APA). (1994). Practice guideline for the treatment of patients with bipolar disorder. *American Journal of Psychiatry, 151* (Suppl., 12), 1–36.

Andreasen, N.C. (1995). Editorial: Posttraumatic stress disorder: Psychology, biology, and Manichaean warfare between false dichotomies. *American Journal of Psychiatry, 152*, 963–965.

Basch, M.F. (1988). *Understanding psychotherapy: The science behind the art*. New York: Basic.

Beaudry, P. (1991). Generalized anxiety disorder. In B.D. Beitman & G.L. Klerman (Eds.), *Integrating pharmacotherapy and psychotherapy*. Washington, DC: American Psychiatric Press.

Beitman, B.D. (1991). Medications during psychotherapy: Case studies of the reciprocal relationship between psychotherapy process and medication use. In B.D. Beitman & G.L. Klerman (Eds.), *Integrating pharmacotherapy and psychotherapy*. Washington, DC: American Psychiatric Press.

Beitman, B.D., Hall, M.J., & Woodward, B. (1992). Integrating pharmacotherapy and psychotherapy. In J.C. Norcross & M.R. Goldfried (Eds.), *Handbook of psychotherapy integration*. New York: Basic.

Beitman, B.D., & Klerman, G.L. (Eds.). (1991). *Integrating pharmacotherapy and psychotherapy*. Washington, DC: American Psychiatric Press.

Burgess, J.W. (1993). The psychotherapy of giving medications: Therapeutic techniques for interpersonal interventions. *American Journal of Psychotherapy, 47*, 393–403.

Busch, F.N., & Gould, E. (1993). Treatment by a psychotherapist and a psychopharmacologist: Transference and countertransference issues. *Hospital and Community Psychiatry, 44*, 772–774.

Chiles, J.A., Carlin, A.S., Benjamin, G.A.H., & Beitman, B.D. (1991). A physician, a nonmedical psychotherapist, and a patient: The pharmacotherapy–psychotherapy triangle. In B.D. Beitman & G.L. Klerman (Eds.), *Integrating pharmacotherapy and psychotherapy.* Washington, DC: American Psychiatric Press.

Cochran, S.D. (1984). Preventing medical noncompliance in the outpatient treatment of bipolar affective disorders. *Journal of Consulting and Clinical Psychology, 52*, 873–878.

Crits-Christoph, P. (1992) The efficacy of brief dynamic psychotherapy: A meta-analysis. *American Journal of Psychiatry, 149*, 151–158.

Donovan, S.J., & Roose, S.P. (1995). Medication use during psychoanalysis: A survey. *Journal of Clinical Psychiatry, 56*, 177–178.

Fawcett, J., Epstein, P., Fiester, S.J., Elkin, I., & Autry, J.H. (1987). Clinical management–Imipramine/placebo administration manual. *Psychopharmacology Bulletin, 23*, 309–324.

Fenton, W.S., & Cole, S.A. (1995). Psychosocial therapies of schizophrenia: Individual, group, and family. In G.O. Gabbard (Ed.), *Treatment of psychiatric disorders.* Washington, DC: American Psychiatric Press.

Frances, A., Clarkin, J., & Perry, S. (1984). *Differential therapeutics in psychiatry: The art and science of treatment selection.* New York: Brunner/Mazel

Frank, J.D. (1973). *Persuasion and healing: A comparative study of psychotherapy* (Rev. ed.). Baltimore: Johns Hopkins University Press.

Gabbard, G.O. (1990). *Psychodynamic psychiatry in clinical practice.* Washington, DC: American Psychiatric Press.

Gabbard, G.O. (1995a). Mind and brain in psychiatric treatment. In G.O. Gabbard (Ed.), *Treatment of psychiatric disorders.* Washington, DC: American Psychiatric Press.

Gabbard, G.O. (1995b), Psychodynamic psychotherapies. In G.O. Gabbard (Ed.), *Treatment of psychiatric disorders,* Washington, DC: American Psychiatric Press.

Goldstein, M.J. (1991). Schizophrenia and family therapy. In B.D. Beitman & G.L. Klerman (Eds.), *Integrating pharmacotherapy and psychotherapy.* Washington, DC: American Psychiatric Press.

Hollender, M.H., & Ford, C.V. (1990). *Dynamic psychotherapy: An introductory approach.* Washington, DC: American Psychiatric Press.

Hollon, S.D., & Fawcett, J. (1995). Depression: Combined medication and psychotherapy. In G.O. Gabbard (Ed.), *Treatment of psychiatric disorders.* Washington, DC: American Psychiatric Press.

Hollon, S.D., Shelton, R.C., & Loosen, P.T. (1991a). Cognitive therapy and pharmacotherapy for depression. *Journal of Consulting and Clinical Psychology, 59,* 88–99.

Hollon, S.D., Shelton, R.C., & Loosen, P.T. (1991b). Research considerations in evaluating combined treatment. In B.D. Beitman & G.L. Klerman (Eds.), *Integrating pharmacotherapy and psychotherapy.* Washington, DC: American Psychiatric Press.

Jamison, K.R. (1991). Manic-depressive illness: The overlooked need for psychotherapy. In B.D. Beitman & G.L. Klerman (Eds.), *Integrating pharmacotherapy and psychotherapy.* Washington, DC: American Psychiatric Press.

Jenike, M.A. (1991). Obsessive–compulsive disorder. In B.D. Beitman & G.L. Klerman (Eds.), *Integrating pharmacotherapy and psychotherapy.* Washington, DC: American Psychiatric Press.

Kantor, S.J. (1993). Analysing a rapid cycler: Can transference keep up? In M. Schacter (Ed.), *Psychotherapy and medication: A dynamic approach.* Northvale, NJ: Jason Aronson.

Karasu, T.B. (1990). Toward a clinical model of psychotherapy for depression, II: An integrative and selective treatment approach. *American Journal of Psychiatry, 147,* 269–278.

Kelly, K.V. (1992). Parallel treatment: Therapy with one clinician and medication with another. *Hospital and Community Psychiatry, 43,* 778–780.

Kennedy, S.H. (1995). Depression. In J. Gray (Ed.), *Therapeutic choices.* Ottawa, ON: Canadian Pharmaceutical Association.

Kennedy, S.H., & Goldbloom, D.S. (1995). Eating disorders: Psychopharmacological treatments. In G.O. Gabbard (Ed.), *Treatment of psychiatric disorders.* Washington, DC: American Psychiatric Press.

Kessler, R.C., McGonagle, K.A., Shanyana, Z., Nelson, C.B., Hughes, M., Eshleman, S., Wittchen, H., & Kendler, K.S. (1994). Lifetime and 12 month prevalence of DSM-III-R psychiatric disorders in the United States: Results from the National Comorbidity Survey. *Archives of General Psychiatry, 51,* 8–19.

Klerman, G.L. (1991). Ideological conflicts in integrating pharmacotherapy and psychotherapy. In B.D. Beitman & G.L. Klerman (Eds.), *Integrating pharmacotherapy and psychotherapy.* Washington, DC: American Psychiatric Press.

Kupfer, D.J. (1991). Long-term treatment of depression. *Journal of Clinical Psychiatry, 52* (Suppl., 5), 28–34.

Lazarus, A. (1994). A proposal for psychiatric collaboration in managed care. *American Journal of Psychotherapy, 48,* 600–609.

Manning, D.W., & Frances, A.J. (Ed.). (1990a). *Combined pharmacotherapy and psychotherapy for depression* (Vol. 26). Washington, DC: American Psychiatric Press.

Manning, D.W., & Frances, A.J. (1990b). Combined therapy for depression: Critical review of the literature. In D.W. Manning & A.J. Frances (Eds.), *Combined pharmacotherapy and psychotherapy for depression* (Vol. 26). Washington, DC: American Psychiatric Press.

Marder, S.R., Johnston-Cronk, K., Wirshing, W.C., & Eckman, T. (1991). Schizophrenia and behavioral skills training. In B.D. Beitman & G.L. Klerman (Eds.), *Integrating pharmacotherapy and psychotherapy.* Washington, DC: American Psychiatric Press.

Marin, D.B., Kocsis, J.H., Frances, A.J., & Klerman, G.L. (1993). Personality disorders in dysthymia. *Journal of Personality Disorders, 7,* 223–231.

Markowitz, J.C. (1994). Psychotherapy of dysthymia. *American Journal of Psychiatry, 151,* 1114–1121.

Mavissakalian, M. (1991). Agoraphobia. In B.D. Beitman & G.L. Klerman (Eds.), *Integrating pharmacotherapy and psychotherapy.* Washington, DC: American Psychiatric Press.

Mitchell, J.E., Pyle, R.L., Eckert, E.D., Hatsukami, D., Pomeroy, C., & Zimmerman, R. (1990). A comparison study of antidepressants and structured intensive group psychotherapy in the treatment of bulimia nervosa. *Archives of General Psychiatry, 47,* 149–157.

Munoz, R.F., Hollon, S.D., McGrath, E., Rehm, L.P., & VandenBos, G.R. (1994). On the AHCPR Depression in Primary Care guidelines: Further considerations for practitioners. *American Psychologist, 49,* 42–61.

Ostow, M. (1979). *The psychodynamic approach to drug therapy,* Toronto: Van Nostrand Reinhold.

Paykel, E.S. (1995). Psychotherapy, medication combinations and compliance. *Journal of Clinical Psychiatry, 56* (Suppl., 1), 24–30.

Persons, J., Thase, M.E., & Crits-Christoph, P. (1996). The role of psychotherapy in the treatment of depression: Review of two practice guidelines. *Archives of General Psychiatry, 53,* 283–290.

Pinsof, W.M. (1983). Integrative problem-centered therapy: Toward the synthesis of family and individual psychotherapies. *Journal of Marital and Family Therapy, 9,* 19–31.

Rosenbaum, J.F., Fava, M., Nierenberg, A.A., & Sachs, G.S. (1995). Treatment-resistant mood disorders. In G.O. Gabbard (Ed.), *Treatment of psychiatric disorders.* Washington, DC: American Psychiatric Press.

Rush, A.J., & Kupfer, D.J. (1995). Strategies and tactics in the treatment of depression. In G.O. Gabbard (Ed.), *Treatment of psychiatric disorders.* Washington, DC: American Psychiatric Press.

Russell, G.F.M., Szmukler, G.I., Dare, C., & Eisler, I. (1987). An evaluation of family therapy in anorexia nervosa and bulimia nervosa. *Archives of General Psychiatry, 44*, 1047–1056.

Schreter, R.K. (1993). Ten trends in managed care and their impact on the biopsychosocial model. *Hospital and Community Psychiatry, 44*, 325–327.

Sotsky, S.M., Glass, D., Shea, J.M., Pilkonis, P.A., Collins, J.F., Elkin, I., Watkins, J.J., Imber, S.D., Leber, W.R., Moyer, J., & Olivieri, M.E. (1991). Patient predictors of response to psychotherapy and pharmacotherapy: Findings in the NIMH Treatment of Depression Collaborative Research Program, *American Journal of Psychiatry, 148*, 997–1008.

Spiegel, D., Bloom, J.R., Kraemer, H.C., & Gottheil, E. (1989). Effect of psychosocial treatment on survival of patients with metastatic breast cancer. *Lancet, 2(8668)*, 888–891.

Strupp, H.H. (1970). Specific vs nonspecific factors in psychotherapy and the problem of control. *Archives of General Psychiatry, 23*, 393–401.

Sullivan, M., Verhurst, J., Russo, J., & Roy-Byrne, P. (1993). Psychotherapy vs. pharmacotherapy: Are psychiatrists polarized? – A survey of academic and clinical faculty. *American Journal of Psychotherapy, 47*, 411–423.

Truax, C.B., & Carkhuff, R.R. (1967). *Toward effective counselling and psychotherapy: Training and practice.* Chicago: Aldine.

Uhde, T.W., & Tancer, M.E. (1991). Social phobia. In B.D. Beitman & G.L. Klerman (Eds.), *Integrating pharmacotherapy and psychotherapy.* Washington, DC: American Psychiatric Press.

Wachtel, P.L. (Ed.). (1982). *Resistance: Psychodynamic and behavioral approaches.* New York: Plenum.

Wiborg, I.M., & Dahl, A.A. (1996). Does brief dynamic psychotherapy reduce the relapse rate of panic disorder? *Archives of General Psychiatry, 53*, 689–694.

Zaretsky, A.E., & Segal, Z.V. (1994). A review of psychosocial interventions in bipolar disorder. *Depression, 2*, 179–188.

12. Guidelines for Psychotherapy with Patients Suffering from Severe and Persistent Mental Illness

Mary Johnston

In the last half of this century, psychiatric practice has been influenced by the development of increasingly effective biological treatments and the phenomenon of deinstitutionalization. Patients with severe and persistent mental illness, however, continue to experience considerable morbidity, and many fall through the cracks of service delivery. Currently, biological therapies and rehabilitation programs are the mainstay for this population, while a variety of psychotherapeutic interventions may facilitate optimum care. This chapter considers the role of psychotherapy in the treatment of persons with severe and persistent mental illness. Using schizophrenia as a model, it addresses issues of definition, efficacy, and practice guidelines.

Who Are the Severely and Persistently Mentally Ill?

Rothbard, Schinnar, and Goldman (1996) have discussed a number of factors which complicate the definition of severe and persistent mental illness. They point out that, from the perspective of service availability, consumers and families may seek a broad definition, while, from the perspective of fiscal accountability, governments may seek a strict definition. Furthermore, the episodic nature of many illnesses and variability in service usage may make it difficult to track those with severe mental health disabilities.

Rothbard et al (1996) define severe and persistent mental illness as the severe and persistent disability which arises secondary to a mental illness. This definition, adopted in this chapter, highlights the individual's experience of illness and the ways in which that illness interferes with his or her ability to live a satisfying life. It should be noted that disability is viewed as being secondary to mental illness in general, not to a specific mental illness. Accordingly, a number of diagnoses may be considered under the general heading of 'severe and persistent mental illness': severe personality disorders; affective disorders; substance abuse; dual diagnosis; organic brain disorders; and psychotic disorders. As it is beyond the scope of this chapter to deal with each of these, the focus will necessarily be restricted.

Schizophrenia is a heterogeneous illness, resulting from environmental and psychological stresses in biologically predisposed individuals. The symptoms of schizophrenia may be more or less controlled by medication, but patients continue to have difficulties with thinking, social interaction, self-care, employment, housing, and other aspects of daily living, all of which have an impact on their quality of life and sense of well-being. As such, a discussion of psychotherapy with persons suffering from schizophrenia includes many of the issues relevant to psychotherapy with persons suffering from severe and persistent mental illness (Deutsch & Munich, 1996).

How Is Psychotherapy Defined in This Context?

Psychotherapeutic treatments for schizophrenia have changed over the years as the theories which inform them and knowledge about the illness itself have grown and developed. Freud (1924/1961) viewed schizophrenia as resulting from the patient's inability to tolerate human contact, or as a regression from object-relatedness to an auto-erotic stage of development. Consistent with this, he believed that patients with schizophrenia were not able to develop transference. Negative symptoms were viewed as withdrawal from reality, and positive symptoms were viewed as the creation of a new and less painful reality. This view complemented Kraepelin's work, which had described schizophrenia as a deteriorating illness with a downhill course. Sullivan, whose emphasis on interpersonal relatedness had an important impact on the development of psychotherapy, emphasized problems in the early child–parent relationship. He believed that anxiety about unmet needs led to psychotic disintegration, but that the capacity for relatedness was always present (Sullivan, 1962). A number of other theorists have contributed to our understanding and misunderstanding of schizophrenia. Some theorists speculated that family dysfunction, in particular, inadequate mothering, caused schizophrenia. More recently, self psychologists have considered schizophrenia as the expression of a struggling self. According to this view, the patient's subjective experience is felt to be real, and the therapist is a functional part of the patient's self (Pollack, 1989). These conceptual developments in the psychoanalytic literature have historically provided and continue to provide a theoretical basis for the psychotherapy of schizophrenia, emphasizing the therapeutic relationship and the individual experience of illness.

Recent knowledge about the biology of schizophrenia has further contributed to our understanding of the illness. From theories of interpersonal relatedness, we move towards a broad conceptualization which includes pharmacotherapy and an awareness of specific neurocognitive deficits of attention, memory, affect regulation, willed action, and the processing and integrating of information (Grotstein, 1995). In keeping with this knowledge base, psychotherapeutic treatments increasingly focus on illness-specific deficits and the difficulties which result.

Overall, recent years have seen significant advances in our understanding of schizophrenia. Current knowledge includes an awareness of neuroleptic medication, the neurophysiological basis of cognitive symptoms, the subjective experience of the illness and its impact on development, and, finally, the significant role of environmental factors on etiology, course, and outcome (Zubin & Spring, 1977; Freeman, 1989). It is commonly held that organic factors interact with environmental factors in individuals who are sensitive to stress so that many aspects of development and daily living are greatly affected by the illness. Accordingly, treatment needs to be comprehensive, encompassing a wide variety of psychosocial modalities in combination with pharmacotherapy (Carpenter, 1986; Jones, 1993).

As the conceptualization of schizophrenia and its treatment broadens, classification of treatment becomes complex. Treatment no longer involves discrete modalities carried out by single caregivers, but a number of caregivers working together as team members with different roles and functions. Specific treatments come in various forms and settings, and the choice of a particular modality at a particular time in a person's life and illness needs to be individually determined. Psychotherapy, then, may refer to specific individual, group, or family treatment modalities (psychodynamic, interpersonal, cognitive, behavioural, supportive, etc.). It may refer to an approach to pharmacological management. It may inform an assertive community outreach program and the work of a number of team members. It may describe a primary relationship between a patient and caregiver which endures over time. Finally, it may describe an approach to treatment which acknowledges the individuality of the person receiving care.

In this chapter 'psychotherapy' refers to a treatment approach which informs and directs an integrated comprehensive treatment plan. It also refers to a number of discrete treatment modalities. The following specific modalities are discussed: individual psychodynamic psychotherapy; family therapy; social-skills training; cognitive/behavioural therapy; psychosocial rehabilitation; and medication.

Efficacy

The psychotherapy of schizophrenia is often practised in the absence of clear guidelines (McGlashan, 1983), which makes its' efficacy difficult to measure. Moreover, as research into schizophrenia has increased, the number of psychotherapeutic treatments available has also increased, so that what is called the 'psychotherapy of schizophrenia' now includes a broad array of treatments, which are often quite different from one another. Increasingly, however, new treatments are being clarified, and their efficacies measured in well-designed outcome studies.

Domains of outcome may be considered using a phase-specific model of illness (Fenton & Cole, 1995; Hogarty et al, 1995). In the acute phase, such issues as symptom control, crisis intervention, family support, and psychoeducation may be addressed. In the maintenance phase, such issues as relapse prevention, medication compliance, housing, vocational pursuits, social skills, relationships, family burden, personal well-being, psychoeducation, and quality of life may be addressed. Alternatively, Buckley and Lys (1996) provide a treatment algorithm based on analysis of symptoms. They suggest that the suitability of a particular treatment modality be based on the individual's response and his or her particular needs at any given time.

Frequently outcome studies measure relapse or rehospitalization. There is often little attention paid to when treatments work best and how they may complement each other. Typically, brief interventions are tested in isolation, which does not reflect the chronic, episodic nature of the illness and the multiple treatment modalities that will be necessary. Rsearch is needed, therefore, on integration and sequencing of different treatments, their optimal timing and duration, and the individualization of treatment over time. Given the chronic nature of this illness and the inevitability of symptom recurrence, there is also a need to shift the focus of research from symptoms and relapse, to functional status and quality-of-life measures.

Six early studies failed to show strongly positive results for the psychotherapy of schizophrenia (Fairweather, Simons, & Gebbard, 1960; Rogers et al, 1967; May, 1968; Grinspoon, Ewalt, & Shader, 1972; Hogarty et al, 1974; Karon & VandenBos, 1981). There were, however, significant problems with these studies: the therapy was poorly described; pharmacotherapy was not controlled; a number of confounding variables were present; therapists were inexperienced; diagnosis tended to be clinical; and the length of treatment was inadequate (Wasylenki, 1992). The seminal work on the psychotherapy of schizophrenia remains the Boston psychotherapy study of Gunderson et al (1984). Patients, who all received standard psychopharmacological management, were assigned to reality-adaptive, supportive (RAS) therapy, or exploratory, insight-oriented (EIO) therapy. While the authors considered the magnitude of differences to be low, RAS did demonstrate preferential effects on rehospitalization and role performance, while EIO exerted preferential, if more modest, effects on ego functioning and cognition. Gabbard (1990) has argued that the two-year data collection, although longer than that of previous studies, was still short by some therapists' standards. He has also addressed the unrealistic expectation of adhering to either an expressive or a supportive modality, since, in practice, therapists frequently shift back and forth from expressive to supportive interventions, depending on the needs of the patient at any particular time. Furthermore, he has argued that random designs do not acknowledge the fit between therapist and patient, a factor which frequently brings them together and keeps them together, particularly in the context of a chronic illness in which exacerbations and remissions are the norm. In clinical practice, patients are not randomly assigned to therapy. Rather, they are assessed, and particular modalities of psychotherapy are prescribed when they are felt to be appropriate.

Some authors have attempted to show that the psychodynamic treatment of schizophrenia is unhelpful, or even harmful (Klerman, 1984; Drake & Sederer, 1986; Mueser & Berenbaum, 1990). Generally, however, one is struck by the competitive rather than collaborative approach to evaluation, the tendency to generalize findings even though the illness is heterogeneous, and the tendency to measure symptoms or relapse rather than quality of life. Given the multiple treatment needs of persons with schizophrenia, it is necessary to measure complementary treatment modalities as they interact together over time.

FAMILY THERAPY

Family therapy looks at practical issues of adaptation to illness, problem solving, and relapse prevention. Many family studies have been based on the work of Brown, Birley, and Wing (1972), later replicated by Leff, Kuipers, Berkowitz, Eberlein-Friess, and Sturgeon (1982), Leff, Kuipers, Berkowitz, and Sturgeon (1985), and Leff, Berkowitz, Shavit, Strachan, Glass, and Vaughan (1988, 1990), on expresed emotion. Expressed emotion is a measure of critical comments, hostility, and overinvolvement. It has been demonstrated that patients from high-expressed-emotion families have a higher relapse rate than patients from low-expressed-emotion families.

A number of studies have delineated brief family-education approaches (McGill, Falloon, Boyd, & Wood-Siverio, 1983; Berkowitz, Eberlein-Friess, Kuipers, & Leff, 1984; Barrowclough & Tarrier, 1987; Smith & Birchwood, 1987; Cozolino, Goldstein, Nuechterlein, West, & Sneider, 1988; Abramovitz & Coursey, 1989). Others have compared the efficacy of family therapy to that of other treatment modalities (Leff et al, 1985, 1988, 1990; Falloon et al, 1985; Tarrier et al, 1989; Hogarty et al, 1991). Duration of treatment in family therapy has been shown to be related to outcome, with nine months of treatment having a more beneficial effect on relapse than briefer interventions (Kottgen, Sonnichsen, Mollenhauer, & Jurth, 1984; Falloon et al, 1985; Leff et al, 1985; Tarrier et al, 1989; Hogarty et al, 1991). Furthermore, gains may be stable up to two years (Leff et al, 1990; McFarlane et al, 1995; Schooler et al, 1997). Multiple family groups may be associated with lower relapse rates than single family groups (McFarlane et al, 1995).

Further work is needed to elucidate the specific criteria responsible for change in family therapy as well as the factors which may help to prevent relapse in patients from low-expressed-emotion families. The focus on expressed emotion has perhaps placed undue emphasis on relapse rate and rehospitalization as markers of therapeutic success. Given the chronicity of schizophrenia, optimal timing, frequency, and duration of the intervention; patient and family perception of illness; patient functioning; family burden; and patient and family ability to request hospitalization when it is needed must also be considered.

SOCIAL-SKILLS TRAINING

A number of controlled studies have concluded that social-skills training is effective in reducing symptoms and increasing social adjustment, but not in decreasing relapse rate (Bellack, Turner, Hersen, & Luber, 1984; Liberman, Mueser, & Wallace, 1986; Hogarty et al, 1986, 1991; Halford & Hayes, 1991; Marder et al, 1996). Hogarty et al (1991) and Bradshaw (1993) demonstrated a positive impact on rehospitalization at one year, but Hogarty's sample showed no impact at two years. The effect on social functioning was also time-limited. Benton and Schroeder's meta-analysis (1990) showed a weak reduction in symptoms, while Corrigan's meta-analysis (1991) showed a large effect. Overall, studies suggest a time-limited effect in most areas measured. Individuals do acquire the targeted skills, but there is no clear evidence that these skills are maintained or generalized.

Work is needed to identify the specific factors responsible for social-skills development and to demonstrate generalization of treatment. It is also important to determine the optimal timing, frequency, and duration of social-skills training. A recent study by Marder et al (1996) suggests that social-skills training may be most beneficial for persons with early onset of illness, so that skills may be learned by these individuals before deficits become too firmly entrenched. Finally, the relationship between cognitive deficits and social-skills attainment needs to be better understood so that complementary treatments may be offered.

COGNITIVE BEHAVIOURAL THERAPY

Some treatments focus on specific cognitive deficits, but it is unclear whether cognitive rehabilitation generalizes to more complex levels of functioning. A number of studies have looked at performance on the Wisconsin Card Sorting Test and have concluded that deficits on this test are remediable (Goldman, Axelrod, & Tompkins, 1992; Green, Satz, Ganzell, & Vaclav, 1992; Metz, Johnson, Pliskin, & Luchins, 1994; Stratta, Mancinia, Mattei, Casacchia, & Rossi, 1994; Vollema, Geurtsen, van Voorst, 1995; Young & Freyslinger, 1995). Two studies looking at vigilance and attention did not support the efficacy of cognitive rehabilitation (Benedict et al, 1994; Kern, Green, & Goldstein, 1995). Integrated psychological therapy is based on the notion that remediation of cognitive deficits will facilitate the acquisition of more complex skills, but, at present, there is no clear data to support this (Brenner, Hodel, Roder, & Corrigan, 1992; Brenner et al, 1995). It is also not clear whether the effects on cognitive skills are specific to the cognitive techniques used, since social-skills training has shown similar effects (Kraemer, 1991). Cognitive behavioural therapy may be helpful in treating hallucinations and delusions (Tarrier et al, 1993; Bentall, Haddock, & Slade, 1994). However, while there is some evidence that cognitive behavioural techniques may help to decrease psychotic symptoms, particularly delusions, there is no evidence that such symptom improvement will generalize.

There is a need to better identify residual cognitive difficulties and their relationship to the symptoms and social difficulties of persons with schizophrenia so that the effects of cognitive therapy may be maximized. There is also a need to study and better appreciate the effects of cognitive deficits on personality development. Such a study could pave the way for more collaborative approaches to treatment in which the full impact of the illness is addressed.

PSYCHOSOCIAL REHABILITATION

Several models of psychosocial rehabilitation have been positively applied to the treatment of schizophrenia and a detailed discussion of these will not be attempted here. Generally, there is a movement towards approaches which are community-based and team-oriented and which emphasize independent living (Santos, 1996). As Bachrach (1996) has pointed out, however, biases and misperceptions on the part of psychiatry and psychosocial rehabilitation frequently lead to the polarization of services and an 'either/or' approach to treatment. She describes the belief system of psychosocial rehabilitation as 'one that insists ... that mentally ill individuals be viewed as persons who have strengths in addition to their illnesses and who necessarily respond to their illnesses in distinctive personal ways' (p. 31). This view highlights the common base of many apparently competing treatment modalities and the need for improved collaboration. Weiden and Havens (1994) have described principles of psychotherapy for use by non-medical team members. Studies are needed to look at collaborative approaches to treatment.

MEDICATION

Although medication is essential for the treatment of schizophrenia, it is only effective as part of an overall treatment approach. Goldstein (1984) has pointed out that aftercare programs and, specifically, drug dosage vary according to length of stay and aggressiveness of inpatient programs. He has considered the role of the community, particularly the family, in assuming the primary caretaker's role. He has also considered what impact community and family involvement have on maintenance drug therapy.

While the value of maintenance drug therapy is clear, the limitation of drugs, as well as their side-effects, have prompted an examination of dose reduction or intermittent use when possible (Hogarty et al, 1979; Kane, Rifkin, Woerner, & Reardon, 1982; Marder et al, 1996). Careful dose reduction may be possible. Targeted intermittent strategies, while feasible in selected cases, may increase the risk of relapse (Schooler, Keith, Severe, & Matthews, 1995). More studies are needed to examine the interaction of various psychosocial treatment modalities with drug dose, compliance and quality of life (Awad, 1995).

Practice Guidelines

INDIVIDUAL PSYCHODYNAMIC PSYCHOTHERAPY

The predisposing, precipitating, perpetuating, and protective factors, from a biological, social, and psychological perspective, are evaluated and integrated in the development of an individually tailored treatment plan which incorporates patient and family preference. Emphasis is placed on the patient's strengths as well as weaknesses, and on the personal meaning and significance of his or her illness and symptoms. For example, if medication is prescribed in order to eliminate voices which the patient experiences as reassuring, compliance may be an issue. Similarly, if medical treatment is experienced as in conflict with religious beliefs, treatment may induce intolerable feelings of guilt.

Wasylenki (1992) underscores the importance of therapeutic listening. Selzer (1983) also highlights the importance of listening and looks at ways in which the hospitalized patient may begin to form a therapeutic alliance by addressing deficits in differentiation of self and other, in reality testing, and in the development of an observing ego. Evidence suggests that the first six months are a critical time for the development of such an alliance (Frank & Gunderson, 1990). Furthermore, the therapeutic alliance has been positively correlated with staying in treatment, complying with medication, improved outcome, and taking lower doses of medication (Frank & Gunderson, 1990).

Persons with schizophrenia frequently fear both relationships and loneliness. At times their symptoms permit withdrawal, and at other times escape. Respect for the illness, as well as maintenance of a comfortable interpersonal distance, therefore, are important principles of alliance formation. Idiosyncrasies of speech, dress, personal appearance, and hygiene may be difficult to tolerate and may be best understood as distance-regulating mechanisms.

The therapist uses the relationship as a base from which a number of supportive treatment modalities may be accessed as required. At times this may mean postponing interpretation until the therapeutic alliance is developed. At others, it may mean the consideration of a variety of complementary treatments, such as medication, stress management, and family intervention. It may also mean appropriate referral to other services – social welfare, housing, or a legal agency. Based on the work of Winnicott, Modell (1976) has described a 'holding environment' for schizophrenic patients in which safety and protection are seen as integral to the therapy.

Far from not forming transferences, patients with schizophrenia frequently form extremely intense transferences. Furthermore, the intensity of feelings, complicated by a distorted perception of reality, may make it difficult to examine transference in the usual way. It has been suggested that fostering positive transference early on (Federn, 1952) and educating patients about transference (Deutsch & Munich, 1996) may be helpful.

Countertransference reactions also tend to be intense. Supervision and collegial support are likely to be necessary and helpful. Gabbard (1990) has highlighted the need for genuineness and openness with patients.

FAMILY THERAPY

Dixon and Lehman (1995) suggest that the most frequently used elements of family intervention are psychoeducation, behavioural problem solving, family support, and crisis management. Most family therapies begin with psychoeducational sessions. These sessions educate patients and families about schizophrenia as an illness – its pathophysiology, course and prognosis, and principles of treatment. They may also include information about community resources and advocacy groups. The number of initial educational sessions ranges from one to six. They may be didactic or interactive. They may involve single or multiple families, both with and without the patient being present. These sessions are mainly for imparting information, and generally lead into more comprehensive interventions.

There are a variety of approaches to long-term family therapy. Lam (1991) has recently reviewed the literature and summarized their common components as follows:

1 A positive and genuine working relationship
2 Structure and stability
3 Focus on the here and now
4 Use of family concepts (i.e., boundaries)
5 Cognitive restructuring
6 Behavioural approaches (i.e., assessing needs and strengths, breaking goals down into smaller steps, and task assignment and review)
7 Improving communication

In general, the therapy is done, not with a sick family, but with a stressed family. Positives are emphasized, and specific concerns around involvement, limit-setting, and personal distance are addressed. Boundaries may also be emphasized in order to clarify interactions and provide structure and support. Relatives are educated to understand and respect both positive and negative symptoms. They are also helped to see the illness in terms of the disease model so that patients are viewed as having an illness rather than a difficult personality. Guilt and blame are discouraged, and emphasis is placed on constructive problem solving in the here and now. Assisting patients with independent-living skills and encouraging separation from families may also be indicated.

SOCIAL-SKILLS TRAINING

Techniques are largely behavioural, although some studies have begun to incorporate cognitive and behavioural methods. Integrated psychological therapy (IPT) is the best described of such approaches and is discussed under cognitive behavioural therapy (Brenner et al, 1992, 1995). Traditional social-skills training generally targets deficits in interpersonal skills. Strategies include: assessment of interpersonal competence; targeting of specific deficits with a view to individualized goal setting; repeated rehearsal of interpersonal strategies (instructions and prompts); role playing and feedback; problem solving; contingent reinforcement; and *in vivo* assignments.

A well-developed treatment which incorporates social-skills training is Hogarty's personal therapy (PT). This systematized, step-wise treatment focuses on affect dysregulation in response to stress. Patients are taught to recognize internal events in order to facilitate better affective control. As patients maintain stability and develop insight into their particular response to stress, more practical skills are taught, with a view to community reintegration. Formats include individual, family, and group (Hogarty et al, 1995).

Liberman and Corrigan (1993) have developed a modular approach to social-skills training based on a three-phase conceptualization of social-skills deficits – receiving, processing, and sending. Goals include: medication management; symptom management; recreation for leisure; conversation; and grooming and self-care. Each module has a videotape, trainer's manual, user's guide, and patient's handbook.

COGNITIVE BEHAVIOURAL THERAPY

In a recent review, Brenner (1994) has organized cognitive therapies into three approaches – direct, indirect, and combined. Direct approaches target specific attentional, mnemonic, and conceptual skills. Patients perform drills and exercises in repetitive fashion. Recently, computerized training programs have also been developed. Indirect approaches are aimed at behaviour modification, while only indirectly effecting cognitive change. Examples are the reframing of delusional thoughts, and self-talking. Combined approaches incorporate both direct and indirect approaches so that specific deficits are addressed in the context of real functional difficulties. An example of the combined approach is integrated psychological therapy, which consists of five subprograms proceeding from cognitive to social-skills training (Brenner, 1995). The subprograms include: cognitive differentiation (attentional skills and conceptualization); social perception (analysis of social stimuli); verbal communication (conversation skills); social-skills (competence in social-skills); and interpersonal problem-solving (application of problem-solving strategies)

The meta-cognitive approach of Perris and Skagerlind (1994), while not yet studied in a controlled fashion, looks at the interaction between biological and psychosocial factors in an effort to appreciate how the illness may influence the individual's view of self. The treatment is based on Beck's principles of cognitive therapy. In a review of the cognitive therapy of schizophrenia, Alford and Correia (1994) cite the following cognitive therapeutic principles:

- the therapeutic relationship (sensitivity to the negative self-concept)
- the intervention (problem identification, self observation, perspective taking)
- the treating of both content and process (i.e., specific distortions, including personalization, arbitrary inference, dichotomous thinking, selective abstraction, as well as the maladaptive delusional content).

The coping-strategy enhancement (CSE) of Tarrier, Harwood, Yusopoff, Beckett, and Bayer (1990) employs cognitive strategies both to identify the symptoms and the behaviour and to develop and practise appropriate coping techniques.

Behavioural interventions are often part of larger treatment designs. Token economy or positive- and negative-reinforcement techniques may be applied in inpatient settings to alter the expression of psychotic symptoms. Humming is a technique based on the hypothesis that movements of the laryngeal muscles are causally related to auditory hallucinations and that interference with these movements should reduce hallucinations (Green & Kinsbourne, in press). Finally, Bentall et al (1994) have developed a cognitive behavioural therapy for auditory hallucinations based on the notion that hallucinations represent failure to attribute internal mental events to the self. Their three stages focus on: physical characteristics of the voices; content of the voices; and related thoughts and assumptions about the voices.

PSYCHOSOCIAL REHABILITATION

Bachrach (1996) has defined psychosocial rehabilitation as 'a therapeutic approach that encourages a mentally ill person to develop his or her fullest capacities through learning and environmental supports' (p. 29). She identifies nine concepts common to rehabilitation approaches: individualized treatment; focus on the environment; focus on the patient's strengths; restoring hope; emphasis on vocational potential; comprehensive care; patient involvement; continuity of care; and therapeutic alliance.

The continuity of care, the integration of multiple services, and the need for long-term intervention, which are required in the treatment of persons with schizophrenia, are often best conceptualized by psychosocial-rehabilitation models. The therapeutic relationship is generally felt to be an integral part of the treatment (Goering & Stylianos, 1988; Mosher & Burti, 1992).

MEDICATION

Patients with schizophrenia frequently take powerful mind-altering drugs which cause debilitating side-effects. Studies demonstrating efficacy of medications have focused on symptom control and relapse rate, with less attention being given to such variables as quality of life or subjective feelings of satisfaction, happiness, or well-being. The experience of psychosis, the post-psychotic depression, chronic feelings of low self-esteem, stigma, and marginalization in society, all need to be addressed. Ironically, as medications improve, the challenge of psychopharmacology moves beyond that of treating symptoms to treating the meaning to the patient of having those symptoms (Kotcher & Smith, 1993).

Important issues of dose, compliance, symptom control, and quality of life are interrelated and can all be influenced by the therapeutic relationship – that is, listening to the patient's experience, appreciating the meaning to the patient of taking medication, allaying fears about loss of control, and giving appropriate and timely information.

Conclusion

In recent years, research into the biology of schizophrenia has contributed greatly to our understanding of the illness. Symptoms, which were once thought to result from inadequate early relationships and family dysfunction, are now attributed to underlying brain pathology. The role of various stresses has also been investigated, and the result is a biopsychosocial or diathesis stress model (Engel, 1982; Mueser & Bellack, 1995). It is now understood that biologically based cognitive deficits interact with environmental factors to influence the development of personality, coping skills, social-skills, relationship skills, etc. It is also understood that individuals with schizophrenia are prone to various stresses which may exacerbate symptoms or precipitate relapse. With this conceptual shift, there has been a corresponding shift in studies looking at treatment. From comparisons of brief therapies, there has been a movement towards the consideration of longer-term and more comprehensive care encompassing a number of treatment modalities (Munetz, Birnbaum, & Wyzik, 1993; Bellack & Mueser, 1993; Hayes, Halford, & Varghese, 1995; Penn & Mueser, 1996). The modalities discussed are summarized in table 12.1.

It is now understood that the disabilities associated with schizophrenia, as an example of serious and persistent mental illness, will be lifelong and that they will vary with such factors as phase of illness, co-

Table 12.1: Psychotherapy of Severe and Persistent Mental Illness: An Overview

Modality	Indications and Contraindications	Mechanism of Change	Setting and Frame	Conclusion
Individual psychodynamic psychotherapy	Gabbard (1990) has suggested the following: *Indications* 1. Intact reality testing. 2. Ability for interpersonal relationship. 3. Ability to integrate the psychotic episode into life. *Contraindictions* Severe disturbance such that danger to the patient or therapist is imminently possible. Using a relationship which moves between the exploratory and supportive poles, individual psychotherapy may be applicable to all phases of illness. As such, it must be flexible, responding to the individual's changing needs over time.	It is generally felt that change parallels the development of the therapeutic relationship and involves the strengthening of ego boundaries. Specific issues may also be addressed: – stress management – problem solving – education about the illness and its treatment – social skills – medication compliance	Generally an office setting, but Gabbard (1990) and Kaplan, Sadock, and Grebb (1994) sugest alternatives may be appropriate (i.e., while walking, over coffee, using an artistic medium, over a recreational pursuit, etc.). The principles of psychotherapy may be useful to all members of a multidisciplinary team.	There is no solid evidence to support individual psycho-dynamic psychotherapy as an alternative to other treatment modalities. There is a need to further explore the additive or interactive effects of different treatment modalities over time.

Table 12.1: (Continued)

Modality	Indications and Contraindications	Mechanism of Change	Setting and Frame	Conclusion
Family therapy	*Indications* Individuals who continue to live with families or equivalent. Not limited to individuals from high-expressed-emotion families. *Contraindications* No identifiable family unit. Family distress, as it has an impact on the patient, must be considered at all phases of the illness.	Family stress is reduced through psycho-education, support, and problem solving. Families are educated about the illness and its treatment. They are assisted in readjusting expectations and demands. They are particularly informed about the role of expressed emotion. The specific therapeutic factors in family therapy are not well understood.	Therapy may occur in an office of *in vivo* at the patient's home or in the community. The patient may be included or excluded. Some studies have looked at multiple family groups. Therapist control of affect intensity is crucial.	Family therapy is associated with reduced relapse rate and reduced expressed emotion. There is no demonstrated benefit to short-term educational packages alone. At least nine months of treatment seem to be required, and gains may be stable over time. There may be a role for long-term family therapy. Optimal frequency, duration, and timing of the intervention need to be determined. Multiple family groups may be of greater benefit to some patients than single family interventions.

Table 12.1: (Continued)

Modality	Indications and Contraindications	Mechanism of Change	Setting and Frame	Conclusion
Social-skills training	*Indications* Deficits in interpersonal, social, and independent living skills. *Contraindications* Symptoms insufficiently controlled so that patients are unable to participate effectively. Patients have adequate social skills.	Sensitivity to environmental stress may exacerbate symptoms. Social-skills training assists patients to develop interpersonal and other coping skills which may serve as a buffer against such stress. It also teaches patients how not to elicit responses from others which are, in turn, stressful. Some approaches use repetitive activities to overlearn behaviours with the understanding that these behaviours will then be used automatically. Others combine a number of therapeutic strategies in a systematized, stepwise fashion, which respects phase of illness and developing skills.	Individual or group. Training rooms should be quiet, respecting the patient's distractability.	Individuals acquire the targeted skills, but there is no clear evidence that they are maintained or generalized. Comprehensive treatments need to be carefully evaluated. Issues such as optimal frequency, duration, and timing of the intervention need to be determined. The temporal and possibly synergistic relationships between social-skills training and other treatment modalities need to be studied.

Table 12.1: (Continued)

Modality	Indications and Contraindications	Mechanism of Change	Setting and Frame	Conclusion
Cognitive/ behavioural therapy a) Remediation of deficits	*Indications* Target symptoms/deficits should be assessed as chronic, since acute symptoms may remit spontaneously. *Contraindications* Patients have insufficient cognitive organization to be able to make use of cognitive techniques. Patients do not have significant cognitive deficits or are not disturbed by them.	Cognitive behavioural interventions are based on the understanding that specific changes in brain structure underlie cognitive deficits. These in turn interact with environmental factors to cause functional disabilities. Some treatments address the deficits; others intervene at the level of problem solving; and still others at the level of self-concept. Most therapies acknowledge the complex interactions that exist between deficit and environment. The specific therapeutic factors in cognitive therapy are not well understood.	A variety of settings but mostly group.	Cognitive behavioural techniques may improve psychotic symptoms, but generalization of symptom improvement is unclear. The distinction between episodic cognitive deficits secondary to psychosis and stable cognitive deficits which predispose to psychosis needs to be clarified so that appropriate treatments may be offered in each case.

Table 12.1: (Continued)

Modality	Indications and Contraindications	Mechanism of Change	Setting and Frame	Conclusion
b) Meta-cognitive approach	*Indications* Patients are motivated and significantly distressed by dysfunctional cognitive working models. *Contraindications* Symptoms are insufficiently controlled so that patients are unable to participate effectively.	Meta-cognitive approaches attempt to restructure dysfunctional cognitive and emotive working models of self and environment (Perris & Skagerlind, 1994).	May comprise milieu, group, and individual therapy.	Not recommended for routine clinical use (*American Journal of Psychiatry* [suppl], 1997).
Psychosocial rehabilitation	*Indications* Problems adapting to illness and accessing and coordinating services. *Contraindications* Patients have adapted adequately to their illness; they have good social support, and psychosocial rehabilitation is not required.	Stress is reduced by addressing daily issues with which persons with schizophrenia have difficulty. Maximization of the individual's strengths in his or her environment, focus on the here and now, and the active collaboration of therapist and patient/client are considered instrumental to the work that is done. The therapeutic relationship is an important therapeutic factor.	Therapy is generally individualized, and team-oriented, and takes place in the community.	The rehabilitation and medical models need to work more collaboratively together.

Table 12.1: (*Concluded*)

Modality	Indications and Contraindications	Mechanism of Change	Setting and Frame	Conclusion
Medication	*Indications* The need for symptom control. *Contraindications* Apart from medical emergencies (i.e., neuroleptic malignant syndrome), guidelines for the treatment of schizophrenia included neuroleptic medication. In the acute phase, goals include symptom control and side-effect management. In the maintenance phase, goals include compliance, dose reduction, quality of life, tardive side-effects, and general medical management.	A number of neurotransmitters are affected, most notably dopamine and seratonin.	Medication management may take place in a number of settings, including clinic, community, and home. Flexibility, particularly among the homeless or hard to serve, is an important principle of care.	Medications are generally felt to have limited efficacy in treating symptoms. Side-effects may be prohibitive, and compliance is often an issue. The psychotherapy of psychopharmacology is an area for future study. The effects of various psychotherapies on medication dose and compliance need to be more thoroughly studied. As neuroleptics become more efficient in the treatment of negative symptoms and cognition, adjunctive psychotherapy treating the experience of illness and the response to improved functioning becomes increasingly important.

morbidity, and changing social network. It is also understood that a number of different treatment modalities is likely to be necessary at different times in the overall course of the illness. The following principles, therefore, are not intended to guide an exclusive treatment modality but, rather, are intended to guide a comprehensive and integrated treatment approach. It is understood that such a treatment is rooted in dynamic principles and acknowledges the centrality of the individual experience of illness.

- Treatment should be based on a biopsychosocial formulation.
- The therapeutic alliance is an essential part of treatment and may take some time to develop.
- Attention to underlying cognitive deficits may help to facilitate more complex therapeutic tasks.
- Social and family stresses may precipitate illness and need to be addressed.
- Treatment should respect patient and family preferences.
- Treatment should be long-term, coordinated, continuous, and comprehensive.
- Treatment should be flexible and individualized to respond to the patient's changing needs over time.

References

Abramowitz, I.A., & Coursey, R.D. (1989). Impact of an educational support group of family participants who take care of their schizophrenic relatives. *Journal of Consulting and Clinical Psychology, 57*, 232–236.

Alford, B.A., & Correia, C.J. (1994). Cognitive therapy of schizophrenia: Theory and empirical status. *Behaviour Therapy, 25*, 17–33.

American Psychiatric Association (APA). (1997). Practice guidelines for treatmentof patients with schizophrenia. *American Journal of Psychiatry, 154*, (Suppl., 4), 00–00.

Awad, A.G. (1995). Quality of life issues in medicated schizophrenic patients. In C.L. Shriqui & H.M. Nasrallah (Eds.), *Contemporary issues in the treatment of schizophrenia* (pp. 735–747). Washington, DC: American Psychiatric Press.

Bachrach, L.L. (1996). Psychosocial rehabilitation and psychiatry: What are the boundaries? *Canadian Journal of Psychiatry, 41*, 28–33.

Barrowclough, C., & Tarrier, N. (1987). A behavioural intervention with a schizophrenic patient. *Behavioural Psychotherapy, 15*, 252–271.

Bellack, A.S., & Mueser, K.T. (1993). Psychosocial treatment for schizophrenia. *Schizophrenia Bulletin, 19,* 317–336.

Bellack, A.S., Turner, S.M., Hersen, M., & Luber, R.F. (1984). An examination of the efficacy of social-skills training for chronic schizophrenic patients. *Hospital and Community Psychiatry, 35,* 1023–1028.

Benedict, R.H.B., Harris, A.E., Markow, I., McCormick, J.A., Nuechterlein, K.H., & Asarnow, R.F. (1994). Effects of attention training on information processing in schizophrenia. *Schizophrenia Bulletin, 20,* 537–546.

Bentall, R.P., Haddock, G., & Slade, P.D. (1994). Cognitive therapy for persistent auditory hallucinations: From theory to therapy. *Behaviour Therapy, 25,* 51–66.

Benton, M.K., & Schroeder, H.E. (1990). Social skills training with schizophrenics: A meta-analytic evaluation. *Journal of Consulting and Clinical Psychology, 58,* 741–747.

Berkowitz, R., Eberlein-Friess, R., Kuipers, L., & Leff, J. (1984). Educating relatives about schizophrenia. *Schizophrenia Bulletin, 10,* 418–429.

Bradshaw, W.H. (1993). Coping-skills training versus a problem-solving approach with schizophrenic patients. *Hospital and Community Psychiatry, 44,* 1102–1104.

Brenner, H.D. (1994). Cognitive therapy with schizophrenic patients: Conceptual basis, present state, future directions. *ACTA Psychiatrica Scandinavica, 90* (Suppl., 384), 108–115.

Brenner, H.D., Hodel, B., Roder, V., & Corrigan, P. (1992). Treatment of cognitive dysfunctions and behavioural deficits in schizophrenia. *Schizophrenia Bulletin, 18,* 21–26.

Brenner, H.D., Roder, V., Hodel, B., Kienzie, N., Reed, D., & Liberman, R.P. (1995). *Integrated psychological therapy for schizophrenic patients.* Bern, Switzerland: Hogrefe & Huber.

Brown, G.W., Birley, J.L.T., & Wing, J.K. (1972). Influence of family life on the course of schizophrenia disorders: Replication. *British Journal of Psychiatry, 121,* 241–258.

Buckley, P.F., & Lys, C. (1996). Psychotherapy and schizophrenia. *Journal of Psychotherapy Practice and Research, 5,* 185–201.

Carpenter, W.T. (1986). Thoughts on the treatment of schizophrenia. *Schizophrenia Bulletin, 12,* 527–539.

Corrigan, P.W. (1991). Social-skills training in adult psychiatric populations: A meta-analysis. *Journal of Behavior Therapy and Experimental Psychiatry, 22,* 203–210.

Cozolino, L.J., Goldstein, M.J., Nuechterlein, K.H., West, K.L., & Synder, K.S. (1988). The impact of education about schizophrenia on relatives varying in expressed emotion. *Schizophrenia Bulletin, 14,* 675–687.

Deutsch, A., & Munich, R. (1996). Psychotherapy with the severely and persistently mentally ill. In S. Soreff (Ed.), *Handbook for the treatment of the seriously mentally ill*. Toronto: Hogrefe & Huber.

Dixon, L.B., & Lehman, A.F. (1995). Family intervention for schizophrenia. *Schizophrenia Bulletin, 21*, 631–643.

Drake, R.E., & Sedener, L.I. (1986). The adverse effects of intensive treatment of chronic schizophrenia. *Comprehensive Psychiatry, 27*, 313–326.

Engel, G.L. (1982). The biopsychosocial model and medical education: Who are to be the teachers? *New England Journal of Medicine, 306*, 802–805.

Fairweather, G.W., Simon, R., & Gebhard, M.E. (1960). Relative effectiveness of psychotherapeutic programs: A multicriteria comparison of four programs for three different patient groups. *Psychological Monographs, 74*, 1–26.

Falloon, I.R.H., Boyd, J.L., McGill, C.W., Williamson, M., Razani, J., Moss, H.B., Gilderman, A.M., & Simpson, G.M. (1985). Family management in the prevention of morbidity of schizophrenia: Clinical outcome of a two-year longitudinal study. *Archives of General Psychiatry, 42*, 887–896.

Federn, P. (1952). *Ego psychology and the psychoses*. New York: Basic.

Fenton, W.S., & Cole, S.A. (1995). Psychological therapies of schizophrenia: Individual, group and family. In G.O. Gabbard, ed., *Treatments of psychiatric disorders*. Washington, DC: American Psychiatric Press.

Frank, A.F., & Gunderson, J.G. (1990). The role of the therapeutic alliance in the treatment of schizophrenia. *Archives of General Psychiatry, 47*, 228–236.

Freeman, H. (1989). Relationship of schizophrenia to the environment. *British Journal of Psychiatry, 155* (5, Supplement), 90–99.

Freud, S. (1961). Neurosis and psychosis. In J. Stachey (Ed. and Trans.), *The standard edition of the complete psychological works of Sigmund Freud* (Vol. 19). London: Hogarth Press (Original work published 1924)

Gabbard, G.O. (1990). Schizophrenia. In *Psychodynamic psychiatry in clinical practice*. Washington, DC: American Psychiatric Press.

Goering, P.N., & Stylianos, S.K. (1988). Exploring the helping relationship between the schizophrenic client and rehabilitation therapist. *American Journal of Orthopsychiatry, 58*, 271–280.

Goldman, R.S., Axelrod, B., & Tompkins, L.M. (1992). Effects of instructional cues on schizophrenic patients' performance on the Wisconsin Card Sorting Test. *American Journal of Psychiatry, 149*, 1718–1722.

Goldstein, M.J. (1984). Schizophrenia: The interaction of family and neuroleptic therapy. In B. Beitman & G. Klerman (Eds.), *Combining psychotherapy and drug therapy in clinical practice*. New York: Spectrum.

Green, M.F., & Kinsbourne, M. (in press). Subvocal activity and auditory hallucinations: Clues for behavioural treatments? *Schizophrenia Bulletin*.

Green, M.F., Satz, P., Ganzell, S., & Vaclav, J.F. (1992). Wisconsin Card Sorting Test performance in schizophrenia: Remediation of a stubborn deficit. *American Journal of Psychiatry, 149,* 62–67.

Grinspoon, L., Ewalt, J.R., & Shader, R.I. (1972). *Schizophrenia: Pharmacotherapy and psychotherapy.* Baltimore: Williams & Wilkins.

Grotstein, J.S. (1995). Orphans of the 'Real': I: Some modern and postmodern perspectives on the neurobiological and psychosocial dimensions of psychosis and other primitive mental disorders. *Bulletin of the Menninger Clinic, 59,* 287–311.

Gunderson, J.G., Frank, A.F., Katz, H.M., Vannicelli, M.L., Frosch, J.P., & Knapp, P.H. (1984). Effects of psychotherapy in schizophrenia, II: Comparative outcome of two forms of treatment. *Schizophrenia Bulletin, 10,* 564–598.

Halford, W.K., & Hayes, R. (1991). Psychological rehabilitation of chronic schizophrenic patients: Recent findings on social-skills training and family psychoeducation. *Clinical Psychology Review, 11,* 23–44.

Hayes, R.L., Halford, W.K., & Varghese, F.T. (1995). Social-skills training with chronic schizophrenic patients: Effects on negative symptoms and community functioning. *Behaviour Therapy, 26,* 433–449.

Hogarty, G.E., Anderson, C.M., Reiss, D.J., Kornblith, S.J., Greenwald, D.P., Javna, C.D., & Madonia, M.J. (1986). Family psycho-education, social-skills training and maintenance chemotherapy, I: One-year effects of a controlled study on relapse and expressed emotion. *Archives of General Psychiatry, 45,* 797–805.

Hogarty, G.E., Anderson, C., Reiss, D., Kornblith, S., Greenwald, D., Ulrich, R., & Carter, M. (1991). Family psychoeducation, social skills training, and maintenance chemotherapy in the aftercare treatment of schizophrenia, II: Two-year effects of a controlled study on relapse and adjustment. *Archives of General Psychiatry, 48,* 340–347.

Hogarty, G.E., Goldberg, S.C., & Schooler, N.R. et al (1974). Drugs and sociotherapy in the aftercare of schizophrenia patients, III: Adjustment of non-relapsed patients. *Archives of General Psychiatry, 31,* 609–625.

Hogarty, G.E., Kornblith, S.J., Greenwald, D., DiBarry, A.L., Cooley, S., Flesher, S., Reiss, D., Carter, M., & Ulrich, R. (1995). Personal therapy: A disorder-relevant psychotherapy for schizophrenia. *Schizophrenia Bulletin, 21,* 379–393.

Hogarty, G.E., Schooler, N.R., & Ulrich, R., Mussare, F., Herron, E., & Ferro, P. (1979). Fluphenazine and social therapy in the aftercare of schizophrenic patients. *Archives of General Psychiatry, 36,* 1283–1294.

Jones, B. (1993). Schizophrenia: Into the next millennium. *Canadian Journal of Psychiatry, 38* (Suppl., 3): 67–69.

Kane, J.M., Rifkin, A., Woerner, M., & Reardon, G. (1982). Low dose neuroleptics in outpatient schizophrenics. *Psychopharmacology Bulletin, 18,* 20–21.

Kaplan, H.I., Sadock, B.J., & Grebb, J.A. (1994). Schizophrenia. In *Synopsis of psychiatry* (7th ed.). Baltimore: Williams & Wilkins.

Karon, B.P., & VandenBos, G.R. (1981). *Psychotherapy of schizophrenia: The treatment of choice.* New York: Jason Aronson.

Kern, R.S., Green, M.F., & Goldstein, M.J. (1995). Modification of performance on the span of apprehension, a putative marker of vulnerability to schizophrenia. *Journal of Abnormal Psychology, 104,* 385–389.

Klerman, G.L. (1984). Ideology and science in the individual psychotherapy of schizophrenia. *Schizophrenia Bulletin, 10,* 608–611.

Kotcher, M., & Smith, T.E. (1993). Three phases of clozapine treatment and phase-specific issues for patients and families. *Hospital and Community Psychiatry, 44,* 744–747.

Kottgen, C., Sonnichsen, I., Mollenhauer, K., & Jurth, R. (1984). Group therapy with the families of schizophrenic patients: Results of the Hamburg Camberwell-Family-Interview Study, III. *International Journal of Family Psychiatry, 5,* 83–94.

Kraemer, S. (1991). Cognitive training and social-skills training in relation to basic disturbances in chronic schizophrenic patients. In C.N. Stefanis (Ed.), *Proceedings of the World Congress of Psychiatry.* Amsterdam: Elseiser.

Lam, D.H. (1991). Psychosocial family intervention in schizophrenia: A review of empirical studies. *Psychological Medicine, 21,* 423–441.

Leff, J.P., Berkowitz, R., Shavit, N., Strachan, A., Glass, I., & Vaughn, C. (1988). A trial of family therapy *v.* a relatives' group for schizophrenia. *British Journal of Psychiatry, 153,* 58–66.

Leff, J.P., Berkowitz, R., Shavit, N., Strachan, A., Glass, I., & Vaughn, C. (1990). A trial of family therapy *v.* a relatives' group for schizophrenia: Two-year follow-up. *British Journal of Psychiatry, 157,* 571–577.

Leff, J.P., Kuipers, L., Berkowitz, R., Eberlein-Friess, R., & Sturgeon, D. (1982). A controlled trial of social intervention in schizophrenia families. *British Journal of Psychiatry, 141,* 121–134.

Leff, J.P., Kuipers, L., Berkowitz, R., & Sturgeon, D. (1985). A controlled trial of social intervention in the families of schizophrenia patients: Two-year follow-up. *British Journal of Psychiatry, 146,* 594–600.

Liberman, R.P., & Corrigan, P.W. (1993). Designing new psychosocial treatments for schizophrenia. *Psychiatry, 56,* 238–249.

Liberman, R.P., Mueser, K.T., & Wallace, C.J. (1986). Social-skills training for schizophrenic individuals at risk for relapse. *American Journal of Psychiatry, 143,* 523–526.

Marder, R., Wirshing, W.G., Mintz, J., McKenzie, J., Johnston, K., Eckman, T.A., Lebell, M., Zimmerman, K., & Liberman, R.P. (1996). Two-year outcome of social skills training and group psychotherapy for outpatients with schizophrenia. *American Journal of Psychiatry, 153,* 1585–1592.

May, P.R. (1968). *Treatment of schizophrenia: A comparative study of five treatment methods.* New York: Science House.

McFarlane, W.R., Lukens, E., Link, B., Dushay, R., Deakins, S.A., Newmark, M., Dunne, E.J., Horen, B., & Toran, J. (1995). Multiple-family groups and psychoeducation in the treatment of schizophrenia. *Archives of General Psychiatry, 52,* 679–687.

McGill, C.W., Falloon, I.R.H., Boyd, J.L., & Wood-Siverio, C. (1983). Family educational intervention in the treatment of schizophrenia. *Hospital and Community Psychiatry, 34,* 934–938.

McGlashan, T.H. (1983). Intensive individual psychotherapy of schizophrenia. *Archives of General Psychiatry, 40,* 909–920.

Metz, J.T., Johnson, M.D., Pliskin, N.H., & Luchins, D.J. (1994). Maintenance of training effects on the Wisconsin Card Sorting Test by patients with schizophrenia or affective disorders. *American Journal of Psychiatry, 151,* 120–122.

Modell, A.H. (1976). 'The holding environment' and the therapeutic action of psychoanalysis. *Journal of the American Psychoanalytic Association, 24,* 285–308.

Mosher, L.R., & Burti, L. (1992). Relationship in rehabilitation: When technology fails. *Psychosocial Rehabilitation Journal, 15,* 11–17.

Mueser, K., & Berenbaum, H. (1990). Psychodynamic treatment of schizophrenia: Is there a future? *Psychological Medicine, 20,* 253–262.

Mueser, K.T., & Bellack, A.S. (1995). Psychotherapy for schizophrenia. In S.R. Hirsch & D.R. Weinberger (Eds.). *Schizophrenia* (pp. 626–648). London: Blackwell.

Munetz, M.R., Birnbaum, A., & Wyzik, P.F. (1993). An integrative ideology to guide community-based multidisciplinary care of severely mentally ill patients. *Hospital and Community Psychiatry, 44,* 551–555.

Penn, D.L., & Mueser, K.T. (1996). Research update on the psychosocial treatment of schizophrenia. *American Journal of Psychiatry, 153,* 607–617.

Perris, C., Skagerlind, L. (1994). Cognitive therapy with schizophrenic patients. *ACTA Psychiatrica Scandinavica, 89* (Suppl., 382), 65–70.

Pollack, W.S. (1989). Schizophrenia and the self: Contributions of psychoanalytic self-psychology. *Schizophrenia Bulletin, 15,* 311–322.

Rogers, C.R., Gendlin, E.G., Kiesler, D.J., & Truax, C.B. (Eds.). (1967). *The therapeutic relationship and its impact: study of psychotherapy with schizophrenics.* Madison: University of Wisconsin Press.

Rothbard, A.B., Schinnar, A.P., & Goldman, H. (1996). The pursuit of a definition for severe and persistent mental illness. In S. Soreff (Ed.), *Handbook for the treatment of the seriously mentally ill.* Toronto: Hogrefe & Huber.

Santos, A.B. (1996). Assertive community treatment. In S. Soreff (Ed.), *Handbook for the treatment of the seriously mentally ill.* Toronto: Hogrefe & Huber.

Scholler, N.R., Keith, S.J., Sever, J.B., & Matthews, S.M. (1995). Maintenance treatment of schizophrenia: A review of dose reduction and family treatment strategies. *Psychiatric Quarterly, 66,* 279–292.

Schooler, N.R., Keith, S.J., Severe, J.B., Mathews, S.M., Bellack, A.S., Glick, I.D., Hargreaves, W.A., Kane, J.M., Ninan, P.T., Frances, A., Jacobs, M., Lieberman, J.A., Mance, R., Simpson, G.M., & Woerner, M.G. (1997). Relapse and rehospitalization during maintenance treatment of schizophrenia: The effects of dose reduction and family treatment. *Archives of General Psychiatry, 54,* 453–463.

Selzer, M. (1983). Preparing the chronic schizophrenic for exploratory psychotherapy: The role of hospitalization. *Psychiatry, 46,* 303–311.

Smith, J., & Birchwood, M.J. (1987). Specific and non-specific effects of educational intervention with families living with schizophrenic relatives. *British Journal of Psychiatry, 150,* 645–652.

Stratta, P., Mancinia F., Mattei P., Casacchia, M., & Rossi, A. (1994). Information processing strategy to remediate Wisconsin Card Sorting Test performance in schizophrenia: A pilot study. *American Journal of Psychiatry, 151,* 915–918.

Sullivan, H.S. (1962). *Schizophrenia as a human process.* New York: Norton.

Tarrier, N., Barrowclough, C., Vaughn, C., Bamrah, J., Porceddu, K., Watts, S., & Freeman, H. (1989). Community management of schizophrenia: A two-year follow-up of a behavioral intervention with families. *British Journal of Psychiatry, 154,* 625–628.

Tarrier, N., Beckett, R., Harwood, S., Baker, A., Yusopoff, L., & Ugareburu, I. (1993). A trial of two cognitive-behavioural methods of treating drug-resistant residual psychotic symptoms in schizophrenic patients, I: Outcome. *British Journal of Psychiatry, 162,* 524–532.

Tarrier, N., Harwood, S., Yusopoff, L., Beckett, R., Baker, A. (1990). Coping strategy enhancement (CSE): A method of treating residual schizophrenic symptoms. *Behavioural Psychotherapy, 18,* 283–293.

Vollema, M.G., Geurtsen, G.J., & van Voorst, A.J.P. (1995). Durable improvements in Wisconsin Card Sorting Test performance in schizophrenic patients. *Schizophrenia Research, 16,* 209–215.

Wasylenki, D.A. (1992). Psychotherapy of schizophrenia revisited. *Hospital and Community Psychiatry, 43,* 123–127.

Weiden, P., & Havens, L. (1994). Psychotherapeutic management techniques in the treatment of outpatients with schizophrenia. *Hospital and Community Psychiatry, 45,* 549–556.

Young, D.A., & Freyslinger, M.G. (1995). Scaffolded instruction and the remediation of Wisconsin Card Sorting Test deficits in chronic schizophrenia. *Schizophrenia Research, 16,* 199–207.

Zubin, J., & Spring, B. (1977). Vulnerability: A new view of schizophrenia. *Journal of Abnormal Psychology, 86,* 103–126.

13. Standards and Guidelines for Psychotherapy Training

Paul Cameron, Molyn Leszcz, Carolyn Rideout, and Martha Wright

Currently standards for psychotherapy training vary considerably among different training centres. This chapter reviews the challenges faced by training programs and proposes a strategy for meeting them. The strategy includes guidelines for: selection and training of supervisors; creation of effective clinical and training structures; curriculum development, including objectives for general psychiatrists and for psychiatrists specializing in psychotherapy; evaluation of trainees; and continuing education. The chapter contains an afterword on personal qualities of medical psychotherapists.

This chapter is not intended as the final word on psychotherapy training. Rather, it is intended to stimulate debate and collaboration between academic course directors and, through this, to improve psychotherapy training and raise its profile within the specialty and the community.

Current Context and General Principles

Although there is current debate about the proper domain, role, and functions of a psychiatrist, every official body examining these questions has emphasized that skills in psychotherapies are considered essential in the repertoire of a competent psychiatrist. This position has been articulated by many of the leading psychiatric associations in the world, including those in the United States (American Psychiatric Association, 1995), Britain (Royal College of Psychiatrists, United Kingdom, 1993), Germany (Hohagen & Berger, 1994), and Canada (Joint Task Force on Standards for Medical [Psychiatric] Psychotherapy, 1995).

The Canadian Psychiatric Association (Katz, 1986) approved a position paper just over a decade ago which stated: 'A psychiatrist must be competent in both psychotherapy and pharmacotherapy' (p. 455). That paper argued for a new research paradigm. This volume summarizes the empirical data in the literature for many of the specific psychotherapies. These data indicate that the psychotherapies have been extensively studied and are definitely effective and useful.

CURRENT POLICIES FOR EDUCATION IN THE PSYCHOTHERAPIES

A survey of Canadian psychiatry program directors (Cameron, 1993) indicated the need for two crucial programs: first, the development of minimum requirements and curriculum for general psychiatrists and for specialists in psychotherapy; second, the development of proper supervisor training, selection, and qualifications. The Royal College of Physicians and Surgeons of Canada (1993) defines very limited expectations regarding psychotherapy. The College's main recommendation is: 'at least two years of one hour per week supervision in short-term and long-term psychotherapy, which may include psychotherapy with children and adolescents as well as adults, is mandatory' (p. 2). The College's training requirements for residents also note that general objectives include 'an opportunity for further development of skills required in making effective relationships with patients'; the acquisition of knowledge of 'the psychotherapies, including behaviour therapy'; and the acquisition of clinical skills of 'competence of both long- and short-term psychotherapy' (p. 2). No provision is made for group therapy, family and marital therapy, interpersonal therapy, and cognitive therapy. These requirements translate into 6 per cent of a resident's time spent in a two-year period, or as little as 3 per cent or less of the total residency time in a four- or five-year residency program, based upon a fifty-hour work week.

A more careful and thorough set of objectives and guidelines was recently developed by the Coordinators of Postgraduate Education in Psychiatry (COPE, 1995). These guidelines describe psychotherapy training as providing a core set of skills central to the psychiatrist's identity. Training includes the imparting of knowledge, skills, attitudes and values, and enabling objectives to promote psychotherapeutic competence. Although training in individual psychodynamic psychotherapy provides a base for training in all other forms of therapy, it is not considered sufficient training in itself for the theoretical and technical aspects of the range of contemporary therapies. These require a particular knowledge base and training opportunity. Enabling objectives include: didactic seminars; observed initial interviews; participation in single and continuous case conferences for broad exposure to different therapist orientations and styles; at least two years of weekly long-term psychotherapy with weekly supervision; and two years of less-intensive, brief therapy with a range of patient types and ages. Family, couple, or group therapy, also with a range of patients, may substitute for some of these clinical requirements.

In the United States, the Association of Academic Psychiatry (AAP) and the American Association of Directors of Psychiatric Residency Training (AADPRT) (Mohl et al, 1990) have both concluded that psychiatrists of the future must be 'deeply and effectively psychodynamically informed and have the opportunity to become psychotherapeutically competent' (p. 13). They add: 'Psychotherapy in which the goal is to explore, understand and alter the inner experience of another human being, is not only the best way, but perhaps the only way to learn and consolidate various core concepts and experiences' (p. 8). They note that intensive dynamic psychotherapy may play less of a role in the future psychiatrist's practice than it has in the past. Nevertheless, they emphasize the importance of psychiatrists' continued ability to understand the full nature of the complexity of the doctor/patient relationship, including the therapist's contribution to the dynamics of the professional relationship in the form of his or her personality and countertransference.

Educators frequently comment about the central importance of the recognition and management of countertransference (Mohl, Sadler, & Miller, 1994), reflecting the potential damage that can arise not only from boundary violations, but also from unexamined and unwitting negative complementary responses to patients and hostile therapeutic reactions (Strupp, 1993). Strupp notes further that, even in structured and manual-based therapies, the therapist's capacity to create an interpersonal context that encourages patient openness and learning is of the greatest importance.

The AAP/AADPRT Task Force suggests a clear rationale for the continued important role of teaching psychotherapy in residency training. They list a number of relevant factors: psychotherapy is an effective treatment for many psychiatric disorders; the practice of psychodynamic psychotherapy provides a unique opportunity for professional growth; competence in the therapy modalities is required for effective administrative management of other practitioners in organizational settings; psychotherapy teaching is the best language for understanding the doctor/patient relationship and mutual contributions to illness and health care; it enhances learning about other dyadic processes such as supervision and administration; it deepens the psychiatrist's understanding about unconscious process as it relates to interviewing, thereby increasing his or her access to relevant materials from patients to aid in diagnosis and treatment; it is a model for learning about ethical concerns and boundary maintenance in psychiatric care; and, finally, it aids in the development of robustness in the understanding of human behaviour in its complexities.

In the United Kingdom, the Royal College of Psychiatrists (1993) has developed a similar process of review and issued a statement from the general psychiatry section, and from the psychotherapy section, articulating psychotherapy training guidelines. They, too, emphasize the need for rigorous psychotherapy training and understanding of the doctor/patient relationship, in order to be able to intervene in a rational and effective psychotherapeutic fashion. They recognize the danger of devaluing the need for rigorous training in the psychotherapies. The British standards appear to be more rigorous and include emphasis on the broad range of the psychotherapies, including family, group therapy, and cognitive/behavioural therapy. To illustrate, in their objectives for the first year of postgraduate training they emphasize: the acquisition of core skills to facilitate the establishment of general rapport and engagement of patients; interpersonal competence within the doctor–patient relationship with empathic awareness of patient distress; knowledge of one's communication style and the importance of non-verbal communication; the capacity to make a psychosocial formulation linking familial contributions to individual illness and health; understanding the conscious and unconscious processes governing personal and social interactions and personality development; understanding concepts of the therapeutic alliance and how to enhance it; understanding countertransference, ethical practice, and boundary maintenance. Later objectives include: the enhanced ability to practise and understand the theory of each modality; knowing the indications and limitations of each modality; and how to supervise co-professionals in psychotherapy, with particular attention paid to team building and organizational dynamics.

They recommend minimum mandatory core training of: one long-term dynamic case; one long-term cognitive behavioural therapy case; two brief dynamic cases; and two brief cognitive behavioural therapy cases. As well, they recommend: some experience in group therapy in either an inpatient or an outpatient setting. Experience in family and marital therapy includes but is not limited to child and adolescent psychiatry, and can potentially be obtained from other patient-related areas in general psychiatry. They also advocate the use of a logbook in order to note clearly the actual patient contact trainees have. In addition to emphasizing the role of supervision and teaching, the Royal College of Psychiatrists report also makes a special notation regarding the role of occupational stress. They recommend that trainees participate in continuous case conferences, seminars, and group supervision where possible, in order to provide both intellectual and emotional support for their difficult work. Both this report and the AAP/AADPRT Task Force report infer that there is a value in personal therapy for trainees, but do not advocate it directly.

In the United Kingdom, Crisp (1992) attempted to define adequate training in his report for the Psychiatric Sub-Committee of the Regional Postgraduate Medical Committee. That report elaborates particular time commitments required and specifies the number of patients to be seen. Crisp's report recommends the following: two patients in one-to-one psychotherapy; three supportive-psychotherapy cases; group exposure in an outpatient or milieu setting with an opportunity for co-leadership; specialty days in the psychotherapies that may include experiential training and crisis-intervention psychotherapy as part of the general psychiatry training. Crisp's committee recommendations are also based upon a fifty-hour work week, and propose that, at the junior level of training, approximately 5 per cent of the residents' time be spent learning dynamic psychotherapy, and 3 per cent learning behavioural psychotherapy, and, at the senior-resident level, 8 per cent and 7 per cent, respectively. Here, too, the total is a range of 8 to 15 per cent, increasing in senior years of training.

It is noteworthy that the Royal College of Psychiatrists has tried to strengthen these recommendations by concluding their report with the restatement of the central role of psychotherapeutic skills in general psychiatric practice, as allied with, and not antagonistic to, other approaches. Psychotherapy is a part of general psychiatry and needs to be taught *both* by specialists in psychotherapy and by general psychiatrists. They also advocate site-approval visits by the College to evaluate the successful achievement of this due rigour, along with greater attention paid to psychotherapeutic issues on the specialty examinations.

In Germany, a similar development occurred in 1992, when the German Council of Physicians revamped psychiatry training to include, for the first time, the central and indispensable role of training in psychodynamic psychotherapy and cognitive/behavioural therapy (Hohagen & Berger, 1994).

In summary, a great deal of activity around the world has identified the need to improve psychotherapy training by articulating and codifying clear standards regarding educational and enabling objectives.

THE ROLE OF PSYCHIATRY

How do the psychotherapies fit with the role of psychiatry in medicine? As outlined in chapter 1, 'The Definition of Psychotherapy,' psychiatry is a medical specialty that is grounded in both biological and psychological knowledge about human nature and development. North American psychiatrists generally endorse a 'biopsychosocial model' that recognizes the interplay of biological, psychological, and social factors in the development of psychiatric disorders and in their treatment.

In order to continue supporting medical (psychiatric) psychotherapy within the health care system, psychiatrists must receive a detailed education in the complex interaction among mind, brain, and body. They need to be aware of the way that medical disorders, developmental and physical changes, and bodily states influence the mind, and how the mind influences the body. The literature demonstrates that combined use of medications and psychotherapy is frequently the most appropriate and effective treatment for a number of disorders in many individual patients (see chapter 11, 'Guidelines for Combining Pharmacotherapy with Psychotherapy'). Because psychiatrists have been trained to care for very ill patients; to manage patients with a wide range of mental disorders; and to use biological treatments, such as electroconvulsive therapy and pharmacological agents, they are best suited for providing treatment that combines pharmacotherapy and psychotherapy.

Psychiatrists have a special role within the field of medicine as the interpreters of social and psychological phenomena for their colleagues and their patients. Psychiatry is the only specialty that can act as a specific reference point for the practice of medical psychotherapy.

For the last several years, the Chief Examiner in Psychiatry of the Royal College of Physicians and Surgeons of Canada, and other examiners in this country, have expressed the view that candidates lack expertise in empathic interviewing and in understanding the meaning for and impact of psychiatric symptoms and disorders on both patients and their families (RCPSC annual report for 1996). In a report to the University of Toronto Department of Psychiatry, Leszcz (1994) pointed out that 'examiners of the Royal College expect candidates to demonstrate their psychotherapeutic skills in the examination.' He confirms that examiners find that 'candidates are often apprehensive about engaging in psychosocial inquiry for fear that it will interfere with the DSM-IV interview.' Leszcz goes on to suggest that 'candidates often fail to focus on the individual and employ a rigid, concrete approach to the interview' (p. 3).

In Britain, the Report of Examiners (RCP 1985) stated that poor formulation was the major reason why candidates failed to obtain specialty qualifications. In North America, Leon Eisenberg (1986) and Z.J. Lipowski (1989) have lamented reductionism and polarization in psychiatry. Eisenberg declared that psychiatry had changed from being 'brainless to being mindless.' Lipowski added that psychiatry could be 'both brainless and mindless.' He concluded that an excessive attempt to reduce complexity is false and unhelpful.

The central role of psychotherapy in the practice of contemporary psychiatry has also been articulated in a strong and clear fashion by the American Psychiatric Association in its recent 'Position Statement on Medical Psychotherapy' (1995).

SURVEYS OF TRAINING IN PSYCHOTHERAPY IN
THE EARLY 1990S IN CANADA

Cameron (1993) surveyed all sixteen program directors in Canada, with 100 per cent response. He found that the types of supervision most commonly utilized are one-to-one (process notes) and discussion with a group of residents. There is little opportunity for residents to be observed or to observe others doing psychotherapy.

A survey of residents conducted by Dr S. Tourjman (1988) at McGill University identified a number of needs, including: better assessment and screening of patients; a graduated competence model of training which recognizes the different needs of junior and senior residents; introductory and advanced seminars with clearly defined learning objectives according to an overall conceptual model; and standards for supervisors.

A Proposed Strategy for Psychotherapy Training

Seven strategies are suggested for improving psychotherapy training:

1 Supervisor selection should be based on qualifications and experience. Supervisors should have had formal training in a psychotherapeutic modality. They must actively practise this form of psychotherapy.

2 A 'pool of supervisors' should be developed to provide ongoing stimulus for the critical evaluation of teaching methods.

3 Clinical research and training programs should be developed, if possible in locations where residents can come in contact with skilled supervisors and selected patients. This allows learning experience in psychotherapy to occur in a step-wise, graduated manner – according to residents' abilities.

4 Curriculum development should include learning objectives established by small groups with competence in specific types of psychotherapy. These objectives must be arranged in sequence according to the level of training and skill of residents.

5 Residents and supervisors should be encouraged to do research and write conceptual papers. Residents often complain that their psychotherapy education is too 'laissez-faire,' seems unrelated to modern psychiatric literature, and includes extremely naïve views about what has been written or achieved in psychotherapy. Supervisors must show an interest in and an ability to keep up with the literature and should make active contributions in order to merit the privilege of supervising residents.

6 An evaluation mechanism must be established, as many program directors are dissatisfied with current methods of evaluating psychotherapy training and of assessing skills acquisition by both residents and supervisors.

7 There should be better collaboration and greater concurrence of training programs with the formation of a 'community' of faculty members devoted to psychotherapy training, to help improve standards of training.

At recent meetings of the Canadian Psychiatric Association, discussions centred on the need to integrate psychotherapy with clinical services, as well as the need for more research, with an emphasis on empirically based therapies (Cameron, Truant, Book, Weerasekera, & Leverette, 1994). The integration of psychotherapy with medical or biological treatments would appear to be a key feature of good psychiatry training programs.

The University of Toronto program (Leszcz, 1994) has prioritized this approach. The policy is as follows:

Ideally, the integrative approach should be the overriding stance of the Department of Psychiatry and the Psychotherapy Program. Theoretically broad understanding of patients and an integrative approach to treatment should be taught and practiced in all clinical teaching settings. This would not preclude training in the individual treatment modalities, rather it requires it as a prerequisite to competent integrated practice. Integration is best considered not so much a specific modality of treatment, but rather an overall stance towards the psychotherapies, their relationship to each other, and their relationship to other modalities of treatment. Putting this into practice requires appropriate attitudes, knowledge of and competence with various therapeutic modalities, as well as theoretical knowledge and clinical skills specific to the task of integration. (p. 1)

SELECTION AND TRAINING OF SUPERVISORS

How should faculty members who supervise residents in psychotherapy be selected? The specialty has reached a position where practitioners must be much more critical about who supervises psychotherapy residents. Training programs need to develop a job description for supervisors in each modality. Cameron (1993) suggests that supervisors should demonstrate:

1 a good working knowledge of current psychiatric literature;
2 adequate training in special therapeutic techniques;
3 the capacity to teach;
4 that they spend a major part of their workday doing psychotherapy;
5 a willingness to attend workshops and to persevere with continuing education and professional development;
6 tolerance towards other viewpoints and the efficacy of therapeutic modalities other than those that they themselves practise.

Supervisor workshops for psychotherapy (Cameron et al, 1994; Frayn, 1991) have been successfully run in Toronto, Edmonton, Hamilton, Ottawa, and Montreal. These workshops were particularly effective in training beginning supervisors. Ideally, faculty members should not start to supervise until they have attained some expertise in supervision. A key group of supervisors, developed in certain centres, can provide a forum for colleagues and peers to examine psychotherapy teaching methods critically.

CREATION OF EFFECTIVE CLINICAL AND TRAINING STRUCTURES

In most subspecialties of psychiatry, there are certain key centres where major psychiatrists attract others who wish to acquire a particular sphere of psychiatric competence. This holds true for child psychiatry, geriatric psychiatry, psychosomatic medicine, psychopharmacology, and forensic psychiatry. However, many have a false perception of psychotherapy, believing that 'everybody does it and anyone can.'

The most effective stimulus for creating well-trained psychotherapists occurs in training centres that contain a core group or critical minimum number of interested experts who collaborate in the same location, as with David Malan's (1976) 'Brief Psychotherapy Workshop' at the Tavistock clinic, Davanloo's (1980) group at the Montreal General Hospital, Sifneos's (1979) group in Boston, and the groups of Bergin (Bergin & Garfield, 1994) in New York, Strupp (1993) in Tennessee, Horowitz (1988) in California, and Luborsky (1984) in Philadelphia.

Many psychotherapists are involved in highly time-intensive work and may resist collaboration or working in groups. This isolationism has hindered the establishment of standards, and often detracted from the profile of psychotherapy. For example, Garfinkel (1992) recently pointed out that research in psychotherapy is underrepresented compared with other areas of medicine.

CURRICULUM DEVELOPMENT

What are the minimum clinical skills a psychiatrist needs in various forms of psychotherapy? What skills should a competent psychiatrist be expected to master at a basic level, or at an advanced level? There is general agreement that the following basic skills are necessary for all psychiatrists:

1 the ability to interview in an empathic manner
2 the capacity to interview using an organized protocol for assessment
3 the ability to complete a formulation according to a variety of methods (Kline and Cameron, 1978; Cameron, Kline, Korenblum, Selzer, & Small, 1978; Cleghorn et al 1983; McDougall & Reade, 1993; Weerasekera, 1993; Fleming & Patterson, 1993; Perry, Cooper, & Michels, 1987;

Perry et al, 1989). This includes a differential and provisional diagnosis, a treatment plan, and a prognosis.

4 an understanding of the principles of supportive psychotherapy

FORMATS OF TEACHING

A mixture of teaching formats is most effective. This includes limited lectures, seminars, continuous case conferences, and journal clubs. Observation of supervision of senior residents by junior residents is a useful format (Robb & Cameron, 1958).

The University of Toronto recently adopted more rigorous minimum requirements (Leszcz, 1994). The minimum core recommendations are as follows: residents would have, at a minimum, three ongoing treatments. For two years, this consists of two long-term treatments and one short-term treatment with ongoing weekly supervision. At least one long-term case should be carried through to supervised termination, in the course of residency training. In two other years of training, one of the long-term treatments should be devoted to acquiring advanced training in group, couple, or family therapy, that is, a multiperson treatment. Similarly, in two other years of training, the time-limited treatment should encompass either cognitive behavioural therapy or interpersonal therapy, and the resident should gain competence in a manual-based treatment over this period. Seminars, continuous case conferences, and observation would account for another one to two hours a week. Residents will graduate with proficiency in long-term dynamic therapy, short-term dynamic therapy, one manual-based therapy, and one multiperson modality, with basic knowledge in the other areas. The percentage of clinical time and supervision required to achieve this is between 14 and 16 per cent of a typical fifty-hour week.

A more detailed list of terminal objectives or exit criteria for competence in psychotherapy necessary for all psychiatrists, or at least all *general* psychiatrists, might be as follows:

1 to be competent in assessing patients as candidates for psychotherapy or psychosocial intervention, either as the treatment of choice or as adjunctive treatment

2 to know the indications, contraindications, benefits, and limitations of various psychotherapies for all *DSM-IV* (APA, 1994) diagnostic categories

3 to know how to combine different therapeutic modalities and be conversant with current ideas about combined effects

4 to know about methods of continuing education in various psychotherapies and psychosocial rehabilitation

5 to know when to refer a patient for a second opinion or to a subspecialist

6 to recognize countertransference

7 to be able to conduct individual psychodynamic psychotherapy – a basic skill that differentiates psychiatrists from other health professionals

8 to know how to conduct a marital and family therapy assessment

9 to know how to assess a patient for behavioural and cognitive psychotherapy in order to suggest an appropriate referral

In developing a curriculum, two basic problems must be addressed: reduced time devoted to didactic lectures, and increasingly less time available for clinical rotation. There is also the abstract problem of choosing the theoretical models for teaching residents. *Here, there is no agreement.* The decision depends on the prejudices and training of the faculty. However, psychiatry can and must develop an objective curriculum for teaching residents the effects of various psychiatric modalities on specific populations. Also, psychotherapy must be recognized as part of the treatment of all patients.

Within each theoretical model, training should expose residents to current research and emphasize the homogeneity of populations. Key clinical skills must be identified within each modality and tied to the theoretical material. One of the issues that concerns program directors is the way that clinical teaching relates theory and empirical data in the current literature.

The total amount of time that residents in Canada devote to psychotherapy, according to Royal College requirements, is estimated to be 3 to 6 per cent (Leszcz, 1994). The recommended time in Britain is 10 to 15 per cent, and, in the United States, 8 to 12.

ADVANCED TRAINING

More intensive training programs should be available for residents who wish to take up careers as specialized psychotherapists or as teachers/researchers in psychotherapy. A few programs in Canada are developing learning objectives for these courses. A subspecialist in psychotherapy should meet the following learning objectives

1 familiarity with the historical and current literature in at least one or more modalities
2 a chosen method for conducting psychotherapy
3 familiarity with the current research in one or more modalities
4 the ability to teach psychotherapy to residents
5 thorough competence in assessing and treating suitable patients in at least one or more modalities

Objectives can be further categorized as knowledge objectives, skill objectives, and attitudinal objectives. Some recommended objectives for consideration are summarized below.

Knowledge Objectives

A subspecialist in psychotherapy should have knowledge of:

1 selection criteria for: individual psychodynamic psychotherapy; couple and family psychotherapy; and behavioural, cognitive, group, and interpersonal psychotherapy;
2 the contraindications for these modalities;
3 medico-legal issues about selecting therapies for certain patients;
4 expected outcomes of psychotherapy;
5 conceptual issues in research methodology and psychotherapy research: (a) outcome; (b) therapist variables; (c) patient variables; (d) process;
6 common concepts in technique, resistance, defences;
7 termination;
8 countertransference;
9 ethics in psychotherapy;
10 psychotherapy modification and outcome for all syndromes in *DSM-IV*;
11 theories of personality development;
12 attachment theory;
13 three major streams of psychoanalytic theory: drive–defence, object relations, and self-psychology;
14 therapeutic alliance – concepts and data;

15 issues that are important in understanding the transcultural approach to psychotherapy;
16 perspectives from sociology, including sociocultural influences on personality development;
17 the current literature regarding gender issues and differences;
18 boundary violations and the current laws (Epstein, 1994).

Skill Objectives

A subspecialist in psychotherapy should have the ability to:

1 assess all patients from a comprehensive perspective – biological, psychological, interpersonal, and social;
2 to prescribe therapy;
3 complete a formulation and revise it;
4 conduct psychodynamic psychotherapy;
5 assess and/or treat: couples, family, groups, and candidates for behavioural and/or cognitive therapy;
6 recognize his or her own contribution to: therapeutic alliance, therapeutic impasse, and process of therapy;
7 know when to seek consultation;
8 assist the development of other people's skills;
9 continue his or her own education;
10 debate the empirical evidence for effectiveness of psychotherapy;
11 develop the capacity for: empathic listening, empathic inquiry, and empathic interventions that are 'experience near';
12 maintain the correct boundary between therapist and patient, and never to abuse patients sexually. As part of the essential process of avoiding boundary violations, students must learn how to deal with their own emotional and sexual feelings that might surface during therapy. They need encouragement to talk with supervisors and colleagues in order to increase the self-awareness that will help to prevent them from acting out such impulses in treatment. They must understand the limits of self-disclosure and extra-therapeutic contact (Leszcz, 1994).
13 understand how to maintain the frame of psychotherapy;
14 use literature from other basic and social sciences, such as sociology, psychology, anthropology, and transcultural psychiatry, to increase his or her understanding of patients.

Attitudinal Objectives

A subspecialist in psychotherapy should be willing to:

1 create a positive understanding of all the factors that influence patients' quality of life: biological, psychological, and social;
2 minimize polarization, prejudice, and bias concerning other 'schools of psychiatry,' i.e., have an open theoretical orientation;
3 maintain an open mind about the prognosis or outlook for many patients;
4 develop an appreciation of the healthy ego function of patients;
5 be aware of the patient's interaction with his or her family, and vice versa;
6 be aware of the different meanings that medical illness can have for different patients;
7 develop a non-judgmental therapeutic attitude;
8 develop clinical distance as a means of avoiding blurred boundaries with patients, prohibit any sexual involvement with patients, and recognize the specific demands of maintaining a therapeutic posture;
9 understand countertransference;
10 appreciate the importance of the therapist–patient fit;
11 appreciate his or her own limitations;
12 be aware of omnipotence and pathological altruism in him- or herself;
13 understand his or her own attitudes towards same- and opposite-sex patients;
14 recognize the interaction between patients and their sociocultural or ethnic group.

Evaluation of Trainees

To be useful, evaluation must be tied to valid, reliable learning objectives and clinical skills. It is crucial to establish teaching methods and achieve consensus about objectives before becoming preoccupied with detailed evaluation forms. Nonetheless, a powerful effect can be achieved by taking evaluations seriously. Provision of ongoing feedback needs to be encouraged (Cameron, 1994; Sakinofsky, 1979; Cameron et al, 1994). Logs of experience, and a formal curriculum of literature, together with requirements to write formulations and present cases, are helpful. A collaborative relationship which provides clear expectations to the resident is important.

The Use of Manuals in Psychotherapy Training

Manuals have been developed in cognitive behavioural therapy, interpersonal psychotherapy, and psychodynamic psychotherapy. The advantage of using a manual is to provide consistent therapist behaviour in research trials that can be checked to validate the psychotherapeutic intervention. Therapists doing therapy according to certain predictable and structured protocols is termed 'adherence.'

Some authors believe that the use of manuals will improve skill acquisition for beginning therapists. However, certain studies point out that increased utilization of psychotherapy manuals offers mixed benefits and disadvantages. Henry, Strupp, Butler, Schacht, and Binder (1993) point out that increased utilization of psychotherapy manuals can demonstrate that therapists behaviours do change. In their study, therapists using a time-limited psychodynamic psychotherapy manual increased the following behaviours: expression of in-session affect, exploration of the therapeutic relationship, an improved participant–observer stance, and use of open-ended questions. However, there was an unexpected deterioration in certain interpersonal and interactional aspects of therapy. Henry, Strupp, et al (1993) showed that, after training, therapists were almost twice as active, and they more frequently introduced a message which was rated as complex and contained an embedded criticism of the patient. This study also demonstrated that therapists used an increased number of messages that were rated as 'hostile.' The authors further state that manualized training results in therapists being judged to be less optimistic and less supportive of the patients' confidence, to spend less time evaluating patients' feelings, and to behave in a more authoritarian manner.

Henry, Schacht, Strupp, Butler, and Binder (1993) argue that treatment manuals have value, but it is unwise to assume only they provide benefit. In this study, the investigators used a one-year manualized training program for time-limited psychodynamic psychotherapy. They discovered that some therapists changed their interventions in line with the treatment manual, but also that there were anticipated changes that ran counter to the intent of training. These changes included increased negative interpersonal transactions between therapists and patients.

Strupp et al (1993b) suggested that extensive previous supervision of a therapist caused him or her to be more resistant to learning manual-guided therapies. He also concluded that researchers and educators should take seriously the proposition that therapists are not inter-changeable units who deliver a standard treatment. Safran (1993) pointed out that Luborsky has demonstrated, in all studies that he reviewed, that the contribution to the outcome of therapy by the indi-vidual therapist overshadows treatment-modality effects. This means that individual therapists have characteristics and behaviours that affect outcome and that manualized training cannot necessarily be used indis-criminantly across large groups of therapists to produce improved out-come. Spontaneity and empathic attunement to moment-to-moment needs of patients can be undermined by the use of treatment manuals.

Continuing Education

A strategy for continuing education for faculty and for the community within which the program is situated is essential. Psychiatrists need to continue their development in psychotherapy after their basic training. This includes reading journals, attending workshops, and participating in peer supervision.

Increasingly, the medical fraternity promotes the idea that doctors need to understand concepts from psychology, sociology, and anthro-pology as well as from traditional medical and psychiatric literature. This broadened approach, plus continuing education, should help psy-chiatrists work in multidisciplinary teams and value the contribution of other health professions.

Afterword: Personal Qualities of Medical Psychotherapists

The practice of psychiatry is under increasing pressure to evaluate the outcome of psychotherapy and the competence of psychotherapists. Personal qualities of psychotherapists are an important component to consider in establishing standards. There has been considerable agree-ment on the qualities of the good psychotherapist. There also seems to be some consensus that the psychotherapist's personality has a consid-erable impact in facilitating a favourable outcome.

Rogers (1957) defined the conditions in the psychotherapist that were considered essential for a positive outcome: 'The therapist should be without major conflict so that he be free to interact genuinely with the patient in order to convey successfully his feelings of respect, unconditional positive regard, and empathic understanding of his predicament' (p. 96).

Several other authors, including Frank (1973) almost twenty years later, agree that the success of the psychotherapist depends in part on a genuine concern for the patient's welfare. Other groups and authors are critical of the values of warmth, empathy, and genuineness. They feel that the ratings of these qualities have not correlated consistently with the outcomes of treatment (Bergin & Jasper, 1969; Kurtz & Grummon, 1972). There are some equally convincing publications that support the view that high levels of empathy, warmth, and genuineness are associated with good outcomes, and that accurate empathy can be reliably rated.

Knobel (1990) describes the significance and importance of personality and experience in the psychotherapist. He stresses that psychotherapists must have unique traits in their dynamic organization. They must have authenticity and the freedom to think and act according to their own ideological principles, and they should possess the creative social ability to take pleasure in living and relating. Psychotherapists must also have the skill and the desire to help. They should have cognitive–affective insight, a therapeutic disposition, and appropriate therapeutic feeling. Knobel quotes Wolberg who described in 1977 the entire equipment that psychotherapists should have at their disposal: essentially, they need an educational equipment that must be formal and systematic and must follow a certain line of thought and theory; a personality equipment that includes sensitivity, objectivity, flexibility, and empathy, and a relative lack of serious emotional problems.

More recently, Aveline (1992) stressed additional qualities required by present-day therapists. Cultural sensitivity and knowledge are especially valuable. Recognizing and accepting the validity of cultural perspectives are crucial. Aveline also states that the essential personal qualities of respect, understanding, decency, tolerance, and self-knowledge must be enhanced through training in order to minimize the risk of patient abuse because of voyeuristic, sadistic, erotic, or power-seeking tendencies in the therapist.

Over the past decade, there has been a movement in medicine and in medical schools towards selecting candidates with a more well-rounded background, candidates who will put a more human face on the practice of medicine and who possess good interpersonal skills. This can be said to be doubly important in the selection of candidates for psychiatric training. Screening must, by and large, take place at the time of candidate selection for postgraduate training in psychiatry and, naturally, throughout the residency period. It should involve pre-acceptance references, candidate interviews, and ongoing evaluation during training. The candidate interview must comprise an in-depth assessment of the individual's psychological functioning and moral/ethical standards. An assessment of the candidate's acceptance of the need for strict adherence to the profession's ethical standards is also vital. The point of the selection process is not to find a perfect candidate – many psychotherapists are able to perform competently despite many vulnerabilities and difficulties – but rather to eliminate those whose psychopathology would interfere with their capacity to relate empathically and might impede strict adherence to the profession's ethical standards. Some candidates will be found unsuitable. For example, candidates with psychotic disorders, antisocial personalities, severe narcissistic disorders are generally unsuited to the practice of psychotherapy. In his work at the Menninger Clinic with psychotherapists who transgress sexual boundaries, Gabbard (1994) found that their psychopathology came under four categories, two of which (psychotic disorders, and psychopathology and paraphilias) fall under the *DSM-IV* classification system. The other two categories relate to the therapists' intrapsychic dynamics.

The acceptable candidate should demonstrate qualities of empathy and understanding, should have a genuine interest in people and their lives and problems, and must demonstrate an absence of major psychopathology and/or character traits inappropriate to the humane and ethical practice of medicine and psychiatry. Evidence of successful resolution of interpersonal/characterological difficulties and awareness of remaining psychological issues are desirable features for a prospective psychotherapist. Personal therapy may be necessary for prospective candidates to achieve sufficient self-awareness and to resolve ongoing difficulties. The American Group Psychotherapy Association (1991) has made group participation a requirement of training in the United States. It is also crucial that a therapist's life be sufficiently well anchored so that he or she does not seek inappropriate or undue gratification from the patients. As well, future psychiatrists/psychotherapists should demonstrate an appreciation for and willingness to develop clinical skills necessary for the competent practice of their specialty. In this era, all psychiatrists/psychotherapists must show an awareness and knowledge of, and sensitivity to, gender and cross-cultural issues. Every candidate should demonstrate a willingness and commitment to practise in an ethical and sensitive manner.

Another question to consider is whether the desirable personal qualities of psychiatrists/psychotherapists vary across different treatment
modalities and different schools of therapy. Although quite different
clinical skills may be required, it seems reasonable to set standards for
the personal qualities of future psychiatrists/psychotherapists regardless of clinical orientation.

In conclusion, there are well recognized and desirable personal qualities and characteristics to look for in anyone wishing to become a psychiatrist or a psychotherapist. Clinical skills can and must be taught,
and the art of psychotherapy can be learned, but all potential psychia-
trists/psychotherapists must possess a personality that has the disposition and potential to be therapeutic.

References

American Group Psychotherapy Association. (1991). *Guidelines for ethics*. New
York: Author.

American Psychiatric Association (APA). (1994). *Diagnostic and statistical manual
of mental disorders* (4th ed.). Washington, DC: Author.

American Psychiatric Association (APA). (1995). Position statement on medical
psychotherapy. *American Journal of Psychiatry, 152,* 11.

Aveline, M. (1992). Training in psychotherapy. *Current Opinion in Psychiatry, 5,*
365–369.

Bergin, A.E., & Garfield, S. (Eds.) (1994). *Handbook of psychotherapy and behavior
change* (4th ed.). New York: Wiley.

Bergin, A.E., & Jasper, L.G. (1969). Correlates of empathy in psychotherapy.
A replication. *Journal of Abnormal Psychology, 74,* 477.

Cameron, P.M. (1993). Psychotherapy training in Canada. *Bulletin of the Canadian
Psychiatric Association, 25,* 21–26.

Cameron, P.M. (1994). *Faculty development: A program to improve teaching of
psychotherapy.* Proceedings of the Sixth Ottawa Conference on Medical
Education.

Cameron, P.M., Kline, S., Korenblum, M., Seltzer, A., & Small, F. (1978). A
method of reporting formulation. *Canadian Psychiatric Association Journal, 23,*
43–50.

Cameron, P.M., Truant, G., Book, H., Weerasekera, P., & Leverette, J. (1994).
Developing Strong Psychotherapy Programs. Symposium at Canadian
Psychiatric Association Meeting, Ottawa.

Cleghorn, J.M., Bellisimo, A., & Will, D. (1983). Teaching some principles of individual psychodynamics through an introductory guide to formulations. *Canadian Psychiatric Association Journal, 28,* 162–172.

Coordinators of Postgraduate Education in Psychiatry (COPE). (1995). Guidelines for Training in Psychotherapy for Psychiatry Residents. (1995).

Crisp, A. (1992). Report of the Regional Postgraduate Medical Committee, United Kingdom.

Davanloo, H. (Ed.). (1980). *Short term dynamic psychotherapy.* New York: Jason Aronson.

Eisenberg, L. (1986). Mindlessness and brainlessness in psychiatry. *British Journal of Psychiatry, 148,* 497–508.

Epstein, R.S. (1994). *Keeping boundaries: Maintaining safety and integrity in the psychotherapeutic process.* Washington, DC: American Psychiatric Press.

Fleming, J.A.E., & Patterson, P.G.R. (1993). The teaching of case formulation in Canada. *Canadian Journal of Psychiatry, 38,* 345–350.

Frank, J. (1973). *Persuasion and healing: A comparative study of psychotherapy.* (Rev. ed). Baltimore: Johns Hopkins University Press.

Frayn, D. (1991). Supervising the supervisors: The evolution of a psychotherapy supervisors group. *American Journal of Psychotherapy 45,* 31–42.

Gabbard, G.O. (1994). Psychotherapists who transgress sexual boundaries with patients. *Bulletin of the Menninger Clinic, 58,* 124–135.

Garfinkel, P. (1992). [Report on Research]. Presented to Canadian Association of Professors of Psychiatry.

Henry W.P., Schacht, T.E., Strupp, H.H., Butler, S.F., & Binder, J.L. (1993). Effects of training in time-limited dynamic psychotherapy: Mediators of therapists' responses to training. *Journal of Consulting and Clinical Psychology, 61,* 441–447.

Henry, W.P., Strupp, H.H., Butler, S.F., Schacht, T.E., & Binder, J.L. (1993). Effects of training in time-limited dynamic psychotherapy: Changes in therapist behavior. *Journal of Consulting and Clinical Psychology, 61,* 434–440.

Hohagen, F., & Berger, M. (1994). The new German specialist for psychiatry and psychotherapy and its consequences for advanced training programs. *European Psychiatry, 9,* 265–271.

Horowitz, M. (1988). *Introduction to psychodynamics: A new synthesis.* New York: Basic.

Joint Task Force on Standards for Medical (Psychiatric) Psychotherapy. (1995). *A report to Council of the Ontario Psychiatric Association and to Executive of the Section of Psychiatry, Ontario Medical Association, on the definition, guidelines and standards for medical (psychiatric) psychotherapy.* Toronto: Author.

Katz, P. (1986). The role of the psychotherapists in the practice of psychiatry. *Canadian Psychiatric Association Journal, 31,* 455–465.

Kline, S., & Cameron, P.M. (1978). Formulation. *Canadian Psychiatry Association Journal, 23*, 39–42.

Knobel, M. (1990). Significance and importance of the psychotherapist's personality and experience. *Journal of Psychotherapy and Psychosomatics, 53*, 58–63.

Kurtz, R.R., & Grummon, D.L. (1972). Different approaches to the measurement of therapist empathy and their relationship to therapy outcomes. *Journal of Consulting and Clinical Psychology, 39*, 106–115.

Leszcz, M. (1994). *Standards for Psychotherapy Training Discussion Paper*, Department of Psychiatry, University of Toronto.

Lipowski, Z.J. (1989). Psychiatry mindless or brainless: Both or neither? *Canadian Psychiatric Association Journal, 34*, 249–254.

Luborsky, L. (1984). *Principles of psychoanalytic psychotherapy: A manual for supportive–expressive treatment.* New York: Basic.

Malan, D.H. (1976). *The frontier of brief psychotherapy.* New York: Plenum.

McDougall, G., & Reade, B. (1993). Teaching biopsychosocial integration and formulation. *Canadian Journal of Psychiatry, 38*, 359–362.

Mohl, P.C., Lomax, J., Tasman, A., Chan, C., Sledge, W., Summergrad, P., & Notman, A. (1990). Psychotherapy training for the psychiatrist of the future. *American Journal of Psychiatry, 147*, 7–13.

Mohl, P.C., Sadler, J.E., & Miller, D.A. (1994). What component should be evaluated in psychiatry residency? *Academic Psychiatry, 18*, 22–29.

Perry S., Cooper, A.M., & Michels, R. (1987). The psychodynamic formulation: Its purpose structure and clinical application. *American Journal of Psychiatry, 144*, 543–550.

Perry, J.C., Luborsky, L., Silberschatz, G. & Popp, (1989). An examination of three methods of psychodynamic formulation based on the same videotaped interview. *Psychiatry, 52*, 302–323.

Rogers, C. (1957). The necessary and sufficient conditions of therapeutic personality change. *Journal of Consulting and Clinical Psychology, 21*, 95–103.

Robb, M., & Cameron, P.M. (1998). Supervision of termination in psychotherapy: A model for teaching. *Canadian Journal of Psychiatry 43*, 397–402.

Royal College of Psychiatrists, United Kingdom (RCP). (1985). Report of Examiners. *Bulletin of Royal College U.K.*

Royal College of Psychiatrists, United Kingdom (RCP). (1993). *Guidelines for Psychotherapy Training as Part of General Professional Psychiatric Training.* London: Author.

Royal College of Physicians and Surgeons of Canada (RCPSC). (1993). *Report of the Examinations Board: Recommendations for Program Directors.* Toronto: Author.

Safran, J.D. (1993). Breaches in the therapeutic alliance: An arena for negotiating authentic relatedness. *Psychotherapy, 30*, 11–24.

Sakinofsky, I. (1979). Evaluating the competence of psychotherapists. *Canadian Journal of Psychiatry, 24,* 193–205.

Sifneos, P. (1979). *Short-term dynamic psychotherapy.* New York: Plenum

Strupp, H.H. (1993). The Vanderbilt psychotherapy studies synopsis. *Journal of Consulting and Clinical Psychology, 6,* 431–433.

Strupp, H., & Binder, J.L. (1984). *Psychotherapy in a new key.* New York: Basic.

Weerasekera, P. (1993). Formulation: A multiperspective model. *Canadian Journal of Psychiatry, 38,* 351–358.

Wolberg, L.R. (1977). *The techniques of psychotherapy.* (3d ed.). New York: Grune & Stratton.

14. Guidelines for Psychotherapy Supervision

Jon Ennis, Paul Cameron, Molyn Leszcz, and Leopoldo Chagoya

Psychotherapy supervision is generally regarded as the most powerful tool for teaching and learning psychotherapy, and constitutes the core of any psychotherapy training program. It is a crucial part of the education that facilitates development of the identity of the trainee as a psychotherapist. The process involves a number of intimate relationships, in which the supervisee reveals the work that he or she has done with patients in the privacy of the office. Supervision takes place in an individual or a group format. It may utilize process notes, audio- or videotape, direct observation, or a combination of these.

Guidelines for psychotherapy supervision will depend on the context of the supervisory process. Psychiatrists supervise trainees in a variety of disciplines and at various levels of training and licensure. Supervision can also take place outside of formal training programs. The major focus of this chapter is the supervision of psychiatric residents as part of their postgraduate training, but many aspects are applicable to supervision of therapists from other disciplines across a broad variety of settings.

These guidelines were developed through a selective review of the literature, incorporating a Medline search using the headings 'Psychotherapy/Education' and 'Psychoanalytic Therapy/Education,' from 1983 to 1995. A number of standard textbooks on psychoanalytic supervision were also consulted. The guidelines have been further augmented through a process of consultation and review by colleagues involved in psychotherapy supervision. Although this chapter focuses on supervision of psychodynamic psychotherapy, it also includes special considerations for the supervision of other modalities.

Role of the Supervisor

According to Searles (1965), the supervisor's usefulness comes from being at a greater psychological distance from the patient's psychopathology, leaving him or her 'relatively free from anxiety and able, therefore to think relatively freely and unconstrictedly' (p. 587). Greben, Markson, and Sadovoy (1973) stress that the general atmosphere should permit a free exchange of opinion between teacher and student, and that this can be enhanced by close informality.

Emphasizing the establishment of a teaching alliance as a precursor to dealing with countertransference issues, Book (1987) states that this 'requires the supervisor to approach the resident with seriousness, respect, tolerance of differences, and a genuine interest in nurturing the autonomous growth and development of that resident, rather than influencing him to become like that supervisor' (p. 556).

In discussing the role of identification with the supervisor, Greben (1991) comments on the development and growth of a professional identity as one of the most important requirements of training. The advantage of meeting with a variety of supervisors during training and experiencing their different attitudes is that this encourages residents to develop their own way of being with patients. He mentions the value of frankness on the part of the supervisor in appropriate discussions of his or her own work, and relevant personal experiences. Supervisors are often deliberately self-disclosing, telling personal anecdotes and discussing their own mistakes. Betcher and Zinburg (1988) caution supervisors to confine the range of personal exploration to issues directly related to the patient's treatment. The issues related to supervisor transparency parallel those of therapist transparency. Self-revelation must always be in the service of the treatment or teaching, not for self-aggrandizement.

In a number of studies in which experienced psychotherapy teachers rated videotapes of supervision sessions, Shanfield and colleagues (Shanfield, Mohl, Matthews, & Hetherly, 1992; Shanfield, Matthews, & Hetherly, 1993) were able to document what 'excellent' supervisors do. Such supervisors were empathic and oriented to the immediate experience of the resident as he or she presented clinical material. They made many synthesizing comments in some depth. Allowing the resident the opportunity to develop the story of the clinical encounter, they consistently tracked the most immediate aspects of the resident's concerns. Their comments, which were usually specific to the material presented in the session, were directed to helping the resident further understand the patient.

Alonso (1985) describes five activities of the supervisor:

1 *Didactic teaching* includes teaching the resident to listen in order to hear subtleties in the patient's communication.
2 *Imparting an appropriate attitude towards patients* implies neutrality; an open-minded curiosity combined with a non-judgmental stance; and the maintenance of an attitude of hovering attention.
3 *Expanding the affective capacity of the therapist* implies the capacity to deliberately feel and contain intense and primitive feelings. In other words, teaching the resident both to empathize and to accept a sense of ambiguity.
4 *Developing the capacity to work in the metaphor of the transference.*
5 *Supporting the therapist.*

The activities of the supervisor will vary according to the needs, interests, and level of training of the resident. For instance, beginning residents are often intimidated by the prospect of starting psychotherapy with a patient for the first time. It is often helpful for the supervisor to suggest that the resident begin the process by discussing patients he or she is treating in clinical settings such as wards or outpatient clinics. The next step is to move on to assessing patients for suitability for therapy. In this way, the resident is introduced to the role of therapist in a graduated fashion. According to Altshuler (1989), beginning residents commonly make the following four types of errors: pressing the past; pushing the transference; inappropriate support; and premature overinterpretation. He believes that these errors reflect the therapists' training 'in the biomedical model in which symptoms demand action and action is taken quickly and aimed at cure' (p. 79). The supervisor's role is to help residents recognize when they are trying too hard and tolerate the uncertainty involved in doing therapy.

Alonso (1985) divides the supervisory work into three main segments: the beginning phase, the mid-phase, and the end phase. In the beginning phase, it is advantageous for both trainee and supervisor to discuss relevant prior experience and therapeutic orientation and philosophy. At this stage they will agree on such parameters of their work as meeting times and method of presentation. During the mid-phase, the processes of incorporation, identification, and integration are facilitated. The end phase focuses on evaluation.

The principles conveyed by the supervisor to the resident should be consistent with the content objectives and skills objectives in the curriculum. This area of training in psychiatry is receiving a new interest and attention (see chapter 13, 'Standards and Guidelines for Psychotherapy Training'). Both the American Association of Directors of Psychiatric Residency Training and the Canadian Association of Directors of Post-graduate Education in Psychiatry recommend a new and augmented curriculum in psychotherapy.

Content issues that supervisors need to address include: providing the resident with a conceptual map of the psychotherapy process; assisting the resident with formulation; alerting the resident to the presence of transference and countertransference; indications for termination; and the handling of special problems. Special situations that require close attention are management of the chronically or acutely suicidal patient; sexualized or erotic transference; continued acting out; and negative therapeutic reactions. The failure to develop a therapeutic alliance or severe fluctuations in this alliance need to be addressed.

Methods of Supervision

The conventional method of supervision involves the resident presenting case material through the use of process notes. This can be supplemented or replaced by video- or audiotapes. In addition, it is occasionally useful for the supervisor to either directly interview the patient with the resident or observe the resident and patient behind a one-way mirror. Betcher and Zinburg (1988) point out that sometimes a meeting or audiotape can clear up a point that has been hard to explicate, thereby setting therapy back on course and providing a common frame of reference for supervisor and trainee. However, they caution that it carries a price and may interfere with the natural rhythms and boundaries of the 'private' therapy situation. They caution that what is gained in accuracy may be offset by a loss in authenticity. In viewing or listening to tapes, one may easily miss the subtle 'feel' of the situation between two people who are face to face.

Although supervision is generally conducted on a one-to-one basis, it can also be carried out in a paired or group format. There are advantages to group supervision, but this format should not be used to the exclusion of individual supervision. Group supervision may have significant advantages for beginning residents, especially if they are able to witness senior residents having success or struggling with a psychotherapy case. Group supervision does require formal rules to regulate competition among residents in the group. Residents highly rated a termination module in which a senior resident discusses the last twelve sessions of a long-term psychotherapy case with a supervisor, witnessed by a group of more junior residents. This specific module of teaching has the advantages of being brief, focused, and directed towards an often ignored phase of psychotherapy supervision (Robb & Cameron, 1998).

The Supervisory Relationship

BOUNDARIES OF THE SUPERVISORY RELATIONSHIP

As it is in psychotherapy, a cooperative personal relationship between supervisor and supervisee is central to psychotherapy supervision. The boundaries of this relationship, however, are different from those in therapy relationships. Although the supervisor's role is to teach the trainee, he or she also has responsibilities to the patient and the administration of the hospital or training institute. This constitutes the 'clinical rhombus,' described by Ekstein and Wallerstein (1972). According to Stone (1994), the nature of supervision has shifted from a simple paradigm in which the supervisor was an autonomous consultant to the trainee, to a complex paradigm in which the supervisor has primary responsibility for the patient. This includes the supervisor's legal liability for the care of the patient. Certainly, in residency training programs, the supervisor is responsible for the resident's actions and decisions. Further, supervisor and trainees are regularly involved in dual relationships These may include collegial relationships such as committee work or other administrative links and planned departmental social contacts.

SUPERVISION VERSUS THERAPY

Although supervision and psychotherapy are different activities, supervisors vary as to where they stand on the continuum between supervision as a purely didactic process, and supervision as a form of therapy. Early in the history of psychoanalytic training, a debate emerged between representatives of two polarized positions. The Hungarian school advocated that the candidate's supervisor also be his or her analyst. In contrast, the Vienna institute favoured the didactic position in which the personal analyst did not supervise the candidate (Ekstein & Wallerstein, 1972). At present this debate focuses on the relative emphasis on examination of countertransference in supervision.

A number of authors (Searles, 1955, Arlow, 1963; Ekstein & Wallerstein, 1972) stress the value of attending to the emotional experience of supervisor and therapist. Searles (1955) proposed that the supervisor could often provide valuable clarification of processes currently characterizing the supervisee–patient relationship by attending to the emotions he or she experienced in the supervisory session. In this 'reflection process,' the supervisor intuitively realizes that the therapist is unconsciously trying to express something about what is going on in the patient. However, due to anxiety, the therapist is unable to describe it. In a similar vein, Ekstein and Wallerstein (1972) described the 'parallel process' where the student-therapist unconsciously uses the patient's material to bring his or her 'learning problems' into the supervision. According to Alonso (1985), in the 'parallel process' the therapist unconsciously selects issues of conflict for both patient and therapist from the patient's material. The trainee then presents these processes directly or indirectly in supervision. Arlow (1963) emphasizes that, during the supervisory session, the therapist, in presenting the material, unconsciously shifts from reporting data of his or her experience with the patient to experiencing the experience of the patient. In other words, during the supervisory session, the therapist transiently acts out an identification with the patient. In the supervisory session, the therapist oscillates between observing the patient and identifying with the patient. The supervisor must empathize (identify) with both therapist and patient. The therapist and patient may share certain fantasy wishes and defensive functions which lead to 'blind spots.' These may be revealed in supervision.

There is a great deal of support for the position that countertransference can be explored without violating the resident's privacy. Writing in the 1970s, Berger and Freebury (1973) differentiate between supervision and therapy. Both processes are anxiety producing and involve periods of regression. In supervision, the therapist's psychodynamics are explored only when they interfere with the learning process. Goin and Kline (1976), in a study using videotaped supervision, found that the majority of supervisors avoided talking about countertransference. They surmised that the supervisors acted out of concern to not act as therapists. This could be accomplished by distinguishing between discussion of the therapist's feelings and their effect on the therapy, on the one hand, and investigation of the origins of those feelings, on the other hand. They advocate a frank and open approach to encouraging the resident to become aware of his or her feelings.

Book (1987) recommends that, prior to dealing with countertransference, the supervisor establish a 'teaching alliance,' characterized by a sense of mutuality, respect, and collegiality. It is most useful to encourage the resident to be curious about and attend to his or her own inner responses while with the patient. It is inappropriate to interpret or comment on the epigenetic roots of a resident's response.

Hunt (1981) views examination of the student's countertransference as highly important for learning because it goes to the core of the therapist–patient relationship. He maintains that this can be done without violating the student-therapist's privacy. The supervisor should maintain a mental set which always asks 'What does this tell us about the patient?' Student-therapists often dismiss their feelings by relating them to something in their personal life, for example, being on call. The supervisor should insist that, however valid this aspect may be, the therapist's emotions in the session are also in some ways responsive to the patient.

Betcher and Zinberg (1988) caution that an overly zealous application of the countertransference model of supervision can interfere with the establishment of rhythms and boundaries essential to therapy and supervision. They warn of the potential for crowding out the therapist's ingenuity and of subtle losses of authenticity as the supervisor's probing infringes on the privacy of therapy and heightens defensiveness. On the other hand, a didactic model runs the risk of supervision becoming more cognitive than affective. If carried out rigidly, it becomes an intellectualized and dry exercise: 'Trainees have more to gain if the dialectic between the personal and the didactic is not fully resolved, so that they have the opportunity to experience the different ways in which a number of supervisors have achieved their own integrations' (p. 801). They emphasize the need for a boundary because 'in a situation where trainees' personal space may be invaded by supervisors, patients, and the institution, they may feel safe enough to learn only if they know that there are limits to the invasion of their privacy' (p. 802).

Alonso (1985) notes that supervision is defined by various authors as: (1) a cognitive and primarily didactic process; (2) an emotional growth experience; and (3) an interpersonal process which focuses on the empathic connectedness between the concerned parties. She points out that, regardless of the supervisor's position on the continuum of didactic versus interpretive, the supervisor's function will vary, depending on the level of experience of the therapist.

Gorman (1997) disputes the distinction made between psychotherapy and supervision, and claims that the concept of a boundary between the two is theoretically insupportable. He prefers to view supervision as a particular kind of focal, time-limited psychotherapy, focusing on therapeutic growth around the supervised case. In this view, supervisory concepts such as parallel process and learning difficulties are merely instances of transference and countertransference. The supervision becomes immeasurably enriched by the tactful interpretation of the countertransferences in the supervised psychotherapy and the transferences and countertransference in the supervision, itself. The dangers that other writers say are inevitable with such a view can be avoided by keeping interpretations within the focus.

Rather than conceptualizing supervision in terms of a polarity between didactic and interpretive, it may be more useful to conceptualize the activities of the supervisor as occurring on a supportive–expressive continuum, as Luborsky (1984) conceptualizes the activities of therapists. In this schema, didactic teaching would be seen as a supportive measure, and interpretation as the expressive end of the continuum. In choosing between a didactic or expressive intervention, the supervisor takes into account a number of factors, which include: the resident's level of training and understanding of the therapy process and techniques; the degree of trust and safety within the supervisory relationship; and the relevance of the supervisor's observations to the understanding of the patient's current difficulties.

SEXUAL RELATIONSHIPS BETWEEN SUPERVISOR AND
SUPERVISEE

The issue of sexual relationships between supervisor and trainee is problematic. Of Canadian psychiatric residents who responded to a survey, 2.5 per cent reported sexual involvement with an educator (Carr, Robinson, Stewart, & Kussin, 1991). Of these reported involvements, only one-quarter involved a psychotherapy supervisor. Although there are currently no regulations concerning this issue in the Canadian Psychiatric Association Code of Ethics, some university departments in Ontario have a written policy prohibiting sexual relationships between supervisors and supervisees. If such a relationship does form, the supervisory relationship should be terminated. The American Psychiatric Association has stated that sexual involvement between trainees and faculty members 'generally takes advantage of inequalities in the working relationship' and therefore may be unethical (APA, quoted in Carr et al, 1991, p. 219). Although the vast majority of residents did not believe that such relationships should be permissible, most believed that they should be permissible after termination of the supervisory relationship. This is the position advocated by the authors of this volume. However, there remains a potential for abuse by the supervisor who chooses to use the supervision as the courtship phase of a sexual relationship.

IMPASSES IN SUPERVISION

In a survey conducted in two university programs (Nigam, Cameron, & Leverette, 1997), residents were asked to describe impasses in psychotherapy supervision. An impasse was defined as a phenomenon which occurred when learning in psychotherapy supervision did not progress for a four-week period. The most common event reported was an impasse between the supervisor and the supervisee. A less-common vignette involved difficulty in understanding the patient. This study demonstrated that a number of residents experienced the relationship with their supervisor as interfering with learning. During impasses the resident experienced the supervisor as intrusive or hurtful. Sometimes it appeared that the supervisor misunderstood the case completely. Frequently the supervisees were unwilling or unable to disclose these experiences. The authors believe that this kind of interference with learning occurs much more often than is readily apparent and that, when impasses are recognized, supervisors can repair them.

Supervision and Specific Psychotherapeutic Modalities

COGNITIVE BEHAVIOURAL PSYCHOTHERAPY

See chapter 15, 'Guidelines for Cognitive Behavioural Psychotherapy Supervision.'

GROUP PSYCHOTHERAPY

The essential aspects of the supervisory relationship outlined in this chapter also pertain to the supervision of group psychotherapy. An educational alliance must be firmly established so that the trainee is not so preoccupied with protecting his or her vulnerable self-esteem that exposure of concerns and difficulties hinder the objective of learning. In addition, there are special considerations related to the supervision of group psychotherapy that reflect unique aspects of the process of group psychotherapy, in particular, for the neophyte or trainee. Leading a psychotherapy group appears to generate considerably more anxiety at the outset than does beginning individual psychotherapy (Leszcz & Murphy, 1994; Murphy, Leszcz, Collings, & Salvendy, 1996). Group therapists have an important role in not only interpreting group phenomenon, but also facilitating the group's becoming interactive and cohesive. Acknowledgment, identification, and addressing the trainee's concerns around exposure, and his or her feelings of shame related to exposure, warrant particular attention. The anxiety may be so great as to elicit a range of countertherapeutic defensive postures (Williams, 1966) in which the group therapist protects him- or herself through a range of collusive or avoidant therapeutic postures. Supervision, therefore, must provide a 'space for thinking' (Mollon, 1989) in which the trainee is able to step back from the emotionally intense and charged treatment situation to begin to process, identify, and make sense of his or her experience as a group leader. Zaslav (1988) has identified the developmental sequence that neophyte group therapists undergo, and it is clear that supervision plays a central role in facilitating this developmental process. The concept of isomorphy (Nicholas, 1989), the parallelism of structure and self-organizational processes among living systems, serves as a useful template for trying to determine in supervision the mutually impactful contributions made by the patients, the group, the therapist, the supervisor, and the system in which the treatment and training occurs.

Supervision may be provided in a range of formats. Dyadic formats consist of one group leader and one supervisor, or an inexperienced cotherapist leading conjointly with a more experienced co-therapist. In triadic supervision, two co-therapists are jointly supervised by a supervisor. In group supervision, a number of group leaders meet together on a regular basis to discuss clinical material from their groups, facilitated by a senior group therapist, who functions as a supervisor. Each model has its strengths and limitations, and there is no research that argues for the superiority of one approach over the others. However, as Dies (1981) notes, since it is often the group process that provides the neophyte trainee with the greatest technical challenges, supervisory formats are enhanced when they provide an opportunity to examine issues relevant to the processes of multilateral relationships and the interpersonal processes of the group leader and supervisor. Of particular importance is the necessity of addressing co-therapy and co-leadership issues in supervision. The absence of the capacity to address and work through this relationship bodes poorly for the overall treatment. In a recent study (Murphy et al, 1996), beginning group therapists reported a remarkably strong correlation between overall satisfaction with their training in group therapy and the experience in supervision. When supervision was experienced as critical, unempathic, or out of tune with the resident, the overall experience in the group was dismal. In contrast, in all instances in which the neophyte group therapists experienced the supervision as supportive, attuned to resident concerns, and able to help make sense of powerful affects and stimuli, the group experience was viewed in a very favourable fashion. An allied finding was that groups led by co-therapists in which there was no vehicle or opportunity to discuss the co-therapy relationship also resulted in negative training experiences. These considerations arise with such regularity that it is essential to anticipate them and to incorporate them into the supervisory process as part of the establishment of the educational or supervisory contract.

COUPLE AND FAMILY PSYCHOTHERAPY

Supervision of couple and family psychotherapy involves a number of specific tasks. Students are taught to apply the theoretical tenets of couple and family therapy to clinical situations. The most important of these involves learning to think in terms of systems, rather than conceptualizing couple and family problems in terms of 'good guys' and 'bad guys.' The supervisor provides the student with a rationale for each technique that the supervisor advises.

The supervisor helps the student tolerate the uncertainty involved in not immediately finding the solution to the couple or family's problems. This involves not rushing to seek closure before understanding the factors contributing to the problems.

Helping the student identify countertransference issues is fundamental to supervision of couple and family therapy. Of particular importance are those reactions in which the therapist behaves in a punitive or disciplinarian manner with the patients. Identifying transference-like phenomena between spouses helps the understanding of countertransference responses in which the student-therapist empathizes with one member of the system and not with the others, or feels impotent and overwhelmed.

In supervision, the student is helped to establish alternating empathy and alternating alliances, so that he or she can be the mouthpiece of different family members or spouses at different times of the session. Empathic equidistance with both spouses or with each family member is the goal.

Supervision of couple and family therapy is enhanced by opportunities for the student to observe the supervisor practising the modality. This can be accomplished by either viewing videotapes or sitting in on sessions conducted by the supervisor.

Supervision Outside of Psychiatric Residency Programs

Psychotherapy supervision is not restricted to the training of psychiatric residents. Psychiatrists supervise therapists of a variety of disciplines and levels of training and licensure, across a variety of settings. These settings include formal psychotherapy programs for all the therapeutic modalities discussed in this volume as well as a number of different schools of therapy within each modality. The psychotherapy programs may be associated with universities, or with established psychotherapy institutes. Many experienced psychotherapists continue to seek individual supervision after completion of formal training. This may be through an ongoing arrangement with a supervisor, or on a consultative basis, following a therapeutic impasse. Supervision of experienced therapists differs not only in terms of supervisory tasks, but also in terms of the legal responsibility for the patient.

In addition to seeking individual supervision, psychiatrists and other therapists engage in peer supervision groups. Such informal groups meet regularly, once or twice a month, and generally consist of six to ten practising therapists. Although most groups are leaderless, some groups also employ senior psychotherapists as facilitators or consultants on an ongoing or occasional basis. An Australian study concluded that 'group peer review contributes significantly to professional accountability and education in well-functioning groups' (Beatson, Rushford, Halasz, Lancaster, & Pragen, 1996, p. 643).

Psychiatrists recognize the importance of psychotherapy supervision as an ongoing activity throughout their professional career. At times, this consists of formal supervision; at other times, it is obtained through peer groups. In addition, well-supervised psychotherapists are continually involved in self-supervision through a process of self-reflection and observation of countertransference and enactment.

Evaluations

Evaluation of the resident's progress is an integral part of the process of supervision. Although training programs include formal evaluations at various intervals, the supervisor gives the resident informal feedback about his or her performance throughout the process.

Residency programs develop formal mechanisms for evaluation. The University of Illinois, College of Medicine, at Chicago, has developed an instrument for evaluating residents (Winer & Mostert, 1988). Every six months, supervisors rate residents on eighteen items and sub-items, using a five-point scale. The sub-items are grouped into the following eight categories: (1) properly establishes a therapeutic situation; (2) facilitates the formation of a therapeutic alliance; (3) recognizes his or her emotional reactions; (4) experiences the patient's feelings temporarily (with respect to quality of feeling rather than degree or quantity), while maintaining his or her separateness and objectivity; (5) communicates his or her empathic understanding in a way that enables the patient to feel understood and recognizes and deals with the situations where the patient does not feel understood; (6) detects multiple meanings when present in a patient's communications; (7) makes interpretations that are plausible, clear, timely, tactful, and evocative of further material; and (8) formulates dynamics.

Written evaluations should be completed at least every six months, and possibly every three months. Ideally an evaluation form should be relatively brief and allow the supervisor to rate the resident according to learning objectives geared to his or her level of training. In reporting to the program director, the supervisor evaluates the resident's specific clinical abilities and avoids discussions of the resident's personality. Evaluation processes should also include informal opportunities for residents to give feedback to supervisors. Formal mechanisms of resident feedback are effective only when residents are secure that negative evaluations will be confidential.

Supervisory Record Keeping

Traditionally, psychotherapy supervisors were not required to record any notes. Under exceptional circumstances such as suicidal crises, erotic transference, or drug side-effects, some supervisors would write a note in the patient's chart. Stone (1994), suggests that the current guidelines may be changing, especially in the United States. He recommends that supervisors document their evaluation and supervision of all cases, including all major decisions by the supervisee. It is prudent for the supervisor to document in the patient's chart that he or she has reviewed the resident's assessment of the patient and treatment plan. In addition, supervisors should record in the chart when there is a major change in the treatment plan or the patient's clinical status.

Supervisors often find it helpful to maintain a separate record which documents the student's progress. A number of considerations apply if such documents are to be kept separate from the patient record. The focus should remain on the student, not on the patient's progress. Confidentiality of patient material must be respected. Finally, the supervisor should be aware that, even though this may be written as an educational record, it is still subject to subpoena in a legal process involving the patient.

Cultural Aspects

See chapter 16, 'Cultural Issues in Psychotherapy.'

Efficacy of Supervision

Sakinofsky (1979) developed a method of evaluating the acquisition of psychotherapy skills. Residents were videotaped in certain simulated situations, and an attempt was made to operationalize a method of evaluating certain basic skills in psychotherapy. In a review of the literature, Holloway and Neufeldt (1995) concluded that there were virtually no studies demonstrating the efficacy of supervision related to the patient outcome. They point out that generally investigators have relied on the perceptions of supervisors and trainees to judge the quality and efficacy of supervision. There has been little attempt to link this with the outcome of the patient's treatment. They discovered that there is no research on standardized training programs for supervisors. They advocate the development of supervision manuals for the training of psychotherapy supervisors. Certainly, determination of the outcome of supervision is not necessarily restricted to a determination of 'success' from the point of view of the patient.

Jones, Krasner, and Howard (1992) designed a questionnaire to measure psychodynamic psychotherapeutic skill in trainees. Skills which trainees tended to perform well included: forming a supervisory alliance; presenting clinical material; recognizing their own affect; empathizing with patients; and maintaining a therapeutic alliance. These abilities may reflect the interpersonal skills required for admission to clinical training programs. However, trainees performed the following tasks less well: recognizing transference; containing the patient's affect; using interpretations; and handling resistance. The authors concluded that these skills are training goals requiring active teaching efforts.

Improving our methods of identifying the acquisition of discrete skills in beginning therapists is important for the development of more effective training.

Institutional Issues

THE ROLE OF THE TRAINING PROGRAM
IN FACILITATING SUPERVISION

Ekstein and Wallerstein (1972) point out that psychotherapy supervision occurs within the 'clinical rhombus,' consisting of patient, therapist, supervisor, and administrator. The functions of the program administrator include protecting the patient, the student, and the supervisor within the system. The clinical setting may facilitate or interfere with the supervision process.

The program administrator can be instrumental in providing orientation to psychotherapy and psychotherapy supervision. Group meetings for beginning residents can address the following issues: assessment of patients; prescription of psychotherapy; and methods of formulation. One of the sessions may be spent discussing what to expect from supervision, including a description of the boundaries of the supervisory relationship. Beginning residents can benefit from observing a faculty member interview a prospective psychotherapy patient or conduct an ongoing case. Group formats can be useful for discussing how supervision works; the importance of the supervisory alliance; and the various treatment models that supervisors use. Discussion of the frame of supervision includes: the contract; the conditions; the method of recording sessions, through notes or tape; and the frequency and length of supervision. The program administrator may discuss policies regarding selection of supervisors and mechanisms of resolving conflict between supervisor and student.

It is essential for the conduct of psychotherapy supervision that supervisor and resident are able to arrange regular weekly meetings. Residents generally have a variety of complex clinical, administrative, and academic demands which can potentially interfere with their ability to maintain regular meetings. Similarly, it is essential that the resident has appropriate physical facilities for both therapy and supervision sessions. It is the responsibility of the institution, through the training director, to ensure that both these conditions are met.

The method of remunerating supervisors has an impact on the educational process. In jurisdictions where third-party payment is used to pay for supervision, it is imperative that ethical billing practices are maintained. For instance, in Ontario psychiatrists may bill for psychotherapy conducted by residents under supervision at the rate of one hour of psychotherapy for every hour of supervision. The supervisor's remuneration is dependent on the patient's attendance in therapy. Residents often report anecdotes of questionable billing practices, usually occurring in 'other hospitals.' Examples include supervisors asking for two patient hours to cover their travelling time, or offering to bill for two hours and split the fee with the resident. Although these practices are certainly anomalous, it is imperative that supervisors not only operate within the law, but communicate this clearly to their residents. The supervisory relationship has the potential to perpetuate unethical practices as well as to promote ethical standards.

It is essential that residents are exposed to a variety of psychotherapy supervisors during their training. According to Betcher and Zinberg (1988), having several supervisors counters the demand on trainees to conform to a rigid outlook and helps them retain their originality. They can appreciate 'that seasoned and well-trained people may arrive at different conclusions, techniques, and perceptions even when operating from the same underlying theoretical base' (p. 801). Greben (1991) states: 'When residents find their supervisors different from one an other, they are encouraged to think that the best way for them to be is their own way, not someone else's way' (p. 309). Residents will benefit from having experience with supervisors of both the same and opposite genders. Similarly residents will benefit from experience with both supervisors who are full-time academics and with supervisors who are community-based.

STANDARDS FOR PSYCHOTHERAPY SUPERVISORS

The following qualifications for supervisors are based on the report of the Joint Task Force on Standards for Medical (Psychiatric) Psychotherapy of the Ontario Psychiatric Association and the Section of Psychiatry, Ontario Medical Association (1995):

1 The supervisor should demonstrate a career commitment to the modality that he or she is teaching.
2 The supervisor should have specialized formal training in the modality as well as a knowledge of other modalities.
3 The supervisor should demonstrate ongoing knowledge of the current literature.
4 The supervisor should demonstrate a continued interest in academic presentations and in writing either research-oriented or conceptual papers in his or her modality.
5 The supervisor should attend a supervisor training group for a minimum of two years. It is preferable that supervisors attend this group for one year before supervising residents so that they become familiar with some of the complexities of the supervision process and some of the literature outlining characteristics of excellent supervision.

Training programs can maintain high standards through the use of groups for supervisors. Frayn (1991) describes the evolution of a supervisors' group at the Clarke Institute for Psychiatry through three formats. The group found the continuous case conference to be the most useful format. The primary goal was discussion concerning the learning of psychotherapy supervision. At The Toronto Hospital, a supervisor's group has been meeting biweekly since 1991. Informal discussion of case material is acknowledged to be the most valuable activity, although some administrative aspects and literature review also take place. Guest lectures, unless focused specifically on supervisory experience, tended to be experienced as intrusive. Although newly appointed supervisors are expected to attend the seminar, all psychotherapy supervisors are encouraged to participate. Cameron (1994) has also described the development of a supervisors' group, outlining some of the resistance and difficulties. The members found the process so useful that the group was unwilling to disband.

References

Alonso, A.E. (1985). *The quiet profession – supervisors of psychotherapy.* New York: Macmillan.
Altshuler, K.Z. (1989). Common mistakes made by beginning psychotherapists. *Academic Psychiatry, 13,* 73–80.

Arlow, J.A. (1963). The supervisory situation. *Journal of the American Psycho-analytic Association, 11,* 576–594.

Beatson, J.A., Rushford, N., Halasz, G., Lancaster, J., & Prager, S. (1996). Group peer review: A questionnaire-based survey. *Australian and New Zealand Journal of Psychiatry, 30,* 643–652.

Berger, D., & Freebury, D.R. (1973). The acquisition of psychotherapy skills: A learning model and some guidelines for instructors. *Canadian Psychiatric Association Journal, 18,* 467–472.

Betcher, R.W. & Zinberg, N.E. (1988). Supervision and privacy in psychotherapy training. *American Journal of Psychiatry, 145,* 796–803.

Book, H.E. (1987). The resident's countertransference: Approaching an avoided topic. *American Journal of Psychotherapy, 41,* 555–562.

Cameron, P.M. (1994). Faculty development: A program to improve teaching of psychotherapy. *Proceedings: The Sixth Ottawa Conference on Medical Education,* 38–41.

Carr, M.L., Robinson, G.E., Stewart, D.E., & Kussin, D. (1991). A survey of Canadian psychiatric residents regarding resident–educator sexual contact. *American Journal of Psychiatry, 148,* 216–220.

Dies, R.R. (1981). Group psychotherapy: Training and supervision. In A.K. Hess (Ed.), *Psychotherapy supervision.* New York: Wiley.

Ekstein, R., & Wallerstein, R.S. (1972). *The teaching and learning of psychotherapy,* 2d ed. Madison, CT: International Universities Press.

Frayn, D.H. (1991). Supervising the supervisors: The evolution of a psycho-therapy supervisors' group. *American Journal of Psychotherapy, 45,* 31–42.

Goin, M.K., & Kline, F. (1976). Countertransference: A neglected subject in clinical supervision. *American Journal of Psychiatry, 13,* 41–44.

Gorman, H.E. (1997). Interpretation of transference in psychoanalytic super-vision. *Free Association, 39,* 394–441.

Greben, S.E. (1991). Interpersonal aspects of the supervision of individual psychotherapy. *American Journal of Psychotherapy, 45,* 306–316.

Greben, S.E., Markson, E.R., & Sadovoy, J. (1973). Resident and supervisor: An examination of their relationship. *Canadian Psychiatric Association Journal, 18,* 473–479.

Holloway, E.L., & Neufeldt, S.A. (1995). Supervision: Its contribution to treat-ment efficacy. *Journal of Consulting and Clinical Psychology, 63,* 207–213.

Hunt, W. (1981). The use of the countertransference in psychotherapy super-vision. *Journal of the American Academy of Psychoanalysis, 9,* 361–373.

Joint Task Force on Standards for Medical (Psychiatric) Psychotherapy. (1995). *A Report to Council of the Ontario Psychiatric Association and to Executive of the*

Section on Psychiatry, Ontario Medical Association, on the definition, guidelines and standards for medical (psychiatric) psychotherapy. Toronto: Author.

Jones, S.H., Krasner, R.F., & Howard, K.I. (1992). Components of supervisors' ratings of therapists' skilfulness. *Academic Psychiatry, 16,* 29–36.

Leszcz, M., & Murphy, L. (1994). Supervision of group psychotherapy. In S.E. Greben & R. Ruskin (Eds.), *Clinical perspectives on psychotherapy supervision.* Washington, DC: American Psychiatric Press.

Luborsky, L. (1984). *Principles of psychoanalytic psychotherapy: A manual for supportive–expressive treatment.* New York: Basic.

Mollon, P. (1989). Anxiety, supervision and a space for thinking: Some narcissistic perils for clinical psychologists in learning psychotherapy. *British Journal of Medical Psychology, 62,* 112–113.

Murphy, L., Leszcz, M., Collings, A.K., & Salvendy, J. (1996). Some observations on the subjective experience of neophyte group therapy trainees. *International Journal of Group Psychotherapy, 46,* 543–552.

Nicholas, M.W. (1989). A systematic perspective of group therapy supervision: Use of energy in the supervisor-therapist–group system. In K.G. Lewis (Ed.), *Variations on teaching and supervising group therapy.* New York: Haworth.

Nigam, T., Cameron, P.M., & Leverette, J. (1997). Impasses in psychotherapy supervision: A resident's perspective. *American Journal of Psychotherapy, 51,* 252–270.

Robb, M., & Cameron, P.M. (1998). Supervision of termination in psychotherapy. *Canadian Journal of Psychiatry, 43,* 397–402.

Sakinofsky, I. (1979). Evaluating the competence of psychotherapists. *Canadian Journal of Psychiatry, 24,* 193–205.

Searles, H.F. (1955) The informational value of the supervisor's emotional experiences. *Psychiatry, 18,* 135–146.

Searles, H.F. (1965) Problems of psycho-analytic supervision. In H.F. Searles, *Collected papers on schizophrenia and related subjects.* New York: International Universities Press.

Shanfield, S.B., Matthews, K.L., & Hetherly, V. (1993) What do excellent psychotherapy supervisors do? *American Journal of Psychiatry, 150,* 1081–1084.

Shanfield, S.B., Mohl, P.C., Matthews, K.L., & Hetherly, V. (1992). Quantitative assessment of the behavior of psychotherapy supervisors. *American Journal of Psychiatry, 149,* 352–357.

Stone, A.A. (1994). Ethical and legal issues in psychotherapy supervision. In S.E. Greben & R. Ruskin (Eds.), *Clinical perspectives on psychotherapy supervision.* Washington, DC: American Psychiatric Press.

Williams, M. (1966) Limitations, fantasies and security operations of beginning group therapists. *International Journal of Group Psychotherapy, 16,* 152–162.

Winer, J.A., & Mostert, M. (1988). Evaluation of resident's dynamic psychotherapy skills. *Journal of Psychiatric Education, 12,* 329–337.

Zaslav, M. (1988). A model of group therapist development. *International Journal of Group Psychotherapy, 38,* 511–519.

15. Guidelines for Cognitive Behavioural Psychotherapy Supervision

Ari E. Zaretsky, Richard P. Swinson,
and Martin M. Antony

Over the past three decades, cognitive behavioural therapy (CBT) has become one of the predominant forces in psychotherapeutic practice (Norcross, 1986). Empirical outcome research suggests that it is arguably the most efficacious psychological treatment for depression (Dobson, 1989) and anxiety disorders (Clark, 1989). Unfortunately, the psychotherapy training of psychiatry residents has dramatically lagged behind CBT's growing acceptance and influence. A recent survey of U.S. psychiatry postgraduate directors (Ritchie & White, 1992) found that only 54 per cent of programs offer any CBT and, even then, most residents treat fewer than five patients, which is grossly inadequate to acquire minimum proficiency in this unique psychotherapy approach. Nonetheless, these trends are slowly changing and, as CBT becomes more accepted, more attention will need to be paid to the supervisory aspect. Until now, although there has been a large contribution in the psychoanalytic and psychodynamic psychotherapy literature dealing with the experience of supervision from the point of view of supervisors and supervisees, the issue of supervision seems to have been sorely neglected in the context of CBT. Given CBT's well-known commitment to empiricism, research into this critical aspect of psychotherapy training is long overdue.

Since there is a limited literature on CBT supervision, what follows is based mainly on the personal experience of the authors, accumulated during several years of work as supervisors and teachers, as well as an integration of previous writing by Shaw (Shaw, 1984; Shaw & Wilson-Smith, 1988) on training of therapists for outcome studies, Perris (1994) on cognitive conceptualization of the supervisory process, and Friedberg and Taylor (1994) on the role of the learning alliance in CBT supervision.

Models of Supervision

The two principal models usually considered when analysing supervision are the model of 'teaching' and that of 'therapy.' Another perspective is to examine supervision in terms of its 'focus on the patient,' 'focus on the therapist,' or 'focus on the process' (Archer & Peake, 1984; Wagner, 1957). In the field of psychodynamic therapy, as well as in the context of CBT, both the teaching and the therapy approaches have their advocates and their critics. Nonetheless, CBT supervision in general focuses more explicitly on a teaching approach than does traditional psychodynamic therapy supervision. It is very important, however, to recognize that many supervisors in CBT do attend to the 'therapist' and the 'process' (Perris, 1994) and view supervision as a modified form of therapy. Lloyd and Whitehead (1976), for example, describe a training program for behavioural therapists in which the same behavioural principles as those used in therapy are systematically applied to the supervision. Similarly, when describing her three-dimensional model of behavioural supervision, comprising goals, procedures, and generalization mechanisms, Linehan (1980) compares psychotherapy supervision to a specialized form of assertiveness training.

Although Wessler and Ellis (1980) clearly emphasize a teaching model, they also point out that, while 'supervision focuses on the patient ... it is advisable at times to transfer the focus of supervision to the therapist,' especially 'when it becomes apparent ... that he or she has a significant problem interfering with the progress of therapy' (p.187). Therefore, in actual practice, CBT supervision may have both a teaching and a therapy component.

Chessick (1971) points out that the focus in supervision greatly depends on the anxiety and skill of the supervisee. Supervision is conceptualized as a hierarchy of tasks over an extended time, and the supervisor is regarded as a person in whom the qualities of teacher and therapist are combined and used according to the specifics of the situation. From a CBT perspective, Perris (1994) has emphasized the importance of reconciling the didactic/therapist dichotomy by taking into account a temporal or developmental dimension to supervision, and regarding the supervisor as neither a teacher nor a therapist, but a person who has succeeded in merging the abilities of the two different roles and is able to use them appropriately in a given context. This, in fact, is the essence of good CBT with patients.

Supervisory Modalities

Psychodynamic therapy supervision has traditionally been based on the verbal report of the supervisee on the contents of one or more therapy sessions, and based on either memory or written process notes. The limitation of this approach has been recognized for some time, and forty years ago Kubie (1958) suggested that the therapeutic session should be tape-recorded because that technique allowed a closer scrutiny of the hidden implications of word exchanges and, in addition, permitted a better grasp of the emotional interactions occurring during the sessions. This would enable the therapist to become more directly aware of his or her own behaviour during the session. More recently, Shaw (1984) has emphasized the advantage of videotaped over audiotaped observations, with the most obvious advantage being that videotapes allow scrutiny of non-verbal data.

In the field of cognitive behavioural psychotherapy, the use of audiotapes or videotapes has, from the very beginning, characterized the practice of therapy, and these records of therapy sessions are believed to be the most suitable basis of supervision, even though they are not a requirement. Although many psychodynamic therapists (Strupp, 1978) criticize the loss of spontaneity and inhibition of emotional disclosure that audiotaping can engender, most CBT supervisors feel that the advantage of being able to directly observe the performance of beginners clearly outweighs the disadvantages. Friedman, Yamamoto, Wolkon, and Davis (1978) have also observed that videotape recording was far more anxiety-inducing for trainees than for their patients, and this study lends support for the need of a supervisor to fully explore, and possibly work through, a supervisee's resistance to the audiotaping or videotaping of therapy sessions.

Focus on Skills in CBT Supervision

In CBT supervision, greater emphasis is placed on conferring specific skills to the novice therapist, and in many ways this emphasis on the development of competence and proficiency parallels the approach of CBT itself to teaching patients specific emotional problem-solving skills to enable them essentially to become their own therapist (Hollon, DeRubeis, & Seligman, 1992). In CBT supervision, the supervisee should develop the skill to be able to:

1 conduct a cognitive behavioural assessment and integrate information generated from the clinical interview with data obtained from the administration of standardized psychometric tests used to assess mood, anxiety, or other pertinent dimensions of psychopathology;
2 generate a specific and sophisticated cognitive/behavioural conceptualization of the patient's problems, integrating dysfunctional thoughts, emotions, and behaviour with deeper meaning structures such as emotionally laden core beliefs and interpersonal schemata derived from earlier life experiences;
3 establish and maintain a solid therapeutic alliance with the patient, based on accurate empathy;
4 socialize the patient to the cognitive behavioural model;
5 socialize the patient to the unique frame of cognitive behavioural therapy and be able to maintain an active, goal-oriented, structured approach throughout treatment;
6 select appropriately, and apply in a timely manner, those therapeutic strategies and techniques best suited to achieving the patient's preferred goals. These may range from a more 'behavioural' emphasis on exposure therapy and response prevention for obsessive–compulsive disorder to the more 'cognitive' identification and challenging of underlying thoughts and dysfunctional beliefs in major depressive disorder;
7 monitor the progress of therapy, and utilize patient records and psychometric scales effectively throughout treatment;
8 critically evaluate the results of therapy and utilize direct feedback from the patient;
9 recognize and evaluate the interpersonal reactions occurring within him- or herself as well as in the patient, and understand how to effectively deal with them during therapy sessions.

The emphasis on skill proficiency in supervision is not meant to imply that technique alone is all that is important in CBT. Persons (1989) has emphasized the pre-eminence of the unique, individualized case formulation as being at the heart of CBT, and specific cognitive or behavioural techniques as being of secondary importance. Burns and Nolen-Hoeksema (1992) have also demonstrated that therapist empathy (independent of technique) had an important influence on response to CBT for patients suffering from depression.

Nevertheless, there is some compelling empirical evidence to suggest that specific technical aspects of CBT also have a significant impact on outcome. For example, in the famous NIMH multi-centre study (Elkin et al, 1989), one explanation for the site differences in the efficacy of CBT for depression was poor therapist adherence to core CBT interventions (Hollon, Shelton, & Loosen, 1991). More recently, Kingdon and colleagues (1996) found that CBT was more effective when performed by competent therapists adhering to the cognitive model. Finally, other studies (Burns & Nolen-Hoeksema, 1992; Neimeyer & Feixas, 1990) have demonstrated that low homework compliance (by either therapist or patient) also adversely influences CBT outcome.

Barriers to Skill Acquisition in CBT Supervision

Supervisee difficulties in learning CBT can be conceptualized as specific and non-specific. Non-specific difficulties in developing a learning alliance with the CBT supervisor refer to common characterological and developmental problems that may be experienced in any type of psychotherapy supervision. For example, many novice supervisees may experience shame and self-doubt about competence, and may therefore be reluctant to participate fully in the supervisory experience and expose their clinical work to their supervisors' scrutiny for fear of humiliation and rejection. Given CBT's special emphasis on more direct observation of the actual therapy session itself, as well as its emphasis on skill training, there is a unique opportunity for CBT supervisors to demystify the process of both supervision and psychotherapy, thereby helping supervisees confront and work through these fundamental issues associated with psychotherapy training. Many CBT supervisors actually begin supervision with the trainee observing the supervisor doing an interview of the patient and conducting a cognitive behavioural assessment.

Supervisee difficulties that are more specific to learning CBT itself include conflict about the cognitive model and problems integrating empathy with structured, change-oriented techniques. Supervisees often learn CBT after they have had some previous exposure to psychodynamic therapy (either as therapists, or sometimes, as patients, if they have been in therapy themselves). These earlier experiences can have a profound effect on influencing and shaping the supervisee's schema of psychotherapy: conceptualization of what psychotherapy really should be and how it should be conducted. A rigid psychotherapy schema can create powerful emotional conflicts about allegiance and may prevent the supervisee from keeping an open mind to alternative approaches. Persons and colleagues (1996) have recently observed that, for many supervisees, resistance to learning CBT is often linked to a perception that: (1) CBT does not emphasize the therapeutic relationship or the use of transference; (2) CBT emphasizes active focused interventions on behaviours rather than feelings; and (3) CBT changes the patient's behaviours, but not the fundamental unconscious conflicts or the 'depth' of the patient.

A view of CBT as being superficial, simplistic, mechanical, and unempathic can seriously interfere with the supervisee's adherence to the cognitive behavioural model. The supervisee may resist being structured or active during a session because of concern about stifling the patient, preventing genuine expression, and being overly controlling and unempathic. Similarly, a supervisee may be reluctant to assign homework or engage the patient in exposure therapy tasks because of concerns about pseudocompliance and being too authoritarian, thereby infantilizing the patient. Reservations about CBT may also lead novice trainees to resort to interpretations instead of using Socratic guided discovery whenever they encounter resistance from the patient in treatment. Concern about interfering with the development of transference can also lead beginner therapists to avoid any transparency and avoid obtaining direct verbal feedback from the patient about the session. A dramatic illustration of this phenomenon can be observed in the example of a novice CBT trainee with extensive training in psychodynamic therapy and a previous personal experience of psychoanalysis. The trainee reported to his CBT supervisor that, the first time that he assigned homework to his patient, he saw the image of his first psychotherapy supervisor looking at him in a disappointed way, indicating to him that the homework assignment was pathetically misguided. These types of concerns about CBT can present emotionally powerful barriers to skill acquisition. To help psychodynamically inclined supervisees overcome obstacles to learning CBT, supervisors need to be acutely aware of these unspoken attitudes and beliefs about CBT and, instead of trying to indoctrinate the supervisee, the supervisor is advised instead to openly engage the supervisee in a discussion of his or her concerns about the cognitive/behavioural approach as it specifically applies to the treatment of the patient who is now in treatment. This allows the supervisee to adopt the role of a 'personal scientist' and empirically evaluate his or her specific concerns or reservations about CBT. It is also very helpful for the supervisor to spend time early on in supervision providing the supervisee with a sophisticated and thoughtful understanding of the many similarities between the psychodynamic and cognitive/behavioural models, while also, at the same time, delineating the clear differences between these models.

A second commonly observed problem for novice supervisees in CBT is a tendency to rigidly and overzealously apply cognitive or behavioural techniques in a mechanical way, to the complete exclusion of any empathic emotional engagement with the patient during the therapy session. This behaviour can be cognitively conceptualized as a type of compensatory strategy to cope with underlying feelings of anxiety. The anxiety in this case may have different causes. It might be caused by the supervisee's lack of self-confidence and fear of appearing incompetent in the eyes of his or her supervisor. In this situation, excessive focus on the technical aspects of CBT is intended to provide the supervisee with the trappings of mastery, proficiency, and apparent fidelity to the cognitive behavioural model. Alternatively, the anxiety may be related to deep uncertainty about CBT's true effectiveness, and conflict about allegiances to a new, more active psychotherapy approach. In this latter type of situation, the supervisee immerses him- or herself in the technical aspects of CBT as a counterphobic manoeuvre, to avoid having to tolerate any uncertainty, conflict, or ambivalence about CBT. Unfortunately, the compensatory immersion in technique can paradoxically result in an intensification of the supervisee's anxiety about competence and allegiance since the patient being treated by the novice therapist often becomes alienated, resistant, and non-compliant with treatment.

An important way for the supervisor to facilitate a 'working through' of this overzealous focus on technique to the exclusion of emotional engagement is to emphasize a cognitive conceptualization of the patient's non-compliance with treatment and to gently point out to the novice therapist that proficient CBT requires an integration of affect with cognitive restructuring and behavioural techniques rather than a dichotomous focus on one at the exclusion of the other. Providing the supervisee with a copy of the Cognitive Therapy Rating Scale (Vallis, Shaw, & Dobson, 1986) can greatly demystify what proficient CBT really implies. It is extremely important to clarify the importance of balancing *adherence* with *appropriateness* and *quality*. 'Adherence' refers to the therapist engaging in behaviours that approximate the cognitive behavioural model with a high degree of fidelity. For example, setting an agenda each session, checking on the patient's symptomatology, and assigning homework would be adhering to the cognitive behavioural model to a high degree. 'Quality' refers to the skill or dexterity that the therapist uses in carrying out these different cognitive and behavioural interventions during the session. 'Appropriateness' refers to the clinical judgment of the therapist in determining if and when a specific cognitive or behavioural intervention should be applied during the session or the course of treatment. An exaggerated illustration of these concepts is a patient coming to a session weeping and reporting to her cognitive behavioural therapist that her father had just died. If the therapist then mechanically says: 'What else would you like to put on today's agenda?' he may score high in terms of adherence at that moment, but the complete callousness and inappropriateness of this intervention (agenda setting) in this context results in a global impression that the therapy provided had been of very poor quality.

Modelling by the Supervisor: A General Strategy to Enhance Learning

In addition to identifying specific problems that impede learning by the novice cognitive behavioural therapist, CBT supervisors can also use modelling as a general technique to enhance the learning alliance and facilitate skill acquisition. In effect, the supervision hour provides the supervisee with a model of the CBT session, and the supervisor–supervisee relationship also serves as a model of the patient–therapist relationship in CBT.

The first thing that the supervisor models to the novice supervisee is a relationship based on mutual respect and collegiality, as well as collaboration and egalitarianism. The supervisor meets with the supervisee to identify the latter's specific goals in the supervision process, and also articulates his or her own goals for the supervisee and the supervision. The supervisee's special interests, experiences, and beliefs about psychotherapy are identified to enhance collaboration and tailor the supervision to the supervisee's needs. The supervisor also respects boundaries and avoids excessive psychological intrusiveness into the supervisee's background in order to foster and reinforce a feeling of security for the supervisee. Bowlby's (1988) concept of a 'secure base' can be applied to the concept of supervision in psychotherapy. The novice supervisee (like the toddler) needs to feel that he or she can depend on the supervisor, and this security gives the supervisee more courage to creatively explore new ways of behaving in psychotherapy and acquire new psychotherapy skills.

The supervisor can also model other important aspects of cognitive behavioural therapy to the novice therapist. By sharing with the beginner therapist his or her own experiences (particularly mistakes made with difficult or challenging patients), and by allowing the supervisee to directly observe his or her own actual clinical work, the supervisor models the concept of therapist transparency, and this in itself helps to demystify psychotherapy, builds the learning alliance, and reduces the supervisee's sense of shame and incompetence.

By collaboratively setting an agenda in the supervision hour, the CBT supervisor can powerfully model to the supervisee how structure can enhance learning and increase a sense of mastery and competence without necessarily being mechanical or stilted. By soliciting frequent feedback from the supervisee throughout supervision, the CBT supervisor can experientially illustrate to the supervisee how feedback can enhance emotional trust and mutual respect in the therapy process itself.

The modelling of CBT techniques can also be applied to teaching the supervisee how to use Socratic questioning effectively and how to utilize a cognitive conceptualization to understand the supervisee's countertransference reactions. Similarly, role-playing how to deal with a difficult patient or patient non-compliance can also be utilized to enhance skill acquisition and to model to the novice therapist how a CBT therapist actively works with a patient. In all of these situations, careful attention needs to be paid to boundaries and informed consent. For example, a CBT supervisor would initiate an exploration into the countertransference reaction of a trainee by asking: 'I wonder if we could look at what was going through your mind when the patient said that? Would you be open to looking at that right now?'

Conclusion

In summary, despite CBT's burgeoning acceptance within today's broad psychotherapy landscape, supervision in CBT has for the most part been sadly neglected. Given the fact that increasingly more therapists are learning CBT, it is critical that the unique elements of supervision in CBT be explored and researched empirically. This is especially important because of the difficulties that inevitably arise when therapists with previous experience with one type of psychotherapy model are trained in a new, more active and structured approach to psychotherapy.

References

Archer, R.P., & Peake, T.H. (1984). Learning and teaching psychotherapy: Signposts and growth stages. *The Clinical Supervisor, 2,* 61–74.

Bowlby, J. (1988). *A secure base.* London: Routledge & Kegan Paul.

Burns, D.D., & Nolen-Hoeksema, S. (1992). Therapeutic empathy and recovery from depression in cognitive-behavioral therapy: A structural equation model. *Journal of Consulting and Clinical Psychology, 59,* 305–311.

Chessick, R.D. (1971). How the resident and the supervisor disappoint each other. *American Journal of Psychotherapy, 25,* 272–283.

Clark, D.M. (1989). Anxiety states. In K. Hawton, P.M. Salkovsky, J. Kirk, & D.M. Clark (Eds.), *Cognitive behaviour therapy for psychiatric problems.* New York: Oxford University Press.

Dobson, K.S. (1989). A meta-analysis of the efficacy of cognitive therapy for depression. *Journal of Consulting and Clinical Psychology, 57,* 414–419.

Elkin, I., Shea, J., Watkins, J.T., Imber, S.D., Sotsky, S.M., Collins, J.F., Glass, D.R., Pilkonis, P.A., Leber, W.R., Docherty, J.P., Fiester, S.J., & Parloff, M.B. (1989). National Institute of Mental Health Treatment of Depression Collaborative Research Program: General effectiveness of treatments. *Archives of General Psychiatry, 46,* 971–982.

Friedberg, R.D., & Taylor, L.A. (1994). Perspectives on supervision in cognitive therapy. *Journal of Rational–Emotive and Cognitive–Behaviour Therapy, 12,* 147–161.

Friedman, C.T.H., Yamamoto, J., Wolkon, G.H., & Davis, L. (1978). Videotape recording of dynamic psychotherapy: Supervisory tool or hindrance? *American Journal of Psychiatry, 135,* 1388–1391.

Hollon, S.D., DeRubeis, R.J., & Seligman, M.E.P. (1992). Cognitive therapy and the prevention of depression. *Applied and Preventive Psychology, 1,* 89–95.

Hollon, S.D., Shelton, R.C., & Loosen, P.T. (1991). Cognitive therapy and pharmacotherapy for depression. *Journal of Consulting and Clinical Psychology, 59,* 88–89.

Kingdon, D., Tyver, P., Seivewright, N., Ferguson, B., & Murphy, S. (1996). The Nottingham study of neurotic disorder: Influence of cognitive therapists on outcome. *British Journal of Psychiatry, 169,* 93–97.

Kubie, L. (1958). Research into the process of supervision in psychoanalysis. *Psychoanalysis Quarterly, 27,* 226–236.

Linehan, M.M. (1980). Supervision of behavior therapy. In A.K. Hess (Ed.) *Psychotherapy supervision: Theory, research and practice.* New York: Wiley.

Lloyd, M.E., & Whitehead, J.S. (1976). Development and evaluation of behaviorally taught practice. In S. Yen & R.W. McIntire (Eds.), *Teaching behavior modification*. Kalamazoo: Behaviordelia.

Neimeyer, R.A., & Feixas, G. (1990). The role of homework and skill acquisition in the outcome of group cognitive therapy for depression. *Behaviour Therapy, 21*, 281–292.

Norcross, J.C. (1986). *Handbook of eclectic psychotherapy.* New York: Brunner/Mazel.

Perris, C. (1994). Supervising cognitive psychotherapy and training supervisors. *Journal of Cognitive Psychotherapy: An International Quarterly, 8* (2), 83–103.

Persons, J.B. (1989). *Cognitive therapy in practice: Case formulation approach.* New York: Norton.

Persons, J.B., Gross, J.J., Etkin, M.S., & Madan, S.K. (1996). Psychodynamic therapists' reservations about cognitive-behavioral therapy: Implications for training and practice. Journal of *Psychotherapy Practice and Research, 5*, 202–212.

Ritchie, E.C., & White, R. (1992). Cognitive therapy training: US psychiatry residency programs. *Academic Psychiatry, 16*, 90–95.

Shaw, B.F. (1984). Specification of the training and evaluation of cognitive therapists for outcome studies. In J.B. Williams & R.L. Spitzer (Eds.), *Psychotherapy research: Where are we and where should we go?* New York: Guilford.

Shaw, B.F., & Wilson-Smith, D. (1988). Training therapists in cognitive–behavior therapy. In C. Perris, I.M. Blackburn, & H. Perris (Eds.), *Cognitive psychotherapy: theory and practice.* Heidelberg: Springer-Verlag.

Strupp, H.H. (1978). Psychotherapy research and practice: An overview. In S.L. Garfield & A.E. Begen (Eds.), *Handbook of psychotherapy and behavior change: An empirical analysis.* New York: Wiley.

Vallis, T.M., Shaw, B.F., & Dobson, K.S. (1986). The Cognitive Therapy Scale: Pychometric properties. *Journal of Consulting and Clinical Psychology, 54*, 381–385.

Wagner, F.F. (1957). Supervision of psychotherapy. *American Journal of Psychotherapy, 11*, 759–768.

Wessler, R.L., & Ellis, A. (1980). Supervision in rational-emotive therapy. In A.K. Hess (Ed.), *Psychotherapy supervision: Theory, research and practice.* New York: Wiley.

16. Gender Issues in Psychotherapy

Rebeka Moscarello, Michael Myers, Norman Doidge, and Jon Ennis

Throughout the twentieth century, there has been an evolution in the role and position of the sexes in society. The psychiatric understanding of gender has been influenced by contributions from anthropology, biology, psychiatry, psychoanalysis, psychology, and sociology. Through awareness and sensitivity, it is essential for psychotherapists to avoid some common biases about sex and gender. (Therapists must be equally sensitive to differences in race, culture, disability, poverty, and religious faith.) In order to enhance their understanding of patients and the patient's understanding of therapists, both male and female therapists must be cognizant of gender differences in the psychological development of men and women. Research continues to contribute new knowledge about the development and behaviour of both genders. The clinician's challenge is to balance empirical findings about gender differences in large groups, and theoretical formulations based on the study of small groups of patients, retaining the need to see each patient as an individual, in whom the expression of gender is likely complex and unique. This chapter explores knowledge, skill, and attitude objectives as applied to gender issues in psychotherapy.

Knowledge Objectives about Gender Issues for Medical Psychotherapists

To have some basic knowledge of the following:

• definitions of sex, gender, gender identity, gender role, and gender-role socialization

- theories about the psychology of men and women
- changing family structures and family breakdown
- gender and psychiatric disorders
- the influence of values and beliefs on psychotherapy
- gender and the process of therapy
- sexual abuse
- gender configurations in individual treatment – four dyads (male therapist–female patient; female therapist–female patient; male therapist–male patient; female therapist–female patient)
- gender and couple therapy

Definitions

Sex: Either of the two major forms that occur in many living things and designated male or female, according to their role in reproduction (*Merriam Webster Dictionary,* 1994).

Gender: One of the salient categories by which people judge and evaluate others. Gender may be defined as culturally, psychologically, and biologically determined cognitions, attitudes, and belief systems *about being masculine or feminine.* Gender is a concept that varies across cultures, that changes through history, and that differs in terms of who makes the observations and judgments (Deaux, 1984). Francoeur (1991) defines gender in its simplest usage as 'one's social role as a sexual person, as opposed to the genital anatomy with which one is born or the social concomitant of being biologically male, female or intersex. Adjectives that describe gender are *masculine* and *feminine.* Adjectives describing sex are *male* or *female.* Gender is a cultural construct applied to the newborn' (p. 238). While gender may be seen as a cultural construct, this in no way implies that it is not influenced by psychological and biological factors.

Gender identity: The internalized sense of being male or female or having ambivalent status, the self-awareness of knowing to which sex one belongs (Francoeur, 1991). Core gender identity begins at birth and, by age eighteen to twenty-four months, the child identifies itself as a boy or a girl (Money & Erhardt, 1972). Gender identity is intimately linked with one's sense of self and body image. Sense of self and body image become distinct during the first two years of life (Notman, Zilbach, Miller, & Nadelson, 1986).

Gender role: Patterns of culturally approved behaviours and attitudes that are regarded as acceptable within a culture for females or males (Worell & Remer, 1992). The public expression of oneself as male or female, masculine or feminine, is not necessarily congruent with gender identity, which is the *inner* conviction that one is a woman or a man.

Gender-role socialization: The way in which biological males and biological females become socialized and portray themselves as men and women in any particular culture (Bishop, 1992). It is the 'scripting or training of children by parents, caregivers and others in behaviour, attitudes and expectations considered appropriate to the child's gender in the society or culture' (Bleier, 1991, p. 66). In any society, men and women may be influenced to adopt the social mores, beliefs, attitudes, and behaviours of their gender throughout life.

Feminist writers argue that the historical power of males in Western industrial society has influenced the values, ethics, and morality of the society, as well as what is accepted as normal and abnormal (Miller, 1986). Although these attitudes are now undergoing considerable change, according to Kushland (1994, March), cultural antagonisms remain.

Theories about the Psychology of Men and Women

For almost a century, psychoanalysts have postulated that differences in the psychologies of men and women rest not only upon constitutional differences, but also upon the different ways that relationships with mothers and fathers develop for boys and girls (Freud, 1905/1953). Research suggests that core gender identity starts to form at birth and that, by age eighteen to twenty-four months, the child self-identifies as a boy or girl (Money & Erhardt, 1972; McEwan, 1991). Children of either sex have different developmental tasks as they move on from intense involvement with the mother in infancy. Chodorow (1978) proposed that girls never fully separate from their mothers, and thus attachment and relationships remain central themes for women. She further stated that 'a quality of embeddedness in social interaction and personal relationships characterizes women's life relative to men's' (Chodorow, 1989, p. 57).

On the other hand, a number of theorists argue that, for most women, the sense of self develops in the context of relationships (Chodorow, 1978; Miller, 1984, 1986; Gilligan, 1982; Gilligan, Lyons, and Hammer,

1990). Traditionally, most women need to maintain relationships through nurturing and caring. In the context of relational theory (Chodorow, 1978; Miller, 1986; Gilligan, 1982; Gilligan et al, 1990), characteristics attributed to women, such as passivity, dependence, and lack of individuality, are re-framed as positive, not negative, characteristics (Broverman et al, 1970).

Gilligan (1982), working with non-clinical samples, states that the morality of women centres on care and responsibility, compared with men, who tend to focus on rights and justice. In relationships, women focus on their attachments and caring for others. In contrast, men have, by and large, been more orientated towards issues of justice, rights, fairness, separateness, and autonomy. Gilligan's group (Brown & Gilligan, 1992; Lohr, Hamberger, & Bonge, 1988; Stapley & Haviland, 1989) also found gender-related differences in the development of self-concept and moral growth of adolescent women and men. Women tend to describe themselves in relational terms. Conversely, men tend to define themselves in terms of personal achievements and work (Vaillant & Milofsky, 1980). Brown and Gilligan (1992) theorize that sociocultural factors influence North American female adolescents not to express thoughts, feelings, or experiences that seem unacceptable to others. This suppression may be reflected in the greater incidence of depression and eating disorders among women (Hsu Lkg, 1987).

Societal expectations for men and women add to the developmental differences. Levinson (1978) argues that many men are raised to value assertiveness, independence, ambition, and will-power or 'strength of will,' and to experience emotionality, dependence, and vulnerability as a lack of self-control.

However, the literature on sex differences in personality is controversial. In particular, the findings by Gilligan (1982) of sex differences and moral development have been criticized (Walker, 1984; Damon & Colby, 1983; Tazris, 1992). In reviewing the literature on sex differences and moral development, Tazris (1992) states: 'In study after study, researchers report no average differences in the kind of moral reasoning that men and women apply' (p. 585).

There is less literature about the psychological development of adolescent men than about that of women. It is suggested that young men suppress or repress feminine aspects of themselves as they strive to fulfil societal expectations of the masculine gender role (Myers, 1991b). One key gender difference is the risk of suicide. Rates of suicide are far higher for adolescent men than for women, although adolescent women are more likely to engage in non-fatal suicidal behaviour/attempts than are males (Klerman, 1986).

Psychotherapists must not allow their knowledge of theoretical differences in the psychologies of men and women to obstruct neutrality and open-mindedness in their clinical work. The major advantage for therapists of being aware of current theories about the psychology of gender is in understanding their own biases, and thus avoiding prejudice in their views of individual men and women. In clinical medicine, the focus is on the individual, not on the group or society. Attention often focuses on problems, disorders, and circumstances that have a very low incidence in society. Therapists must be able to appreciate behaviours that occur infrequently and understand their adaptive or maladaptive nature, as distinct from their statistical normality.

Changing Family Structures and Family Breakdown

The pattern of family structures within society has changed markedly during this century. Although the traditional extended family and the nuclear family still predominate, within these families non-traditional sex roles are increasingly common. Single-parent families have burgeoned, as have reconstituted or second-marriage families. Gay and lesbian couples, living with or without children, are increasingly visible.

A body of research evidence is accumulating on the impact of family breakdown on both children and adults. 'An analysis of thirty-two studies, most of them conducted during the past fifteen years, reveals that adult children of divorced parents have more problems and lower levels of wellbeing than adults whose parents stayed married. They are depressed more frequently, feel less satisfied with life, get less education, and have less prestigious jobs. One study included 2,460 men and women from both divorced and intact families who were living in their own households. It confirmed that the impact of divorce endures throughout a person's lifetime' (Beal & Hochman, 1991, p. 73). The protective effect of marriage against affective disorders is confirmed in much of the epidemiologic literature (Robins & Reiger, 1991).

Through non-judgmental listening, therapists must be able to work with people in various new living modes, acknowledging the changes both to themselves and to their patients. New understanding through research will continue to throw light on the stresses, conflicts, and vulnerabilities experienced by individuals in a variety of family arrangements.

Gender and Psychiatric Disorders

Epidemiological and clinical studies demonstrate differential rates of psychiatric disorders between the sexes (American Psychiatric Association [APA], 1994; Robins & Reiger, 1991). Studies reveal a higher incidence among women of the following Axis I disorders: major depression; eating disorders; panic disorder with and without agoraphobia; dissociative identity disorder; and somatization disorder. The following disorders have a higher incidence among men: attention deficit disorder; substance abuse disorders; and paraphilias. For Axis II disorders, borderline personality disorder is more prevalent among women, while antisocial personality disorder, obsessive–compulsive personality disorder, and narcissistic personality disorder are more frequently diagnosed in men. Although, in clinical settings, histrionic personality disorder and dependent personality disorder are diagnosed more frequently in females, the sex ratio is not significantly different from the sex ratio of females within the respective clinical setting. For both these disorders, studies report similar prevalence rates among males and females. In discussing the gender features of personality disorders, *DSM-IV* cautions: 'Although these differences in prevalence probably reflect real gender differences in the presence of such patterns, clinicians must be cautious not to overdiagnose or underdiagnose certain Personality Disorders in females or in males because of social stereotypes about typical gender roles and behaviors' (APA, 1994, p. 632).

Women tend to seek treatment, especially psychotherapy, more frequently than do men. Men appear to have more severe psychiatric disorders, and are hospitalized more than are women.

Values, Beliefs, and Their Influence on Psychotherapy

An individual therapist's gender role and sociocultural background can affect his or her concept of what seems 'acceptable as average behaviour' and may influence the perception, diagnosis, and treatment of mental disorders (Nadelson & Notman, 1977, 1986; Person, 1983). The classic study of Broverman et al (1970) found that both male and female psychotherapists' descriptions of mature healthy persons, either male or female, reflected what was expected of mature *males* in Western society. Loring and Powell (1988) found that traditional viewpoints continue to influence concepts of gender role among therapists.

Either directly or indirectly, therapists may unintentionally communicate to patients their values about the selection of material to question or comment upon, their affective reactions to what the patient says, and the timing of interpretations.

The risk of 'contaminating' the psychotherapeutic process with a therapist's values and beliefs is a serious problem. Therapists, like everyone else, have personal beliefs and opinions about gender issues, as well as many other issues that affect the lives of patients in therapy, such as abortion, extramarital sex, welfare, tax fraud, and religious practices. It is essential that therapists strive to maintain technical neutrality with patients through non-judgmental listening and awareness of their own biases and preferences. The goals of therapy have little to do with imposing 'normality' or expectations of socially acceptable 'average behaviour' on patients.

Gender and the Process of Therapy

Integral to the process of therapy are issues related to transference, countertransference, choice of therapist, sexualization, and aggressivization of therapeutic relationships. Patients often perceive their therapists as powerful. Although this is a manifestation of transference, it may be intensified by the therapist's behaviour. In certain situations, patients may perceive their therapists as weak, which can also be a manifestation of transference.

According to Nadelson and Notman's (1991) classic conceptualization of transference, patients 'transfer' feelings and unconscious attitudes derived from their crucial early relationships to the therapist, regardless of the therapist's gender, values, and attributes. A patient in properly conducted psychiatric treatment may project either male or female transference images onto a therapist of either gender. The influence of the therapist's gender on transference has been explored by Lester (cited in Nadelson & Notman, 1991). She suggests that the gender of the analyst can be critical in the development of transference in certain cases. Nadelson and Notman (1986) argue that gender can influence the initial relationship and early transference, particularly sexualized transference. They claim that the therapist's gender may also alter the sequence in which therapeutic issues are presented by the patient, the speed at which therapy progresses, and the sequence of transference developments.

Countertransference issues may also be influenced by a therapist's gender or sociocultural background. Unacknowledged values, preferences, and prejudices can have a negative effect upon therapy.

The choice of therapist depends on conscious as well as unconscious motives. Some of the reasons for the choice may reflect patients' gender stereotypes. Women may express a variety of reasons for seeking a woman therapist, for instance, a belief that women are 'more nurturing' while men 'perpetuate patriarchal values,' a search for a role model who is an effective manager of both career and home life (Notman & Nadelson, 1978), or a hope that a woman might more readily 'empathize' with wishes for self-actualization. A woman might select a male therapist because she believes that this will be advantageous for working through her relationship with her father and/or interpersonal relationships with men. A man may choose a male therapist as a role model to work through his relationship with his father, or to receive male caring and understanding (Myers, 1991b). Concurrent with such conscious reasons for seeking a therapist of a particular gender, patient choices may be defensively determined, to avoid dealing with painful material. For instance, a man may choose a female therapist, believing that he can control her and fearing that a male therapist would control him. Both men and women may avoid therapists of either sex to protect themselves from painful feelings associated with involvements with people of that gender. There is no scientific evidence to support an advantage for the use of therapists of a particular gender with any patient population. When a patient expresses a preference for a therapist of a particular gender, it is worthwhile to explore the meaning of the stated wish. Although a psychiatrist may not choose to facilitate the patient's request, there is no justification for interfering with the patient's choice.

The sexual orientation of either therapist or patient may also influence a patient's choice of therapist. Homosexual patients frequently request homosexual therapists, in the belief that the therapist will be more understanding. A patient may be disappointed or angry and devalue the therapist if the choice was used to avoid major issues, or if the patient's expectations and fantasies about the therapist's 'magical qualities' were not fulfilled (Nadelson & Notman, 1986).

Erotic transference, as defined by Person (1985), refers to 'some mixture of affectionate, tender, erotic and sexual feeling that a patient experiences in reference to his or her analyst' (p. 161) and, as such, forms part of a positive transference. Erotic transference or transference love occurs in four treatment dyads (female patient–male therapist, male patient–female therapist, female patient–female therapist, male patient–male therapist). Blum (1973) distinguished erotized transference from erotic transference, describing it as 'an intense, vivid, irrational erotic preoccupation with the therapist, characterized by overt, seemingly ego-syntonic demands for love and sexual involvement with the therapist ... Through projection and denial they [patients] can assume their analyst indeed loves them' (p. 63).

Sexual Abuse

Therapists should be knowledgeable about the epidemiology, and the immediate and long-term psychological and physical sequelae resulting from the sexual abuse of children, adolescents, and adults. Factors that contribute to the severity of the psychological trauma include abuse at an early age, the duration of abuse, the context in which the abuse occurred, and the depth of betrayed trust. Sex abuse may be intrafamilial, extrafamilial, or stranger or date/acquaintance or marital rape. There may be repeated abuse or revictimization. Sexual abuse by professionals requires special attention. Sexual abuse is accompanied by intense fear, helplessness, or horror, acutely damaging the self. The relationship between the self and the world is traumatized; attachment bonds are fractured; internal schema are altered; and negative self-images are evoked, possibly accompanied by neurophysiological changes that lead to post-traumatic stress disorder (Horowitz, 1986; Kaufman, 1986; Janoff-Bulman, 1992; Epstein, 1991).

Currently, there is considerable controversy regarding the authenticity of memories of abuse recovered in therapy. Although therapists must be willing to explore with patients any memories of sexual abuse, it is unacceptable to suggest to a patient that he or she was abused if the patient does not remember abuse. However when patients describe experiences of sexual or physical abuse, there is usually no justification for therapists to question the truth of such reports (see chapter 2, 'General Guidelines for the Practice of Psychotherapy' and the Position Statement of the Canadian Psychiatric Association [Blackshaw, Chandarana, Garneaus, Merskey, & Moscarello, 1996])

SOME PRINCIPLES OF TREATMENT FOR VICTIMS OF
SEXUAL TRAUMA

The experience and sequelae of sexual trauma are intense and complex. Traumatized individuals experience emotions ranging from helplessness, intense fear or horror, to impotent rage, shame, prematurely awakened sexual sensations, and guilt (Levine, 1990). The recovery processes are based on reconnection with others as the victim regains a sense of self (Herman, 1992). As witnesses to the intense emotions of the patient's trauma, therapists may experience feelings of helpless terror, grief, and rage along with wishes to deny, blame, rescue, and punish their patient. Understanding or recognizing the extremely disturbing nature of the trauma, therapists may benefit from an ongoing support system to deal with their countertransference reactions.

Recovery processes occur in three main stages: establishment of safety; integration of memories and affects associated with the trauma; re-establishment of the self and social reconnection with others (Herman 1992). Traumatic experiences are varied and complex, some occurring suddenly, others transpiring over years. Recovery is particularly complex for those who experienced sexual trauma at an early age and over a lengthy period. In assessing a traumatized patient, it is essential to determine which tasks have been accomplished and what the patient is ready to do.

In the immediate aftermath of a traumatic experience, attention must be directed to establishing safety, that is, control of the body and control of the environment. The focus is on basic health needs such as sleep, nutrition, exercise, and the control of self-destructive behaviours. Safe living conditions are mandatory – including enough money, work, and safe accommodation. This stage may require non-addictive medication, stress management, and cognitive strategies, aiming for the gradual formation of reliable attachments in therapy. Stress-management techniques may be useful, as often the victims of sexual trauma feel compelled to maintain constant vigilance in order to feel safe. Social strategies to provide safety and containment may include self-help groups, social agencies, and the formal mental health care system, such as drug and alcohol detoxification, day treatment, inpatient admission, and emergency services.

Only when basic safety needs are met may it be advantageous to begin in-depth psychotherapeutic exploration of the traumatic experience. For some patients this may begin almost immediately. Other patients may require considerable time to feel safe enough to explore issues therapeutically. Therapists may err through premature and over-zealous psychotherapeutic exploration. Or a therapist may maintain a focus on the patient's safety rather than exploring the trauma, to protect the therapist from distress. Within the therapeutic alliance, the purpose is to integrate the trauma through careful exploration of dissociated or repressed aspects of memory, cognition, and affects. Once the victim becomes aware of the full extent of his or her losses, a major depression may ensue. The victim is sustained through this painful process by the therapeutic alliance, peer support, and the hope of restoring or building non-coercive relationships, as well as an ability to view the trauma with new meaning and acceptance.

The third stage is the establishment or re-establishment of social connections. Group psychotherapy may assist this stage, allowing the resolution of secrecy, shame, and stigma in a manner that is not possible in individual therapy. It is only at this final stage that confrontation of the abuser or families might be undertaken. Patients' motives for confrontation are mixed and complex. When they involve revenge or the anticipation of an apology or acknowledgment of the abuse by the abuser, or abusers, the outcome may well be unsatisfactory. One positive benefit of a frank discussion of the trauma is that it may alter family relationships (Gelinas, 1993). If the patient chooses to bring up the fact of sexual abuse with the perpetrator, this may – depending on the patient – be therapeutic if it is not a substitute for working through. However, in all cases, the decision to confront must be made by the patient; otherwise it is a repetition of coercion and, in that sense, a repetition of abuse.

Outcome studies on the use of particular forms of therapy during each of the three stages of the recovery process are required. Imaginal exposure and stress management may be effective strategies for overcoming post-traumatic stress disorder (Foa, Rothbaum, Riggs, & Murdock, 1991). A review of thirty-five studies reported in 1997 finds psychotherapy has a beneficial impact on some severe mental disorders including borderine personality disorder (Gabbard, Lazar, Hornberger, & Spiegel, 1997). Further research could explore the utility of psychoeducational groups during the first stage of recovery, the indications for individual and group psychodynamic therapies, and other related issues.

In summary, for victims of sexual trauma, multiple forms and models of psychotherapy are used in different stages of the recovery process.

Gender Configurations in Individual Treatment: Four Treatment Dyads

1 *Male therapist–female patient:* This is both the most common and the most studied dyad. Despite concerns about potential problems in cross-gender psychotherapy, outcome studies demonstrate that this configuration can be highly efficacious. In fact, some women who have experi-

enced abuse in previous relationships with male figures seek out male therapists to work through those issues. Therapist empathy can be enhanced by knowledge of recent theories about the psychological development of girls and women, and of the changing social roles for women and men.

This most frequent dyad is also the one about which we have the most information concerning sexual boundary violations. Therapists who have sex with patients often include those with narcissitic, perverse, and antisocial personalities (Twemlow & Gabbard, 1989); depressed therapists, during or after divorce or relationship losses; and those who have become psychotic. Acting on an erotic countertransference leads to 'a complete defeat for the treatment' (Freud, 1915/1958, p. 166). However, awareness of the erotic countertransference is extremely helpful in recognizing and understanding what is emerging in the patient during treatment. Acting out the erotic countertransference deprives the patient of a chance to analyse her own erotic transference and related difficulties. Hence, a thorough understanding of the role of countertransference, including eroticism, feelings of inferiority or intimidation, omnipotence, and defensive hostility, can reduce boundary violations.

Therapists of both sexes, working in depth with patients, have learned to spot both maternal and paternal transferences (Klein, 1945; Winnicott, 1955; Bowlby, 1958; Meyers, 1986; Chasseguet-Smirgel, 1988). Because males, in the course of their development (at least in part), have to disidentify with their mothers to form a male identity, some male therapists may have difficulty in identifying with the patient's maternal transferences (Liebert, 1986), leading them to miss important therapeutic opportunities.

Countertransference pitfalls can emerge in a climate in which male–female reactions are discussed in very ideological terms that tend to absolutize gender differences as irreconcilable. Both patient and therapist may steer clear of any discussion about contentious gender issues, fearing to disrupt the therapeutic calm. Or gender issues can be discussed defensively by both parties, as a cover for dealing with other issues.

Some women patients insist on a male therapist, and then idealize or devalue him in transference repetitions. Those who idealize their male therapists may be subtly devaluing themselves. Feeling flattered in the countertransference, some therapists may be tempted to take this idealization at face value without analysing the woman's sense of inferiority or self-devaluation.

Or a patient may devalue a male therapist by insisting he is psychologically incapable of understanding her *because* he is male. These devaluations may be pre-emptive accusations that cover a woman's fear of rejection, fear of closeness, or feelings that she is weak, unlovable, bad, or competitive. In the countertransference, the male therapist may accept the devaluation at face value. It may awaken his own doubts about his male identity. He may feel impotent, or try to prove the accusations unfounded, and retaliate, rather than collaboratively exploring the motives for the devaluation and the associated transference.

2 *Female therapist–female patient:* As increasing numbers of women enter the fields of medicine and psychiatry, there are now more women practising medical psychotherapy. Some women prefer to be treated by female psychiatrists, believing that a female therapist has more knowledge and empathic understanding of female problems, such as premenstrual dysphoria; menopause; therapeutic abortion; breast disease; sexual dysfunction; adult sequelae of childhood sexual abuse; lesbianism; and the life-balancing dilemmas of paid work and family. It is common for a female patient to idealize her female therapist as someone who has achieved both professional success and a happy personal life. Although in this way the therapist provides a positive role model, envy can be an important affect to explore in the transference.

Countertransference issues for female therapists in treating women include overly gratifying the patient's needs; not setting appropriate limits (i.e., an unrealistic 'need to be liked'); accepting projected patient idealization; overidentification with the patient (because of female gender); colluding in the idealization of women and the devaluation of men in order to ward off heterosexual anxieties; and boundary violations (e.g., socializing with the patient; not charging fees for missed appointments).

3 *Male therapist–male patient:* This is also a common dyad. Potential difficulties may surface when men treat men about issues such as intellectualization; competition; power struggles; denial of affective issues; fear of homosexual feelings; role-blurring; and discomfort. Some male therapists may experience more difficulty expressing sensitivity, kindness, and compassion to male patients than to female patients. An empathic attitude is beneficial not only for understanding patients, but also for modelling another way of relating to others. This can help male patients to overcome any misunderstandings they may harbour about non-erotic tenderness between men.

Conflicts about control and power dynamics commonly emerge in this dyad. Male patients often fight regression in the transference and ward off feelings of dependency and inferiority when being treated by men (Dickstein et al, 1991). Hence, they may stop therapy or avoid dealing with deeper issues, especially 'shameful' matters such as relationship failures, sexual abuse, or assault (Myers, 1989), erectile dysfunction, and homosexual or bisexual issues. Or, they might adopt a highly intellectualized stance about such troubles and fail to express feelings that accompany them.

Countertransference issues common to the four dyads in psychotherapy, highlighted in the male–male dyad include competition (to demonstrate power or skill), intellectual defences against powerful and often frightening feelings that may arise in treatment (rage, jealousy, shame, love for a male patient), not noticing maternal transference, and boundary violations (therapists accepting investment tips, engaging in collusive behaviour, becoming involved sexually).

4 *Female therapist–male patient:* This is probably the least common dyad. Some male patients may believe that a female therapist will provide extraordinary empathy and nurturing. For instance, a man may seek a female therapist, hoping she may have greater sensitivity about issues such as sexual orientation, sexual trauma, or sexual dysfunctions. Transference feelings may have a dependent cast. Some men develop erotic feelings for their therapist, or they may try to control the female therapist.

Countertransference issues can present challenges such as dealing with aggression or the need to be in control; experiencing some male patients as sexist; managing (and therapeutically using) erotic transference; accepting and understanding erotic countertransference; guarding against overly gratifying a patient's dependency needs; anticipating, and not avoiding, male sexual fantasies; and watching for boundary violations.

Gender and Couple Therapy

There are three broad gender issues in couple therapy: (1) the content and substance of the couple's complaints; their conflicts may be rooted in gender values, expectations, roles, and their own socialization process; (2) the gender and sexual orientation of each member of a couple, e.g., heterosexual, homosexual (gay or lesbian); and (3) the gender and sexual orientation of the therapist. Co-therapists may be same-sexed or opposite-sexed. Together with the diversity of couples requesting treatment, gender issues can lead to varied alliances and incongruities.

With respect to gender roles, women more readily seek therapy than do men. Many women assume that it is their 'problem,' while their male partners (who appear strong and independent on the surface) may try to avoid therapy (Dickstein, 1991). Therapists who recognize the gender gap – namely, that girls are often socialized to 'take care of others' and that boys are socialized to deny vulnerability and be autonomous – may be more willing to take on couple therapy. Dual-career couples come to therapy with a range of conflicts, including some related to changing sex-role expectations, either at work or at home (Alger, 1991).

Heterosexual couples may have both competitive and complementary attitudes. There may be some sex-role reversal and fluidity, which enhances the couple's solidarity and richness (for example, *she* may do some mechanical repairs, while *he* cooks). The therapist's role is to explore couple conflicts in order to understand openly and objectively what generates the problems.

If one member of a couple has experienced some type of past trauma by a central male or female figure, he or she may enter treatment fearing repeat injury. Therapists must be particularly attuned to this possibility when they treat couples in which one or other has been sexually abused, physically assaulted abandoned, or sexually abused in previous therapy (Nadelson & Polonsky, 1991).

Same-sex relationship problems are more similar than different to those of heterosexual couples. However, there are some noteworthy specifics. In male homosexual couples there are often communication barriers owing to an inability to be 'in touch' with feelings, inability to express them openly to one's partner, and a tendency to act out conflicts sexually rather than communicating concerns verbally. Male homosexual couples may have conflicting attitudes towards sexual fidelity. In the male homosexual couple, competition may reflect the dynamics of a father–son relationship. Both may struggle to varying degrees with their homosexual identity. They may disagree on how 'out' each should be with his homosexuality. There may be conflict with families of origin and children. In some couples, living with HIV is an ongoing and severe stress (Friedman, 1991). In lesbian couples, problems include a sense of 'accommodation and nurturance,' with a tendency towards fusion or merger; issues of independence, differentiation, and individual development; acceptance of emotional intimacy and affection (with reduced emphasis on sexual expression); lack of social support or endorsement for the relationship; conflicts about childbearing or joint parenting of children (as a couple); and, in some cases, living with HIV (Kirkpatrick, 1991).

The gender of the therapist or therapists can play a crucial role in couple therapy. One member of the heterosexual couple may be comforted by having a same-sex therapist, while the other may be fearful. Opposite-sex co-therapists might be welcomed by heterosexual couples, but same-sex co-therapists may cause anxiety. Therapists must strive to recognize concerns of *both* the man and the woman. Understanding homophobia is essential for working with same-sex couples (Myers, 1991a).

Skill and Attitude Obectives Regarding Gender Issues

- To be aware of one's own gender-role socialization and its impact upon oneself, patient relationships, and the therapeutic process.
- To employ language and behaviour that is respectful and sensitive to the impact of gender-role socialization on the individual.
- To avoid the use of gender-role stereotypes, which can obscure understanding of the individual patient.
- To evaluate the literature critically in order to be aware of and identify gender bias, as well as bias towards race, ethnicity, sexual orientation, age, and ability.
- To be aware of and respectful towards the trust placed by patients in the therapist, also acknowledging the potential for abuse of power in therapist–patient relationships.

References

Alger, I. (1991). Marital therapy with dual-career couples. *Psychiatric Annals, 21*, 455–458.

American Psychiatric Association (APA). (1994). *Diagnostic and statistical manual of mental disorders* (4th Ed.). Washington, DC: Author.

Beal, E.W., & Hochman, G. (1991). *Adult children of divorce*. New York: Delacorte.

Bishop, J. (1992). Guidelines for a non-sexist (gender-sensitive) doctor–patient relationship. *Canadian Journal of Psychiatry, 37*, 62–65.

Blackshaw, S., Chandarana, P., Garneaus, Y., Merskey, H., & Moscarello, R. (1996). Position statement: Adult recovered memories of childhood sexual abuse. *Canadian Journal of Psychiatry, 41*, 305–306.

Bleier, R. (1991). Gender ideology and the brain: Sex differences research. In M.K. Notman & C.C. Nadelson (Eds.), *Women and men: New perspectives on gender differences*. Washington, DC: American Psychiatric Press.

Blum, H.P. (1973). The concept of erotized transference. *Journal of the American Psychoanalytic Association, 21*, 61–76.

Bowlby, J. (1958). The nature of the child's tie to his mother. *International Journal of Psycho-Analysis 39*, 350.

Broverman, I., Broverman, D., & Clarkson, F., Rosenkrantz, P.S., & Vogel, S.R. (1970). Sex role stereotypes and clinical judgements of mental health. *Journal of Consulting and Clinical Psychology, 34*, 1–7.

Brown, L.M., & Gilligan, L. (1992). *Meeting at the crossroads: Women's Psychology and Girl's Development*. Cambridge, MA: Harvard University Press.

Chasseguet-Smirgel, J. (1988). Archaic matrix to the Oedipus complex: Theory, technique. *Psychoanalytic Quarterly, 57*, p. 505.

Chodorow, N.J. (1978). *The reproduction of mothering*. Berkeley: University of California Press.

Chodorow, N.J. (1989). *Feminism and psychoanalytic theory*. New Haven, CT: Yale University Press.

Damon, W., & Colby, A. (1983). Listening to a different voice: A review of Carol Gilligan's 'In a Different Voice.' *Merril Palmer Quarterly, 29*, 475.

Deaux, K. (1984). From individual differences to social categories: Analysis of a decade's research on gender. *American Psychologist, 39*, 105–116.

Dickstein, L.J. (1991). Marital therapy with university students in the 1990s. *Psychiatric Annals, 21*, 471–478.

Dickstein, L.J., Stein, T.S., Pleck, J.H., Myers, M.F., Lewis, R.A., Duncan, S.F., & Brod, H. (1991). Men changing social roles in the 1990s: Emerging issues in the psychiatric treatment of men. *Hospital and Community Psychiatry, 42*, 701–705.

Epstein, S. (1991). The self-concept, the traumatic neurosis and the structure of personality. In D. Ozer, J. M. Healy, Jr, & R.A.J. Stewart (Eds.), *Perspectives on personality* (Vol. 3). Greenwich, CT: JAI.

Foa, E.B., Rothbaum, R.O., Riggs, D.S., & Murdock, T.B. (1991). Treatment of post-traumatic stress disorder in rape victims: A comparison between cognitive-behavioural procedures and counselling. *Journal of Consulting and Clinical Psychology, 59*, 715–723.

Francoeur, R.T. (1991). *A descriptive dictionary and atlas of sexology*. New York: Greenwood.

Freud, S. (1905/1953). Three essays on the theory of sexuality. In J. Strachey (Ed. and Trans.), *The standard edition of the works of Sigmund Freud* (Vol. 7, pp. 125–245). London: Hogarth Press. (Original work published 1905)

Freud, S. (1915/1958). Observations on transference love. In J. Strachey (Ed. and

Trans.), *The standard edition of the works of Sigmund Freud* (Vol. 12, pp. 157–173). London: Hogarth Press. (Original work published 1915)

Friedman, R.C. (1991). Couple therapy with gay couples. *Psychiatric Annals, 21,* 485–490.

Gabbard, G.O., Lazar, S.G., Hornberger, G., & Spiegel, D. (1997). The economic impact of psychotherapy: A review. *American Journal of Psychiatry, 151,* 147–155.

Gelinas, D. (1993). Relational patterns in incestuous families: Malevolent variations and specific variations with adult survivors. In P.L. Paddison (Ed.), *Treatment of adult survivors of incest.* Washington, DC: American Psychiatric Press.

Gilligan, C. (1982). *In a different voice: Psychological theory and women's development.* Cambridge, MA: Harvard University Press.

Gilligan, C., Lyons, P., & Hammer, T.J. (Eds.). (1990). *Making connections: The relationship worlds of adolescent girls at Emma Willard School.* Cambridge, MA: Harvard University Press.

Herman, J.L. (1992). *Trauma and recovery.* New York: Basic.

Horowitz, M. J. (1986). Psychological response to serious life events. In D. Hamilton & D.M. Warburton (Eds.), *Human stress and cognition: An information processing approach* (pp. 237–265). Chichester, England: Wiley.

Hsu Lkg. (1987). An overview of the eating disorders. In J.D. Noshpitz (Ed.), *Basic handbook of child psychiatry* (Vol. 5, pp. 374–386). New York: Basic.

Janoff-Bulman, R. (1992). *Shattered assumptions: Towards a new psychology of trauma.* New York: Free Press.

Kaufman, G. (1985). *Shame: the power of caring* (Rev. ed.). Boston: Schenkman.

Kirkpatrick, M. (1991). Lesbian couples in therapy. *Psychiatric Annals, 21,* 491–496.

Klein, M. (1945). The Oedipus complex in the light of early anxieties. *International Journal of Psycho-Analysis, 26,* p. 11.

Klerman, G.L. (Ed.). (1986). *Suicide and depression among adolescents and young adults.* Washington, DC: American Psychiatric Press.

Kushland, D.E., Jr. (1994, March). Science: Women in science. *Comparisons across Cultures, 263,* 1355.

Levine, H. (Ed.) (1990). *Adult analysis and childhood sexual abuse.* Hillsdale, NJ: Analytic Press.

Levinson, D.J. (1978). *Seasons of man's life.* New York: Knopf.

Liebert, R. (1986). Transference and countertransference issues in the treatment of women by a male analyst. In H. Meyers (Ed.), *Between patient and analyst.* Hillsdale, NJ: The Analytic Press.

Lohr, J.M., Hamberger, L.K., & Bonge, D. (1988). The relationship of factorially validated measures of anger-proneness and irrational beliefs. *Motivation and Emotion, 12,* 171–183.

Loring, M., & Powell, B.J. (1988). Gender, race and DSM-III: A study of objectivity of psychiatric diagnostic behaviour. *Journal Health and Social Behavior, 29*, 1–22.

McEwan, B.S. (1991). Sex differences in the brain: What they are and how they arise. In M.T. Notman & C.C. Nadelson (Eds.), *Women and men: New perspectives on gender differences*. Washington, DC: American Psychiatric Press.

Merriam Webster Dictionary. (1994). Springfield, MA: Merriam-Webster.

Meyers, H. (1986). Analytic work by and with women. In H. Meyers (Ed.), *Between patient and analyst*. Hillsdale, NJ: The Analytic Press.

Miller, J.B. (1984). *The development of women's sense of self (Work in progress no. 12).* Wellesley, MA: Stoner Center Working Paper Series.

Miller, J.B. (1986). *Towards a new psychology of women* (2d ed.). Boston: Beacon.

Money, J., & Erhardt, A.A. (1972). *Man and woman, boy and girl: The differentiation and dimorphism of gender identity from conception to maturity.* Baltimore: Johns Hopkins University Press.

Myers, M.F. (1989). Men sexually assaulted as adults and sexually abused as boys. *Archives of Sexual Behaviour, 18*, 203–215.

Myers, M.F. (1991a). Marital therapy with HIV-infected men and their wives. *Psychiatric Annals, 21*, 466–470.

Myers, M.F. (1991b). Men's unique development issues across the lifecycle. In A. Tasman & S.M. Goldfinger (Eds.), *American Psychiatric Association Press review of psychiatry* (Vol. 10). Washington, DC: American Psychiatric Press.

Nadelson, C.C., & Notman, M.T. (1977). Psychotherapy supervision: The problem of conflicting values. *American Journal of Psychotherapy, 31*, 275–283.

Nadelson, C.C., & Notman, M.T. (1986). Psychotherapy and women: Changing issues. In J.H. Masserman, & F.L. Orlando (Eds.), *Current psychiatric therapies* (Vol. 23, pp. 13–25). Orlando: Grune & Stratton.

Nadelson, C.C., & Notman, M.T. (1991). The impact of new psychology of men and women in psychotherapy. In A. Tasman & S.M. Goldfinger (Eds.), *American Psychiatric Association Press review of psychiatry* (Vol. 10). Washington, DC: American Psychiatric Press.

Nadelson, C.C., & Polonsky, D. (1991). Childhood sexual abuse: The invisible ghost in couple therapy. *Psychiatric Annals, 21*, 479–484.

Notman, M.T., & Nadelson, C.C. (1978). *Sexual and Reproductive Aspects of Women's Health Care: Vol. 1. The Woman Patient.* New York: Plenum.

Notman, M.T., Zilbach, J.J., Miller, J.B., & Nadelson, C.C. (1986). Themes in psychoanalytic understanding of women: Some reconsiderations of autonomy and affiliation. *Journal of American Academy of Psychoanalysis, 14*, 241–253.

Person, E.S. (1983). The influence of values in psychoanalysis: The case of female psychology. Psychiatry update. In L. Grinspoon (Ed.), *The American Psychiatric Annual Review* (Vol. 2). Washington, DC: American Psychiatric Press.

Person, E.S. (1985). The erotic transference in women and in men: Differences and consequences. *Journal of the American Academy of Psychoanalysis, 13,* 159–180.

Robins, L., & Reiger, D. (Eds.). (1991). *Psychiatric disorders in America: The epidemiologic catchment area study.* New York: Free Press.

Stapley, J., & Haviland, J. (1989). Beyond depression: Gender differences in normal adolescents' emotional experiences. *Sex Roles, 20,* 295–308.

Tavris, C. (1992). *The mismeasure of women: Why women are not the better sex, the inferior sex or the opposite sex.* New York: Simon & Shuster.

Twemlow, S.W., & Gabbard, G.O. (1989). The lovesick therapist. In G.O. Gabbard (Ed.), *Sexual exploitation in professional relationships.* Washington, DC: American Psychiatric Press.

Vaillant, G.E., & Milofsky, E. (1980). Natural history of male psychological health, IX: Empirical evidence for Erikson's model of life cycle. *American Journal of Psychiatry, 137,* 1348–1359.

Walker, L.J. (1984). Sex differences in the development of moral reasoning: A critical review. *Child Development, 55,* 677–691.

Winnicott, D.W. (1955). Transitional objects and transitional phenomena. *International Journal of Psycho-Analysis, 34,* p. 89.

Worell, J., & Remer, P. (1992). *Feminist perspectives in therapy: An empowerment model for women.* Chichester, England: Wiley.

17. Cultural Issues in Psychotherapy

Ronald Ruskin and Morton Beiser

According to one of the field's authorities (Wolberg, 1967), psychotherapy is 'treatment, by psychological means, of problems of an emotional nature in which a trained person deliberately establishes a professional relationship with the patient with the object of 1) removing, modifying, or retarding existing symptoms, 2) mediating disturbed patterns of behaviour, and 3) promoting positive personality growth and development' (p. 3).

This thirty-year-old definition articulates important goals for practice. However, radical changes in Canadian and U.S. society are challenging what once seemed unassailable philosophical tenets – the tenets of psychotherapeutic practice among them.

During the past two decades, immigration has transformed Canada from a country dominated by citizens of Euro-American stock into a mosaic of cultures, languages, and expectations. 'In place of Europe and the U.S. – traditional sources of immigration from the time of Confederation until 1960 Asia, Africa, the Middle East and Latin America now account for more than 75% of Canada's new settlers' (Beiser, Dion, Gotowiec, Hyman, & Vu, 1995, p. 68).

The mother tongue of nearly 50 per cent of the population of contemporary Metropolitan Toronto is a language other than English. Legislation, including the Canadian Charter, the Health Care Act, and the Multiculturalism Act, enshrines a pledge to honour diverse cultural heritages and to ensure ethnoculturally blind equity in health care access.

Although the United States has not adopted a multiculturalism policy like Canada's (in fact, no other country has), the cultural transformation of the world's most powerful nation is equally undeniable.

Despite legislation that should guarantee equity, immigrants and ethnic minorities in Canada underutilize the mental health care system in comparison with members of the majority culture (Beiser, Gill, & Edwards, 1993; Munroe-Blum et al, 1989; Canadian Task Force on Mental Health Issues Affecting Immigrants and Refugees, 1988). The trend also exists in the United States.

Service underutilization probably stems in part from attitudes held by potential consumers and in part from blocks within the mental health care system. In a study in Seattle, Sue and Morishima (1981) demonstrated that Asians were far less likely than Caucasians to follow through on a referral for mental health consultation.

The stigma of mental illness leads many Asians to avoid mental health care (Nguyen, 1984; Lin, Tardiff, Donetz, & Goresky, 1978; Lin & Lin, 1978). Consumer attitudes are only part of the problem; treatment system barriers also play a role. For example, even though research has suggested that psychotherapy is as likely to benefit blacks as whites (Rosenthal & Frank, 1958), blacks with mental health problems receive more somatic treatment (Glazer, Morgenstern, & Doucetre, 1994) and less of other kinds of care (Solomon, 1988). Premature termination of therapy occurs more commonly among Asians than among Caucasians (Sue & Morishima, 1981).

'Ethnic groups in Canada avoid the mental health system because they feel that barriers impeding access to appropriate services are often insurmountable. They also feel that, even if they sometimes succeed in overcoming barriers, the treatment they receive is inappropriate or ineffective. These feelings are not confined to small communities or recent arrivals. Large cultural groups who have been in Canada for generations also feel disenfranchised from care' (Canadian Task Force, 1988, p. 37).

Social and cultural factors not only contribute to the patient's state of health or disorder, but affect each phase of the help-seeking behaviours, resource utilization, treatment, therapist selection, and outcome.

Culture and Psychotherapy

According to Foulks (1980), 'culture plays a major role in shaping how we think, behave, feel. Culture determines how and by whom children are raised, how they are fed ... how they acquire rules of behaviour, how they are punished, and how they learn about sex, gender roles, and marriage. Culture may affect personal psychology and shape character. Culture provides standards and values according to how one evaluates one's self, one's group, and outsiders. Culture provides guidelines and rules for recognizing and diagnosing emotional illness, for its management, and at times, its treatment' (p. 812)

Culture shapes the attitudes of both therapists and healers. It is, however, important to recognize that culture is not a monolith: each of the participants in the healing encounter belongs to, and is influenced by, more than one culture, as well as by individual history and circumstance.

Psychotherapists are the products of a professional culture as well as of their own unique backgrounds. Psychiatry or medical psychotherapy is a sociopolitical system with unique, often implicit ideologies. 'Mental health professionals use normative criteria to define mental health and illness ... normalcy and deviancy are seen through the cultural lens of the dominant group in society' (Casimir & Morrison, 1993, p. 548). Criticism has been often directed at psychiatrists who fail to explore or confront the role of culture in the diagnosis of mental illness (Fernando, 1991; Pinderhughes, 1989). Similar criticisms might be levelled at psycho-therapists who remain blind and deaf to cultural factors that influence themselves, their patients, their psychotherapeutic approach, and the institutional systems in which they work (Gibbs, 1985).

A Cultural Framework for Psychotherapy

Most cultures have rituals that rely on psychological and social means to alleviate symptoms and promote personal growth. The Euro-American–inspired ritual of psychotherapy is a variant on a universal theme of psychologically and socially induced healing, its particular form and process shaped by local traditions and values.

In some cultures, the therapeutic potency of ritual depends in part on its mystery. The healer knows esoteric, sometimes supernatural, secrets that are hidden from most people; he or she is expected to guard that knowledge from everyone except privileged disciples. This is less true for healers in North America, a culture that values science, empiricism, and pragmatism. The recent contraction of health care resources combined with the supremacy of scientific discourse has resulted in demands for the demystification of psychotherapy, for clear articulation of its principles, and for explicit rationales for practice.

This chapter addresses the role of culture with respect to some of the major elements of psychotherapeutic practice. These include assessment, the therapeutic contract, explanation, myth, metaphor, and meaning, transference/countertransference, therapist matching and outcome, boundary issues, teaching, training, and research.

ASSESSMENT

Accurate assessment – by both clinician and patient – is a prerequisite for successful therapy. The therapist's assessment is the most explicit, but not the only one to take place during a therapeutic encounter. A trained therapist elicits patient symptoms and experiences, searching for patterns that will lead to a diagnosis.

Although it is only one of a number of influences, culture affects patient reports of symptoms. According to Draguns (1987), 'the way a person expresses and experiences psychopathology is the joint result of the disorder in question, the person's personality, and the culture in which it occurs.' (p. 59). The balance in Draguns's formulation is important. On the one hand, he calls attention to the influence of cultural context in shaping symptom expression; on the other hand, the statement provides a caution against the sometimes excessive claims of cultural relativists (e.g., Obeyesekere, 1985). Culture alone cannot explain the phenomenology of illness: processes inherent in a particular disorder and personal idiosyncrasy are also important determinants of psychopathological expression.

Although many theoreticians working in cross-cultural psychiatry have focused their attention on culturally unique expression, contemporary research tends to demonstrate more cross-cultural similarity than difference in many disorders, including schizophrenia (World Health Organization [WHO], 1973), and major depressive disorder (MDD) (Beiser, Cargo, & Woodbury, 1994). Human physiology probably limits the range of expression of human suffering.

Culture does, however, exert a profound effect on explanations and categorizations of psychiatric disorders. For example, even though Asians probably experience MDD in the same way as North American Caucasians (Beiser et al, 1994), they are, as a whole, far less likely to voluntarily disclose their symptoms (Cheung, Lau, & Waldman 1980–1981). Because they do not consider depressive symptoms appropriate currency for a health care encounter (Tung, 1980), many Asians emphasize their somatic, rather than their psychic, symptoms. The popular but misleading aphorism 'Asians somatize and North Americans psychologize' (Kleinman, 1980; Tseng, 1975) has resulted from mistaking a culturally determined style of reporting distress for a culturally shaped difference in its experience.

In an initial clinical encounter, clinicians elicit symptoms, and then incorporate these into a diagnostic formulation that includes judgments about the most appropriate treatment and the most likely prognosis. Ethnoracial and class distinctions can vitiate the reliability and validity of the diagnostic process (Kramer, 1969; WHO, 1973; Beiser, 1985; Fernando, 1991; Loring & Powell, 1988). Black patients are at greater risk of receiving erroneous diagnoses – including schizophrenia – than whites (Adebimpe, 1981, 1994; Jones & Gray, 1986; Lawson, 1986; Glazer et al, 1994), Italians of being perceived through the distorting lens of stereotypes regarding their emotionality and tendency to dramatize (Zola, 1963, 1973).

Official North American psychiatric nomenclatures, from the American Psychiatric Association's first *Diagnostic and Statistical Manual of Mental Disorders* (*DSM-I* (American Psychiatric Association [APA], 1952) through its third incarnation, the *DSM-III-R* (APA, 1987), paid scant attention to culture. *DSM-IV* (APA, 1994), improves the situation by incorporating discussion about cultural variations in the clinical presentations of disorders described in the manual. Because it exoticizes cultural considerations rather than making them integral to every clinical encounter, an appendix that describes cultural-bound syndromes is of dubious value. However, future publication of a casebook describing the process of cultural formulation may help redress the situation.

Although diagnosis is usually thought of as a one-way process in which a physician observes, questions, and evaluates a patient, this is only part of the story. As John Donne (Coffin, 1952) observed over three hundred years ago, 'I observe the physician with the same diligence as he the disease.'

Cultural difference affects patient perceptions: 'While therapists diagnose their patients, the clients are deciding whether their potential therapist is likely to help them. Premature termination of treatment is a major problem. Many ethnic patients do not continue treatment after their first mental care contact and as many as half drop-out before five contacts. The most common reason for dropping out of treatment is because of negative feelings towards therapists. Clients often suspect that their therapist is racist. Unfortunately, clients rarely discuss these feelings with the therapist or anyone else' (Canadian Task Force, 1988, p. 40).

ESTABLISHING A THERAPEUTIC CONTRACT

No psychotherapist, no matter what form of therapy he or she practises, could fail to agree on the fundamental importance of establishing a therapist–client relationship of comfort and trust. Conviction and good intention, however, can guarantee neither comfort nor trust.

Structural aspects of psychotherapy may create relationship problems. For example, although Wolberg's (1967) definition takes for granted that the relationship will be a dyad, many African, Asian, Middle Eastern, and First Nations patients would expect to be seen together with their families. Many of Canada's ethnocultural communities do not subscribe to the model of the person as an individual and do not place great store in the value of individualism, two concepts that are implicit components of traditional psychotherapy. In sociocentric, as opposed to egocentric, societies, the person does not exist apart from the social group. Individual identity is always subsumed under the mantle of family.

Drawing on her experience with the West Coast Salish, Jilek-Aall (1976) comments that, during an Indian healing ceremony, the family members, relatives, neighbours, and friends take part in the procedure. The sick person experiences the support of all these people, but in Western psychotherapy he or she is alone and feels unprotected.

Therapist–patient differences in expectation militate against the establishment of a relationship. Although Western-trained psychotherapists expect to carry out talking therapy, their patients may have different views about the proper conduct of a health care encounter. Kinzie (1981), for example, points out that Southeast Asian patients expect all physicians, including psychiatrists, to take a careful medical history and to perform a physical examination. Fulfilling this expectation enhances the therapist's credibility. Touching may be comforting to patients who fear they may have an incurable disease or who feel disfigured. Many First Nations, as well as Southeast Asian, patients expect quick symptom relief. They are not prepared to accept the therapeutic dictum that problems that have taken a long time to develop may take a long time to resolve. A number of authorities (Kinzie, 1981; Tseng, 1975; Jilek-Aall, 1976) recommend the judicious use of medication to help fulfil a patient's hope for quick relief. Having established an initial rapport, the therapist may then be able to persuade the patient to explore relationships between the occurrence of symptoms and stressful circumstances or other psychodynamic issues.

Empathy is a *sine qua non* for a meaningful relationship. The capacity of the medical psychotherapist to narratively contextualize and empathically respond to the patient's distress is a crucial element in reducing suffering (Laub & Auerhan, 1985; Ornstein, 1995). However, a patient who describes experiences that a therapist has difficulty imagining, let alone has shared, taxes empathic ability. Exposure to extreme phenomena in clinical work requires the psychotherapist to draw closer to the experience of the other, to see, to know, even when traditional diagnostic categories may be of dubious value. Survivors of atrocities in Nazi concentration camps were for some time denied appropriate treatment and compensation because the examining psychiatrists were unable to comprehend the enormity of their suffering. Niederland (1964) for example, cites the chief psychiatrist in a German university clinic who, after examining a concentration camp survivor, concluded that the patient was 'quite young when he experienced the persecution and that he therefore could hardly have recollection of this period' (p. 461).

This anecdote was not, unfortunately, an isolated instance of attentional fatigue. Although post-traumatic stress disorder is now widely recognized, many diagnosticians of an earlier generation who assessed Holocaust survivors suffered from a failure of *imagination of individual suffering*. Refugees who have fled horrors in Cambodia, El Salvador, Bosnia, or Rwanda, and North American victims of circumstance such as street people and battered women, challenge the imaginative capacity of contemporary psychiatrists. Danieli (1985) suggests that traditional mental health training 'does not usually prepare professionals to deal with *massive, real, adult traumata* and their life-long effects' (p. 31). In a similar tone, Parson (1985) writes: 'therapeutic work towards mastery of traumatic stress reactions and disorders with ethnic group persons is a painstaking process for both therapist and patient ... Therapists are encouraged to study, seek supervision, re-examine their own ethnocentrism, and maintain an openness to learn from their clients ... it is virtually impossible to make patients feel understood and empathically confirmed if the therapist does not comprehend the patient's cultural-behavioural norms. This is especially true when the patient has been traumatized' (p. 333).

Courageous self-examination can help clinicians surmount empathic barriers produced by clinician–patient differences in experience and culture. Empathic communication can also help correct inappropriate judgments about suitability for therapy. Pinderhughes (1989) appropriates two acronyms from earlier work to describe psychotherapy selection biases: YAVIS, young, attractive, verbal, intelligent, and sophisticated patients, are the group most likely to be considered 'appropriate' for therapy, while QUOID, the quiet, ugly, old, indigent, and *dissimilar*, are the least likely to be selected. A rigid fixation on the primacy of insight, verbal expressiveness, personal agency, reflection on past events, and individualism, rather than approaches centred in the present and focused on discrete behavioural change within the group, family, and community, can be used to justify current, but perhaps short-sighted, decisions about who would or would not benefit from psychotherapy.

EXPLANATION

Sick and distressed individuals always ask the questions 'Why me?' and 'Why now?' and 'Who (or what) is to blame?' Both patient and clinician will inevitably search for an explanation that draws upon cultural conceptions of illness and the body, individual experience and training, and cultural views about what healers do. The result, what Kleinman (1980) calls an 'explanatory model of illness,' guides the clinician's response to his or her patients' sometimes unspoken questions about their illnesses, as well as the patients' readiness to accept explanations they are offered.

Patient and clinician explanatory models do not always match. For example, although Western physicians' explanatory models focus on disease, that is, on biological events, patients often focus on illness, the psychocultural construction of a biological upset (Beiser, Flavel, & Collomb, 1975; Kleiman, 1977; Manson, Shore & Bloom, 1985). Kleinman (1982) used structured interviews and strict *DSM-III* (APA, 1980) criteria to assess patients in Hunan, China, who had been locally diagnosed as neurasthenic. Based on the structured clinical assessments, Kleinman was able to rediagnose many patients as depressed, thereby justifying their treatment with tricyclic antidepressants. Although many experienced some relief, they continued to complain of symptoms. Kleinman felt that at least three-quarters of the patients in his sample were using sick-role behaviour to negotiate a change in what they considered an intolerable work situation. Until the situation altered, the patients could not accept an explanation centred on internal feeling states.

Explanatory models are not immutable. For example, for almost twenty years, Kinzie (1981) has directed an outpatient service for Southeast Asian refugees in which psychotherapeutic practice follows principles of exploring and resolving conflict operative in most so-called mainstream services. First-generation Southeast Asian immigrants do not, on the whole, initially come to therapy sharing their treatment clinicians' assumptions about the nature of psychological symptoms. Kinzie's highly successful work with Southeast Asians involves a sensitive process that begins with creating rapport by attempting to meet patient expectations, then drawing on cultural brokers and staff sensitivity to bridge gaps between explanatory models held by patients and by professionals.

Explanatory models usually remain a covert part of the clinical encounter. Building on the work of Kleinman, Weiss et al (1992) have developed an explanatory model interview to aid in their elicitation. The interview covers topics such as the patient's preferred name for his or her condition, assumptions about cause, explanations for how and why the condition began, sources of fear about the illness, and expectations for its professional management.

Mutual understanding of differing constructions of a disorder is part of the therapeutic contract. Therapists and clients must also be in agreement about how they will work together.

Disagreements create obstacles, but not necessarily insurmountable ones. One of the authors of this chapter (M.B.) had the opportunity to observe the psychotherapeutic approach taken by a Navaho psychiatric social worker on her home reservation. Although Dorothy Red Bird had graduated from a psychoanalytically oriented training program in a major U.S. city, she respected and valued the knowledge handed down by tribal tradition as well as academic authority. Ms Red Bird was concerned about what she perceived to be a high prevalence of depression among patients attending Indian Health Services hospitals and clinics. She attributed this to aborted or incomplete mourning for people who had died, a consequence of cultural practice. Shortly after a death occurs, traditional Navahos burn the dwelling of the deceased, together with his or her possessions, and never mention the name again. M.B. was surprised to learn that, in psychotherapy with a depressed individual, Ms Red Bird focused on bereavements and unresolved mourning issues. Wasn't this a violation of a cultural taboo? Could this Navajo social worker have become so professionalized that she was now insensitive to her own cultural mores?

Dorothy Red Bird was not insensitive. She was highly creative. In establishing a therapeutic contract with her patients, she acknowledged the danger inherent in discussing a dead person. Talk of this kind could attract the 'chi'idi,' or spirit of the dead, and the consequences could be catastrophic. However, she pointed out to her patients that life was never free from risk. In fact, two of the greatest warriors in Navajo legend had to undergo terrible risks and trials in order to save their fellow human beings from destruction. Their triumph would have been impossible without risk. Talking about the dead was indeed a risk. By pointing out the choice between being safe but unhappy or taking a risk that might lead to relief and improved functioning, Ms Red Bird helped many clients to engage in therapy and to work through previously unresolved grief. She provides an important example of how disparate systems for explaining behaviour can be creatively and respectfully synthesized.

MYTH, METAPHOR, AND MEANING

Freud (1904/1973) would probably have approved of Dorothy Red Bird. Early in his career, the father of psychoanalysis pointed out that 'psychotherapy is in no way a modern method of healing. On the contrary, it is the most ancient form of therapy in medicine ... in order to effect a cure a condition of "expectant faith" was induced in sick persons, the same condition which answers a similar purpose for us today' (p. 258). He added, 'There are many ways and means of practicing psychotherapy. All that lead to recovery are good' (p. 259). Jerome Frank (1974) pointed out that the condition of expectant faith depends upon the therapist's and patient's sharing a belief system encompassing not only the explanation for a disorder, but the appropriate methods for its alleviation. More recently, Moerman (1979) has posited that 'the system of meaning of a healing discipline is decisive in its effectiveness, as important as any other "actual," "physical," "pharmaceutical elements"' (p. 60).

Majority-culture North American therapists and clients typically share a body of assumptions, including a belief that disturbed early relationships, problems in the development of autonomy, conflicts about sexuality, and exposure to massive trauma, memories of which become embedded in the unconscious, often lead to difficulties in adult life. It is a core belief that remembering conflicts and 'working through' their contemporary elaborations and repetitions can alleviate symptoms and promote growth. Since Euro-American culture stresses the value of personal privacy, therapy is a personal affair, usually involving only two people.

Many people from Asia, Africa, the Middle East, and First Nations communities value privacy far less than do their majority-culture North American counterparts. Family, and sometimes the entire community, is an integral part of the ritual of healing. Too rigid adherence to one's own values in the face of cultural challenge can impede a therapist's effectiveness.

Assumptions about cause may prove culture-bound. For example, it is probably true that the lack of satisfactory early attachment leads to later behavioural aberration. However, cultural lenses can distort judgments about whether or not successful attachment was ever achieved. 'The development of the mother is not a biopsychosocial process isolated from the cultural values and social patterns of the community; on the contrary, mothers and other caregivers are deeply influenced by culture specific norms in the preference that guide their interaction with babies and set goals for their behavioural development' (LeVine, quoted in Harwood, Miller, & Irizarry, 1995). Harwood et al point out that group C (anxious/resistant) and A (anxious/avoidant) attachments are considered suboptimal. Group A attachments are more prevalent in western European countries, whereas Group C is more common is Israel and Japan. A possible explanation, arrived at by contextualizing attachment behaviour, is that infants from *kibbutzim* in Israel see relatively few strangers. In Japan, infants rarely experience separation from their mothers. Cultural context thus can influence explanations for, as well as determinants of, behaviour.

Therapy involves myth and metaphor. The problem is that myths and metaphors do not always translate across cultures. Freud was able to use the myth of Oedipus as part of his therapeutic approach because the idea that people could develop conflicts about possession and competition made sense within a culture that emphasized acquisition, possessions, and competitiveness. For a traditional Navajo, the ritual of talking about conflicts over independence is likely to make as much sense as a 'Yei Bi Chei' would to a majority culture observer who knew nothing about Navajo culture. The key to comprehending the 'Yei Bi Chei' healing ritual lies in understanding the metaphorical basis of illness. To the Navajo, illness occurs when someone falls out of harmony with a universal order. The out-of-harmony, sick individual is not unique. His or her affliction is a repetition of something suffered in earlier times by one of the figures in Navajo history.

Elaborate 'sand paintings' that figure prominently in healing rituals are not art, but metaphors of illness and heroism. Before beginning a ceremony, the healer and his or her attendants use sand of different colours to create a picture that covers most of the earth floor of the medicine *hogan*. The painting depicts an episode in history when someone became ill in a context similar to the one in which the contemporary patient is involved. The conflict is re-enacted and resolved during an elaborate ritual that lasts many days and nights, and is attended by family and community. By the ceremony's conclusion, the individual's struggle will have been placed in its proper social and historical context, and the sand painting destroyed.

Psychotherapists cannot become shamans, and they should not try. However, the practice of culturally sensitive psychotherapy calls for a re-examination of one's culture-bound assumptions about the context in which therapy should take place, the involvement of family, and the tools and metaphors of communication.

The literature contains an ever-increasing number of descriptions by therapists about the ways in which they have adapted the tools in their psychotherapeutic armamentaria in order to effect culturally sensitive care (e.g., Akhtar, 1995; Amati-Mehler, Argentieri, & Conestri, 1993; Beiser, 1985; Bergin, 1980; Boehnlein, 1987; Borins, 1995; Brantley, 1983; Cabaniss, Oquendo, & Singer, 1994; Casimir & Morrison, 1993; Cavenar & Spaulding, 1978; Comaz-Diaz & Jacobsen, 1987; Dahl, 1989; Dale, Witztum, Mark, & Robinowitz, 1992; El-Sherbini & Chalebry, 1992; Fischer, 1971; Gerber, 1994; Gorkin, 1986; Greengold & Ault, 1996; Grinberg & Grinberg, 1989; Harwood et al, 1995; Holmes, 1992; Howard, 1991; Kirmayer, Young, & Robbins, 1994; Luk, 1993; Malgady, Costantino, & Rogler, 1990; Malgady, Rogler, & Costantino, 1987; Marsella, 1993; Munoz, 1986; Myers, 1988; Niederland, 1964; Noon & Lewis, 1992; Obendorf, 1954; Ornstein, 1985; Rogler & Cortes, 1993; Saris, 1995; Schacter & Butts, 1968; Shamasundar, 1993; Shapiro & Pinkser, 1973; Ticho, 1971; Varghese, 1983; Wang, 1994; Westermeyer, Vang, & Neider, 1983; Wilkeson, 1982; Williams, 1995; Wittkower & Warnes, 1974; Wohl, 1989; Wong, 1978). To cite one example, Shamasundar (1993) describes the incorporation of South Asian myths into therapy. In a similar vein, Saris (1995) writes of illness narratives, and Howard (1991) reports on the use of narrative structures, or 'cuentos,' when dealing with Hispanic patients. Jilek-Aall (1976) emphasizes that talking is not the only medium of communications possible. In her work with the Coast Salish, Jilek-Aall uses the patient's drawings for mutual understanding of areas of conflict and to help identify possible solutions.

TRANSFERENCE AND COUNTERTRANSFERENCE

Transference is a process in which a patient attributes characteristics and expectations to the therapist that derive from significant relationships in the past. To a greater or lesser degree, resolution of the transference is an important part of therapy. Some authors feel that cross-cultural encounters complicate transference issues, and should be addressed only gently, if at all (Obendorf, 1954). Many others, however, advise confronting intercultural issues quickly, and treating them as one would any other aspect of transference. Fischer (1971) observed that 'racial differences between analyst and analysand involve issues of unconscious meaning at many levels. These issues and meanings must be recognized and utilized, for there are serious hazards in either overestimating or ignoring them' (p. 737). After describing the successful psychotherapeutic treatment of a white male by a black female, Cavenar and Spaulding (1978) concluded that interracial therapy can be as productive as any other psychotherapy: 'The same conflicts must be worked through in this kind of interracial therapy – as in any other treatment, the sequence of the unfolding of the conflict may be altered by racial issues. Differences in race may serve as a scaffold for multiple projections by the patient. Projections pertaining to race must be dealt with early in the treatment by helping to appreciate these are unconscious conflicts' (p. 1086).

Brantley (1983) recommended that racial issues not be minimized. In a similar vein, Varghese (1983) described 'failure to appreciate the impact of racial differences can impede therapeutic progress, while sensitive confrontation may be a valuable tool in the recognition and communication of emotionally charged feelings in therapy' (p. 329).

Countertransference has received more attention than transference in the psychotherapeutic literature. Poussaint asserts the harmful effects of racially based countertransference distortions: 'as a psychiatrist who has supervised and consulted with trainees in all the mental health disciplines ... biases and ignorance of ethnocentrism or culturally one-dimensional therapists have not only hindered treatment, but have, all too often, harmed clients. Clinicians who evince their unrealized prejudices or view their clients stereotypically as members of a particular ethnic group can unwittingly abuse their patients, rendering them powerless to cope with the practitioners' conscious or unconscious regarded superiority' (Poussaint, quoted in Pinderhughes, 1989, p. ix).

Writing about highly charged encounters between Jewish therapists and Arab patients in Israel, Gorkin (1986) describes common countertransference responses. These include excessive ambivalent curiosity, defensive avoidance of cultural divergence, manifestations of guilt, and aggressive superiority. Gorkin suggests that direct acknowledgment of such issues may be helpful and therapeutic. Closer to home, Western therapists' relative ignorance of Muslim culture may dispose them to cultural stereotyping of such patients, which disrupts therapeutic relationships. Clinical data in this area are conspicuous by their absence. More recently, Myers (1988) has opined that a patient or supervisee may use racial or cultural differences to counter awareness of underlying transference/countertransference issues or latent psychodynamic content. Holmes (1992) cautioned that a therapist may not fully interpret intrapsychic conflicts in the 'face of racial explanations offered by patients [*if they*] induce white therapist guilt, black therapist overidentification with the downtrodden particular form of countertransference problem and ward off aggression in that therapist' (p.1; italics added).

In a review of cultural aspects of transference and countertransference, Ticho (1971) observed that self-stereotyping may sometimes be a neurotic defence. She cited as an example black patients who hide their difficulties behind cultural stereotypes of oppression and disenfranchisement. The broad acceptance of the oppressed black may tempt a therapist to ignore individual psychodynamic elements that may be contributing to a patient's depression. Ticho also raised the important question of whether it was better for like to treat like, that is, whether ethnic matching is more likely to lead to successful therapy. She suggested that ethnic matching does not obviate prejudice. A therapist working with a patient from his or her own culture may not explore prejudices because of an erroneous assumption that they are shared beliefs.

Therapist Matching and Treatment Outcome

It seems a reasonable hypothesis that matching patients with therapists from a similar cultural background would help obviate transference and countertransference issues, thereby improving therapy. However, as far back as 1973, Shapiro and Pinsker asserted that 'historical and clinical evidence does not support the proposition that common ethnicity is critical for successful psychotherapy' (p. 1540). Even earlier, Rosenthal and Frank (1958) found no differences between black and white improvement rates after completing a course of psychotherapy. The study took place at the Henry Phipps Clinic, where the majority of therapists were white and a substantial proportion of the patient population was black.

Patients may be more concerned about therapist sensitivity to cultural issues than to ethnoracial matching. Jones (1982) studied black and white patients, evenly divided by race, who were seen in individual psychotherapy. Half the patients in each group were in racially similar therapist–patient matches, and half in racially dissimilar pairings. Assessments of treatment outcome were obtained from therapists after termination. White therapists generally rated their clients, especially their black clients, as psychologically more impaired than did black therapists. However, contrary to expectations, there were no differences in psychotherapy outcome as a function of client–therapist racial match. According to Sue (1988), 'empirical evidence has failed to consistently demonstrate differential outcomes for ethnic and White clients' (p. 301).

In a recent study, Sue, Fujino, Hu, and Takeuchi (1991) investigated services received, length of treatment, and treatment outcomes among 600,000 Asian-American, African-American, Mexican-American, and white clients between 1973 and 1988 in Los Angeles. The investigators tested the hypothesis that therapist–client matches in ethnicity and language were beneficial. Based on their respective numbers in the general population, Asian Americans and Hispanics were underrepresented, and African Americans overrepresented, in the mental health system. However, African Americans were highly likely to drop out of treatment. With the exception of Mexican Americans, ethnic matching did not predict treatment outcome. Patients ethnically matched with therapists tended to stay in treatment longer than patients in unmatched dyads. For the subgroup of clients whose primary language was not English, ethnic matching was associated with a low drop-out rate, and with better outcome.

Ethnic matching may be particularly valuable for non–English speakers. For many other patients, cultural sensitivity overrides ethnic matching in importance. This is hardly reassuring to psychotherapists who rightfully despair of ever learning enough about the many diverse cultural groups currently living in North America to ensure that they will always be sensitive. However, Sue (1988) has argued that it may not be necessary to know everything about another's culture. *Proximal* factors – factors that can be captured by assessment tools such as the explanatory model interview and that directly influence the conduct of therapy – affect outcome much more strongly than general knowledge about the patient's culture: 'in the treatment of ethnic minority clients, a therapist's knowledge of the client's culture is *distal* to outcome in the sense that the cultural knowledge must somehow be translated into concrete behaviours in the therapy session. These culturally based behaviours may enhance the process of credibility (e.g., the client's belief that the therapist is understanding, knowledgeable, and competent), which is more proximal to therapy outcome and effectiveness. Distal variables are likely to exhibit a weaker relationship to outcome than are proximal variables' (p. 306).

Therapists should recognize the limits of their cultural competence and be open to consultation from colleagues, culture brokers, and the patients themselves.

Boundary Issues and Cultural Difference

Patients from some cultural groups may expect contact with healers of a sort that may be at variance with the North American guidelines for physician conduct. In Ontario, for example, physical touching or body contact between therapist and patient is actively discouraged and may, in fact, be the source of disciplinary action by the College of Physicians and Surgeons.

Certain authors (e.g., Kinzie, 1981) suggest that physical examination of the patient by the psychiatrist is both therapeutic and necessary. Although there may be arguably valid reasons for physical contact, the current climate of medico-legal uncertainty about patients' rights and boundary violations dictates therapist caution.

In many cultures, people expect to express positive feelings by giving a gift. Should a therapist accept patients' gifts? Is this an aspect of transference that must always be interpreted? Is a gift a bribe? Giving a gift to a therapist may be a culturally appropriate expression of gratitude and respect. Depriving the patient of this culturally sanctioned process may invoke feelings of hurt pride, shame, or anger that interfere with the therapy. Inviting the psychiatrist to family ceremonies and special occasions may at first seem inappropriate, but is not at all unusual. In such instances, the therapist may be well advised to consult with other therapists or culturally literate colleagues before making a decision.

Although individually oriented psychotherapists may feel ill at ease seeing other family members at the behest of the identified patient, it is important to recognize that, in sociocentric families, influence and organization lies within the extended-family kinship system. The family leader, and not the identified patient, may be the locus of decision making regarding therapy.

Teaching, Training, and Research Issues

The opportunities to acquaint medical psychotherapists with cultural issues first occur in medical undergraduate training. Subsequent teaching at the level of the postgraduate residency programs in the area of psychotherapy and culture teach the student basic concepts. Classroom and small-group teaching can introduce specific cultural issues, and present psycho-diagnostic challenges and treatment dilemmas, yet the most relevant area for learning comes from direct clinical experience with patients, colleagues from other cultures, and locums in different cultures (Greengold & Ault, 1996). The experience of the psychiatric resident working in two cultures and two languages is invaluable (Ruskin, 1994). The psychotherapy supervisor is in a crucial and formative relationship with the supervisee to not only examine the patient's symptoms and therapeutic interaction with the supervisee, but also explore the cultural contribution that patient, trainee-therapist, supervisor, and institution bring to the supervisory relationship (Ruskin, 1994). Since a large proportion of psychiatry residents are themselves foreign medical graduates and have different cultural backgrounds, the openness and respect with which the supervisors, staff, and teachers approach the area of culture may facilitate an attitude which invites exploration of cultural difference as part of a mature integration of psychotherapy technique and practice.

Special workshops, lectures, and continuing medical education programs in culture and psychotherapy serve to develop a critical awareness of needs and sensitivities of ethnic groups within the community. Efforts to explore what types of psychotherapeutic treatments are effective with what type of therapist to produce positive outcomes with ethnic groups remain an area for considerable research work.

A Final Word about Culture in Psychotherapy

Some clinicians mistakenly think of culture as something to be gotten over or gotten around in order to get on with the real business of therapy. However, it can never be gotten over or around. Culture creates the context for therapy, helps determine the response of clinician and patient to each other, and provides meaning for the interpretive work of therapy. Rather than being obstacles, cultural factors can provide creative leads for therapeutic work. For example, a patient's discovery that he or she is more tied to a historical cultural past than he or she may have realized can be salutary (Meyer, 1974). Recognition of the way culture affects the therapeutic transaction is part of the process of mutual discovery that is the essence of psychotherapy.

References

Adebimpe, V.R. (1981). Overview: White norms and psychiatric patients. *American Journal of Psychiatry, 138,* 279–285.

Adebimpe, V.R. (1994). Race, racism, and epidemiological surveys. *Hospital and Community Psychiatry, 45,* 27–31.

Akhtar, S.A. (1995). Third individuation: Immigration, identity, and the psychoanalytic process. *Journal of American Psychoanalytic Association, 43,* 1051–1084.

Amati-Mehler, J. Argentieri, S., & Conestri, J. (1993). *The Babel of the unconscious: Mother tongue and foreign languages in the psychoanalytic dimension.* New York: International Universities Press.

American Psychiatric Association (APA). (1952). *Diagnostic and statistical manual of mental disorders.* Washington, DC: Author.

American Psychiatric Association (APA). (1980). *Diagnostic and statistical manual of mental disorders* (3d ed.) Washington, DC: Author.

American Psychiatric Association (APA). (1987). *Diagnostic and statistical manual of mental disorders* (3d ed., revised). Washington, DC: Author.

American Psychiatric Association (APA). (1994). *Diagnostic and statistical manual of mental disorders* (4th ed.). Washington, DC: Author.

Beiser, M. (1985). The grieving witch: A framework for applying principles of cultural psychiatry to clinical practice. *Canadian Journal of Psychiatry, 30,* 130–141.

Beiser, M., Cargo, M., & Woodbury, M.A. (1994). A comparison of psychiatric disorders in different cultures: Depression typologies in Southeast Asian refugees and resident Canadians. *International Journal on Methods in Psychiatric Research, 4,* 157–172.

Beiser, M., Dion, R., Gotowiec, A., Hyman, I., & Vu, N. (1995). Immigrants and refugee children in Canada. *Canadian Journal of Psychiatry, 40,* 67–72.

Beiser, M., Flavel, J.L., & Collomb, H. (1975). Illness of the spirit among the Serer of Senegal. *Journal of Nervous and Mental Disease, 154,* 141–151.

Beiser, M., Gill, K., & Edwards, R.G. (1993). Mental health care in Canada: Is it accessible and equal? *Canada's Mental Health, Summer,* 2–7.

Bergin, A.E. (1980). Psychotherapy and religious values. *Journal of Consulting and Clinical Psychology, 1,* 95–105.

Boehnlein, J.K. (1987). Culture and society in post-traumatic stress disorder: Implications for psychotherapy. *American Journal of Psychotherapy, 41,* 519–530.

Borins, M. (1995). Native healing traditions must be protected and preserved for future generations. *Canadian Medical Association Journal, 153,* 1356–1367.

Brantley, T. (1983). Racism and its impact on psychotherapy. *American Journal of Psychiatry, 140,* 519–530, 1605–1608.

Cabaniss, D.L., Oquendo, M.A., & Singer, M.S. (1994). The impact of psychoanalytic values on transference and countertransference: A study in transcultural
psychotherapy. *Journal of the American Academy of Psychoanalysis, 22*, 609–621.

Canadian Task Force on Mental Health Issues Affecting Immigrants and
Refugees (1988). *After the door has been opened: Mental health issues affecting
refugees and immigrants in Canada. Report of the Canadian Task Force on Mental
Health Issues Affecting Immigrants and Refugees.* Ottawa: Multiculturalism and
Citizenship Canada.

Casimir, G.I., & Morrison, B.J. (1993). Rethinking work with multicultural populations. *Community Mental Health Journal, 29*, 547–559.

Cavenar, J., & Spaulding, J.G. (1978). When the psychotherapist is black.
American Journal of Psychiatry, 135, 1084–1087.

Cheung, F.M., Lau, B.W.K., & Waldman, E. (1980–1981). Somatization among
depressives in general practice. *International Journal of Psychiatric Medicine, 10*,
361–373.

Coffin, C.M. (1952). *The complete poetry and selected prose of John Donne.* New York:
Modern Library.

Comas-Diaz, L., & Jacobsen, F.M. (1987). Ethnocultural identification in psychotherapy. *Psychiatry, 50* (5), 232–241.

Dahl, C.I. (1989). Some problems of cross-cultural psychotherapy with refugees
seeking treatment. *American Journal of Psychoanalysis, 49*, 19–32.

Dale, N., Witztum, E., Mark, M., & Rabinowitz, S. (1992). The belief in transmi-
gration of souls: Psychotherapy with a Druze with severe anxiety. *British
Journal of Medical Psychology, 65*, 119–130.

Danieli, Y. (1985). The treatment and prevention of long-term effects and intergenerational transmission of victimization: A lesson from Holocaust survivors and their children. In C. Figley (Ed.), *Trauma and its wake: The study and
treatment of post-traumatic stress disorder* (pp. 295–313). New York: Brunner/
Mazel.

Draguns, J.G. (1987). Psychological disorders across cultures. In P. Pedersen
(Ed.), *Handbook of cross-cultural counseling and therapy.* Westport, CT: Praeger.

El-Sherbini, E., & Chalebry, K. (1992, March). Towards a cultural specific psychotherapy [letter]. *British Journal of Psychiatry, 160*, 425.

Fernando, S. (1991). *Mental health, race, and culture.* New York: St Martin's Press.

Fischer, N. (1971). An interracial analysis: Transference and countertransference
significance. *Journal of the American Psychoanalytic Association, 19*, 736–745.

Foulks, E.F. (1980). The concept of culture in psychiatric residency education.
American Journal of Psychiatry, 137, 811–816.

Frank, J.D. (1974). *Persuasion and healing.* New York: Schocken.

Freud, S. (1973). On psychotherapy. In J. Strachey (Ed. and Trans.), *The standard edition of the complete psychological works of Sigmund Freud* (Vol. 7, pp. 257–268). London: Hogarth Press. (Original work published 1904)

Gerber, L. (1994). Psychotherapy with Southeast Asia refugees: Implications for treatment of Western patients. *American Journal of Psychotherapy, 48,* 290–293.

Gibbs, J.T. (1985). Can we continue to be color-blind and class bound? *The Counseling Psychologist, 13,* 426–435.

Gorkin, M. (1986). Countertransference in a cross-cultural psychotherapy: The example of Jewish therapist and Arab patient. *Psychiatry, 49,* 69–79.

Glazer, Q.M., Morgenstern, H., & Doucetre, J. (1994). Race and tardive dyskinesia among outpatients at a CMHC. *Journal of Clinical Psychiatry, 54*: 133–139.

Greengold, N.L., & Ault, M. (1996). Crossing the cultural doctor–patient barrier. *Academic Medicine, 171,* 110–112.

Grinberg, L., & Grinberg, R. (1989). *Psychoanalytic perspectives on migration and exile.* New Haven, CT: Yale University Press.

Harwood, R., Miller, J.G., & Irizarry, N.L. (1995). *Culture and attachment.* New York: Guilford.

Holmes, D.E. (1992). Race and transference in psychoanalysis and psychotherapy. *International Journal of Psycho-Analysis, 73,* 1–11.

Howard, G.S. (1991). Culture tales: A narrative approach to thinking. Cross-cultural psychology and psychotherapy. *American Psychologist, 48,* 187–197.

Jilek-Aall, L. (1976). The Western psychiatrist and his non-Western clientele. *Canadian Psychiatric Association Journal, 21,* 353–359.

Jones, B.F., & Gray, B.A. (1986). Problems in diagnosing schizophrenia and affective disorders among Blacks. *Hospital and Community Psychiatry, 37*: 61–65.

Jones, E. (1982). Psychotherapists' impressions of treatment outcome as a function of race. *Journal of Clinical Psychology, 33,* 722–731.

Kinzie, J.D. (1981). Evaluation and psychotherapy of Indochinese refugee patients. *American Journal of Psychotherapy, 35,* 251–261.

Kleinman, A. (1977).Depression, somatization, and the 'New cross-cultural psychiatry.' *Social Science and Medicine, 11,* 3–10..

Kleinman, A. (1980). *Patients and healers in the context of culture.* Berkeley: University of California Press.

Kleinman, A. (1982). Neurasthenia and depression: A study of somatization and culture in China. *Culture, Medicine and Psychiatry, 6,* 117–190.

Kirmayer, L., Young, A., & Robbins, J. (1994). Symptom attribution in cultural perspective. *Canadian Journal of Psychiatry, 39,* 584–595.

Kramer, M. (1969). Cross-national study of diagnosis of the mental disorders: Origin of the problem. *American Journal of Psychiatry, 125* (Suppl), 1–11.

Laub, D., & Auerhan, N.C. (1985). Prologue: On knowing and not knowing. *Psychoanalytic Inquiry, 5,* 1–8.

Lawson, W.R. (1986). Racial and ethnic factors in psychiatric research. *Hospital and Community Psychiatry, 37*, 50–54.

Lin, T.Y., & Lin, N.C. (1978). Service delivery issues in Asian–North American communities. *American Journal of Psychiatry, 135*, 454–456.

Lin, T.Y., Tardiff, K., Donetz, G., & Goresky, W. (1978). Ethnicity and patterns of help seeking. *Culture, Medicine and Psychiatry, 2*, 3–14.

Loring, M., & Powell, B. (1988). Gender, race, and DSM-III: A study of the objectivity of psychiatric diagnostic behaviour. *Journal of Health and Social Behavior, 29*, 1–22.

Luk, S.-I. (1993). Adolescent identity disorder: A case presenting with cultural identification problem. *Australian and New Zealand Journal of Psychiatry, 27*, 108–114.

Malgady, R.G., Costantino, G., & Rogler, L.H. (1990). Culturally sensitive psychotherapy for Puerto Rican children and adolescents: A program of treatment outcome research. *Journal of Consulting and Clinical Psychology, 58*, 704–712.

Malgady, R.G. Rogler, L.H., & Costantino, G. (1987). Ethnocultural and linguistic bias in mental health evaluation of Hispanics. *American Psychology, 42*, 228–234.

Manson, S.M., Shore, J.H. & Bloom, J.D. (1985). Depressive experience in American Indian communities: A challenge for psychiatric theory and diagnosis. In A. Kleinman & B. Good (Eds.), *Culture and depression: Studies in the anthropology and cross-cultural psychiatry of affective disorders*. Berkeley: University of California Press.

Marsella, A.D. (1993). Counselling and psychotherapy in Japanese Americans: Cross-cultural considerations. *American Journal of Orthopsychiatry, 63*, 200–238.

Meyer, G. (1974). On helping the casualties of rapid change. *Psychiatric Annals, 4*, 24–26.

Moerman, D.E. (1979). Anthropology of symbolic healing. *Current Anthropology, 20*, 59–80.

Munoz, J.A. (1986). Countertransference and its implementation in the treatment of a Hispanic adolescent boy. *Psychiatry, 49*, 169–179.

Munroe-Blum, H., Boyle, M.H., Offord, D.R., & Kates, N. (1989). Immigrant children: Psychiatric disorder, school performance, and service utilization. *American Journal of Orthopsychiatry, 59*, 510–519.

Myers, W.A. (1988). Some issues involved in the supervision of interracial and transcultural treatments. In J.M. Ross & M. Myers (Eds.), *New concepts in psychoanalytic psychotherapy* (pp. 140–148). Washington, DC: American Psychiatric Press.

Nguyen, S.D. (1984). Mental health services for refugees and immigrants. *Psychiatric Journal of the University of Ottawa, 9*, 85–91.

Niederland, W.G. (1964). Psychiatric disorders among persecution victims: A contribution to the understanding of concentration camp pathology and its after-effects. *Journal of Nervous and Mental Disorders, 139,* 458–474.

Noon, J.M., & Lewis, J.R. (1992). Therapeutic strategies and outcome perspectives from different cultures. *British Journal of Psychiatry, 65,* 107–117.

Obendorf, C.P. (1954). Selectivity and option for psychiatry. *American Journal of Psychiatry, 110,* 745–758.

Obeyesekere, G. (1985). Depression, Buddhism, and the world of culture in Sri Lanka. In A. Kleinman & B. Good (Eds.), *Culture and depression: Studies in the anthropology and cross-cultural psychiatry of affective disorders* (pp. 134–152). Berkeley: University of California Press.

Ornstein, A. (1985). Survival and recovery. *Psychoanalytic Inquiry, 5,* 99–130.

Parson, E.R. (1985) Ethnicity and traumatic stress: The intersecting point in psychotherapy. In C. Figley (Ed.), *Trauma and its wake: The study and treatment of post-traumatic stress disorder* (pp. 314–337). New York: Brunner/Mazel.

Pinderhughes, E. (1989). *Understanding race, ethnicity, and power.* New York: Free Press.

Rogler, L., & Cortes, D.E. (1993). Help-seeking pathways: A unifying concept in mental health care. *American Journal of Psychiatry, 150,* 554–561.

Rosenthal, D., & Frank, J.D. (1958). The fate of psychiatric clinic outpatients assigned to psychotherapy. *Journal of Nervous and Mental Disorders, 127:* 330–343.

Ruskin, R. (1994). Issues in psychotherapy supervision when participants are from different cultures. In S.E. Greben & R. Ruskin R. (Eds.), *Clinical perspectives on psychotherapy supervision* (pp. 53–72). Washington, DC: American Psychiatric Press.

Saris, A.J. (1995). Telling stories, life histories, illness narratives, and institutional landscapes. *Culture, Medicine and Psychiatry, 19,* 39–72.

Schacter, J.S., & Butts, H.F. (1968). Transference and countertransference in interracial analysis. *Journal of the American Psychoanalytic Association, 16,* 792–808.

Shamasundar, C. (1993). Therapeutic wisdom in Indian mythology. *American Journal of Psychotherapy, 47,* 443–450.

Shapiro, E.T., & Pinsker, H. (1973). Shared ethnic scotoma. *American Journal of Psychiatry, 130,* 338–341.

Solomon, P. (1988). Racial factors in mental health service utilization. *Psychosocial Rehabilitation Journal, 11,* 3–12.

Sue, S. (1988). Psychotherapeutic services for ethnic minorities. Two decades of research findings. *American Psychologist, 43,* 301–308.

Sue, S., Fujino, D.C., Hu, L., & Takeuchi, D.T. (1991). Community mental health services for ethnic minority groups: A test of the cultural responsiveness hypothesis. *Journal of Consulting and Clinical Psychology, 39,* 533–540.

Sue, S., & Morishima, J.K. (1981). *The mental health of Asian Americans: Contempo-*

rary issues in identifying and treating mental problems. San Francisco: Jossey-Bass.

Ticho, G. (1971). Cultural aspects of transference and countertransference. *Bulletin of the Menninger Clinic, 35*, 313–326.

Tseng, W.S. (1975). The nature of somatic complaints among psychiatric patients: The Chinese case. *Comprehensive Psychiatry, 16*, 237–245.

Tung, T.M. (1980). *Indochinese patients*. Falls Church, VA: Actions for Southeast Asians.

Varghese, F.I. (1983). The racially different psychiatrist – Implications for psychotherapy. *Australian and New Zealand Journal of Psychiatry, 17*, 329–333.

Wang, C. (1994). Cross-cultural training in medical education [letter]. *Academic Medicine, 69*, 359.

Weiss, M.G., Doongaji, S., Wypij, S.D., Parthare, S., Bhatawdekor, M., Bhave, A., Sheth, A., & Fernandes, R. (1992). The explanatory model interview catalogue (EMIC): Contribution to cross-cultural research method. *British Journal of Psychiatry, 160*, 819–830.

Westermeyer, J., Vang, T.F., & Neider, J. (1983). Refugees who do and do not seek psychiatric care: An analysis of premigratory and postmigratory characteristics. *Journal of Nervous and Mental Disease, 171*, 86–91.

Wilkeson, A.G. (1982). A resident's perspective in cross-cultural psychiatry. In A. Gaw (Ed.), *Cross-cultural psychiatry* (pp. 285–299). Boston: John Wright.

Williams, L. (1995, 7 April). Psychiatry and cultural issues. Residents' forum. *Psychiatric News*, 15.

Wittkower, E.D., & Warnes, H. (1974). Cultural aspects of psychotherapy. *American Journal of Psychotherapy, 28*, 566–573.

Wolberg, L.R. (1967). *The technique of psychotherapy* (2d ed.). New York: Grune & Stratton.

Wohl, J. (1989). Integration of cultural awareness into psychotherapy. *American Journal of Psychotherapy, 43*, 343–353.

Wong, N. (1978). Psychiatric education and training of Asian and Asian-American psychiatrists. *American Journal of Psychiatry, 133*, 1525–1529.

World Health Organization (WHO). (1973). *Report of the International Pilot Study of Schizophrenia, 1*. Geneva: Author.

World Health Organization (WHO). (1983). *Depressive disorder in different cultures*. Geneva: Author.

Zola, I.K. (1963). Problems of communication, diagnosis, and patient care: The interplay of patient, physician, and clinical organization. *Journal of Medical Education, 38*, 829–838.

Zola, I.K. (1973). Pathways to the doctor – From person to patient. *Social Science and Medicine, 7*, 677–689.

18. Guidelines for Consent in Psychotherapy

Michel Silberfeld and Arthur Fish

The clear consensus of legal, ethical, and clinical opinion is that a therapist is ordinarily obligated to obtain his or her patient's informed consent to psychotherapy prior to initiating treatment. (Appelbaum & Gutheil, 1991; Sharpe, 1987; *Zinermon v. Burch*, 1990; *Fleming v. Reid and Gallagher*, 1991). Yet, although the obligation itself is clear, its basis and purpose are less so, and in practice it may sometimes be difficult to satisfy. The purpose of this chapter is to highlight and describe the obligation; to sketch the tensions or difficulties that it embodies; and to offer a concise, practical outline of what is involved in obtaining a consent to psychotherapy.

The obligation to obtain a patient's prior consent to treatment originates in law and it remains primarily a legal obligation. The general elements of the obligation are remarkably uniform from place to place, but the details vary widely, and the reader must consult his or her local laws and practices before fixing a clinical approach to obtaining consent. We have based this chapter on the consent statute that applies in the Canadian province of Ontario, for this statute (or at least the parts of it that we emphasize) is broadly representative of its kind and concisely states the main elements of a valid consent (Health Care Consent Act [HCCA], 1996). Readers who wish to understand the principles governing specialized areas of practice, for example, obtaining consent from a civilly committed patient or a prisoner, should consult one of the excellent general guides to law and psychiatry that are now available (e.g., Appelbaum & Gutheil, 1991; Melton, Petrila, Poythress, & Slobogin, 1987; Bloom & Bay, 1996). Positively stated, this chapter is aimed primarily at regulated health practitioners (e.g., physicians, psychologists, and social workers) who treat willing patients in a private office or some other clinical setting.

Consent to Treatment in Outline

In essence the doctrine of consent stipulates that it is the mentally competent patient's – not his or her therapist's – right to decide whether to accept or refuse a therapy, even when it is overwhelmingly in the patient's best interest to receive it (Lidz, Applebaum, & Meisel, 1988). Negatively put, the law of consent forbids therapists to treat patients without a prior consent. The following general elements comprise a valid consent:

1 The consent relates to the treatment.
2 The consent is informed.
3 The consent is voluntary.
4 The patient is mentally capable of giving the consent, or, if he or she is not, it has been given on his or her behalf by someone with the legal authority to do so (HCCA, s.11; Melton et al., 1987; Appelbaum & Grisso, 1995; *Canterbury v. Spence*, 1972; *Hopp v. Lepp*, 1980; *Reibl v. Hughes*, 1980; Rozovsky, 1990).

The legal requirement of prior consent to treatment protects the patient's right to make treatment decisions, and the elements of a legally valid consent are intended to ensure that the patient's decisions are a meaningful reflection of his or her wishes. We consider each of these elements in more detail below, but, prior to doing so, we will briefly discuss the purposes of the doctrine.

Purpose of Consent

The legal doctrine of consent originates in the right to be free from unwanted touching, that is, assaults and batteries, from which starting-point it expanded into a general right: 'every human being of adult years and sound mind has a right to determine what shall be done with his body ...' (*Canterbury v. Spence*, 1972; *Reibl v. Hughes*, 1980). In the 1960s and 1970s a series of American and Canadian cases established beyond doubt that the body includes the mind, and so a consent is needed prior to the administration of psychiatric treatment (Appelbaum, 1994; Grunberg 1990; *Fleming v. Reid and Gallagher*, 1991). As the scope of the doctrine has expanded, so, too, has the basis on which it rests. The right is now often said to rest in a general right of 'autonomy' or 'privacy,' that is, not simply in the sanctity or integrity of the body, but rather in each individual's right to make his or her own decisions regarding him- or herself (hereinafter we refer to this general principle as 'self-determination') (*Cruzan v. Director; Missouri Health Department*, 1990; *Malette v. Shulman*, 1990; *Nancy B. v. Hôtel-Dieu de Québec*, 1992; *Rodriguez v. British Columbia*, 1993). The overwhelming opinion of commentators on the subject is that consent is required prior to the initiation of psychotherapy. Moreover, many consent statutes (and civil commitment laws) specifically require that a consent be obtained before administering psychiatric treatment (Appelbaum, 1994; Horowitz, 1984).

In the literature, six main arguments are advanced to support the requirement that consent be obtained prior to the administration of treatment.

1 Obtaining prior consent shows due respect for the individual's right of self-determination (*Canterbury v. Spence*, 1972; *Fleming v. Reid and Gallagher*, 1991).
2 Giving the patient the opportunity to accept or refuse treatment is sensible because the individual is the best judge of his or her own needs and values, and is the ultimate arbiter of whether he or she requires therapy or not (Lidz et. al, 1984; Marta & Lowy, 1993).
3 Obtaining consent establishes a relationship of mutual respect between therapist and patient, and so facilitates therapy (Grossman, 1994).
4 The process of receiving information and providing (or refusing) consent is itself therapeutic (Katz, 1984; Winick, 1993).
5 Obtaining prior consent protects the therapist from legal liability (Melton et al, 1987; Rozovsky, 1995).
6 Obtaining prior consent gives the therapist and his patient an opportunity to negotiate the ground rules of their relationship. (Bray, Shephard, & Hays, 1985; Jensen, Josephson, & Frey, 1989).

It is undoubtedly true that therapists should approach the process of obtaining consent in a positive spirit and with a view to developing a mutually respectful relationship with their patients. But this does not mean that the doctrine itself can reasonably be characterized as 'therapeutic.' Indeed, even enthusiastic proponents of this view recognize that, for some groups of people, for example, the actively psychotic, it is not (Winick, 1993). Moreover the right to decide includes the right to refuse, and it is difficult to accept the argument that a refusal of needed treatment is in itself therapeutic. Indeed, the law of consent permits individuals to make decisions that are foolish, self-destructive, or otherwise countertherapeutic. In short, the doctrine brings – and is *meant* to bring – a certain amount of conflict to the relationship between therapist and patient, and involves a certain deprecation of expert, that is, clinical or therapeutic, knowledge. It is important to grasp this basic truth (which is much clearer in the earlier writing on the subject than it is in the more recent), for in doing so the therapist will be prepared for the conflict that the process of obtaining consent *may* arouse. In practice the therapist's task is to recognize that the law *requires* that consent be obtained, that this legal imperative may hinder therapy, and that it is important to consider how best in practice to reconcile the conflict between the therapist's desire to treat and the patient's right to say no.

The Elements of Consent

WHO

It is the obligation of the therapist who provides treatment to ensure that a prior consent has been obtained from the patient. This does not mean that the therapist him- or herself must always obtain the consent personally, and the law on this question varies from place to place. Under Ontario's law, one 'health practitioner' may delegate the task of obtaining consent to another (HCCA, s.13; Rozovsky, 1995). Delegation may permit an efficient division of clinical labour, and it may also diminish or eliminate the problems that can arise when a therapist fully informs his or her own patient about the risks and benefits of, and the alternatives to, a proposed psychotherapy. So, when a patient is assessed by one clinician who recommends therapy and makes an appropriate referral, it may be appropriate for the assessing clinician to obtain a consent prior to making the referral, especially if the assessment and the therapy are done within the same institution, for example, in an assessment clinic (Horowitz, 1984).

WHEN

Consent must be obtained prior to the initiation of therapy, and preferably at the first meeting between a therapist and a prospective patient.

However, it is misleading to think of consent as an event, that is, that a moment arrives at which consent somehow materializes in the relationship between therapist and patient, and thereafter remains. Rather, consent is a *process* that involves dialogue between the therapist and patient, and therapists may have to explicitly raise the issue of consent at various points or stages in therapy, for example, as the patient's diagnosis, prognosis, or treatment changes (Rozovsky, 1995; Wenning, 1993). Ontario's consent statute specifies that a consent is presumed to include 'variations or adjustments in the treatment, if the nature, expected benefits, material risks and material side effects of the changed treatment are not significantly different' from those attendant on the original one (HCCA, s.12).

EXPRESS OR IMPLIED CONSENT

In many places a consent may be either express or implied. An express consent is one that is openly and formally given, and an implied consent is one inferred from the patient's conduct (Appelbaum, Lidz, & Meisel, 1987; Veatch, 1987, 1991; HCCA, s.11[4]) However, an implied consent is valid only if given after the patient has been adequately informed about the treatment that he or she is to receive. Implied consent is to be distinguished from a *waiver* of consent, which is an informed decision to forgo the right to be informed about the treatment. More precisely, a waiver is valid only if it is given by someone who understands that he or she has the right to obtain a consent and chooses to forgo it (Buchanan & Brock, 1989; Lidz, Appelbaum, & Meisel, 1988; *Pittman Estate v. Bain*, 1994). In many places such a waiver is not legally valid, and legal advice should be sought before relying on one.

WRITTEN OR ORAL CONSENT

Many therapists wonder whether they should document the patient's consent in writing. The short answer is yes, but there is no uniquely best format for doing so. The range of practice varies from a therapist's note on the patient's chart through elaborate prepared forms that the patient is asked to read and sign. Ordinarily, when forms are used, a copy of each one signed by the patient is placed in the chart and a copy is given to the patient for his or her own records. On the question of how to document consent, it is essential to consult an experienced local colleague and to consider local laws and practices. But it should be said that too often clinicians invest a kind of talismanic force in consent forms. It is not the form that represents the consent, but rather that decision which the patient's signature on the form documents. Even so, a written record of a patient's consent may serve one or more of four important purposes:

1 It is an *aide de mémoir* for the busy therapist who, if questions arise years after the event, may not recall that a consent was obtained or what information was conveyed to the patient in obtaining one.
2 It is a convenient reference for the patient on the terms of the therapeutic relationship. It brings home to him or her the importance of the decision he or she is making, and it may forestall unwarranted claims that no consent was obtained.
3 Written materials may be used to convey information to the prospective patient, even prior to a first meeting with the therapist, and so give him or her an opportunity to formulate questions.
4 The preparation of written materials allows therapists to pool their collective experience, and to adequately consider and summarize the literature on treatment.

In short, even where a consent need not be documented in writing, it is highly advantageous to do so.

INFORMED CONSENT: RELATED TO THE TREATMENT

The requirement that a consent relate to the treatment is another way of saying that a valid consent must be an informed one, that is, that the patient must know what he or she is consenting to. It also entails the obligation to renew the patient's consent if his or her diagnosis, prognosis, or treatment changes materially (e.g., if new risks become apparent in the course of treatment).

STANDARDS TO BE MET

There are two main legal standards used to distinguish a legally valid consent:

1 Standard of the profession, that is, what therapists generally agree a patient should be told before agreeing to accept treatment.
2 'Reasonable person' standard, that is, what a reasonable person in the patient's position would wish to know prior to consenting to treatment.

There is a third standard (the information subjectively desired by the patient), but this tends to be expressed not as a sole standard, but rather as an addition to the 'reasonable person' standard; it requires that, in addition to receiving the 'standard' information, the patient must be given the opportunity to ask questions and receive answers to them. In practice, the two main standards tend to overlap. This chapter addresses the 'reasonable person' standard.

The 'Reasonable Person'

Ontario's consent legislation contains a succinct statement of those matters that a patient must be informed of before consenting to treatment. These are:

1 *The nature of the treatment:* Some writers suggest that patients have a right to be informed of their diagnosis and about the diagnostic system used by the therapist. It would be unfortunate if this were construed to mean that therapists must communicate using technical jargon rather than plain language that the patient is likely to understand. The purpose of the exercise is to enhance the patient's understanding, not to mystify him or her, and even where a diagnostic term is well known (e.g., depression), the clinical and common meanings of the term may not be identical.
2 *The expected benefits of the treatment:* Patients should be given some understanding of what people with their particular difficulty can reasonably expect to achieve from treatment. Without such information, patients are not in a position to decide whether the risks or disadvantages of treatment are worth accepting. Moreover, writing on consent tends to dwell on the negative aspects of therapy, and this is as much an error as is withholding negative information from patients. The goal of informing the patient is to allow him or her to make a decision about treatment with a full understanding of what the decision entails, and so the patient is entitled to be told, for example, that the treatment is likely to materially improve his or her life in foreseeable ways if this is, in fact, the case (Inglefinger, 1980).
3 *The material risks of the treatment:* A material risk is one that might affect a reasonable patient's willingness to accept treatment, and includes both common risks that are not particularly serious, and uncommon ones that may cause considerable harm (*Canterbury v. Spence,* 1972; *Hopp v. Lepp,* 1980; *Reibl v. Hughes* 1980; Silberfeld, 1992). The literature suggests that the risks of psychotherapy include treatment failure, as a result of

which the patient may end up worse off than he or she was at the outset of treatment, and intermediate worsening of the patient's condition as painful or warded-off feelings and experiences are reopened. The literature also suggests that therapists have an obligation to warn patients of the risk that confidential information revealed in therapy may be disclosed to third parties. This risk has four aspects:

1 The therapist may have to provide information to either public or private medical insurers.
2 The patient may in some circumstances (e.g., when applying for disability insurance) have to reveal that he or she has been diagnosed with a psychiatric condition or has received psychiatric treatment.
3 The therapist may be required to reveal clinical information in the course of legal proceedings (e.g., if the patient is charged with a crime or divorces his or her spouse and seeks custody of their children).
4 The therapist will alert the appropriate authorities or initiate civil commitment of his or her patient if it becomes apparent that the patient may harm another or him- or herself (Bray et al, 1984; Wenning, 1993; *Tarasoff v. Regents of the University of California*, 1976; *Wenden v. Trikha*, 1991).

Although the literature clearly identifies the existence of the risk that confidentiality will be breached, it does not provide therapists with clear guidance on whether a warning about potential breaches is always necessary, or what form the warning should take. Moreover, the risk to confidentiality that arises in the context of psychotherapy should not be exaggerated. The first three 'risks' described above are present in any physician–patient relationship, yet physicians are not required to routinely disclose that their records may be open to third-party inspection. And although therapy often involves intimate self-disclosure, so, too, do many other physician–patient relationships. As for the fourth risk (disclosure of dangerousness to self or others), requiring the disclosure of this possibility to every patient who enters therapy would be akin to informing every new patient of a family practitioner about the risks attendant on antibiotics before determining that the patient is ill. On balance, the authors' view is that a warning about the potential for breaches of confidentiality should not routinely be given to new patients. Rather, the risk should be disclosed:

a. where therapy is initiated in circumstances that give rise to a concern about confidentiality (e.g., the patient's care is provided as part of a managed-care plan in which the physician is required to regularly report on the patient's progress to a third party); where the patient is referred for a medico-legal assessment; where the patient is in the midst of legal proceedings at the outset of the therapy; or where the patient has a history of civil commitment or criminal behaviour;

b. where circumstances arise in the course of therapy indicating that disclosure may become necessary;

c. where the patient questions the therapist about the circumstances in which confidentiality might be breached.

4 *The material side-effects of the treatment:* It is often difficult to distinguish a side-effect from a risk, and, in practice, the two categories overlap. Still there is some utility in distinguishing the two categories, and for the purposes of discussion we define a side-effect as a foreseeable risk of harm to the patient that accompanies successful therapy or the effect that successful therapy may have on third parties who play an important role in the patient's life. The truth about this sensitive area is that it is often impossible to predict the effect that psychotherapy will have on third persons, although it is very common for a patient's social functioning to improve with therapy (see chapter 4, 'Empirical Evidence for the Core Clinical Concepts and Efficacy of the Psychoanalytic Psychotherapies: An Overview'). Another problem arises solely in relation to multiparty therapy (e.g., couples or group therapy) in which mere participation will involve disclosure of information to persons who are not bound by a legal or (professional) ethical duty of confidentiality.

5 *Alternative courses of action:* Where the current state of therapeutic knowledge suggests that there is more than one legitimate approach to a particular condition (e.g., pharmacology or cognitive therapy versus insight-oriented psychotherapy for the treatment of depression), the patient has the right to know that this is so, and to make his or her own choice (Silberfeld, 1994). In discussing treatment options, the therapist may, indeed should, state his or her reasons for thinking that one approach is better than another for a particular patient, but should be careful to provide accurate and reasonably complete information about the alternatives. With the seemingly increased prevalence of therapeutic eclecticism, one may reasonably hope that the question of informing patients about alternatives will become less heated. In any event, each therapist has an obligation to consider the array of treatment options reasonably open to a given patient based on the state of current thera-

peutic knowledge and to communicate this information to the patient (Stone, 1984; Klerman, 1990; Wenning, 1993). We hope that the availability of a consensus document, such as this volume, will make it easier for practitioners of different therapies to comply with the obligation to identify and disclose alternatives.

6 *The likely consequences of not having treatment:* Just as the patient is entitled to know about the risks and benefits of treatment, he or she is also entitled to know what will likely happen if he or she refuses treatment altogether.

7 *Answering the patient's questions:* Having provided the requisite information, the therapist must also give the patient an opportunity to ask questions and receive answers about it and any related matters. As well, in general, the therapist should strive to recognize the patient's individual needs, desires, and circumstances (i.e., to individualize the provision of information, as much as this can possibly be done). In some jurisdictions the law requires this individualized approach, but, even where it does not, it will likely make it easier for the patient to understand otherwise abstract information about a proposed treatment.

ANCILLARY MATTERS

The literature suggests that therapists ought to inform patients about a variety of housekeeping matters while providing the other information needed to obtain a valid consent. These include the frequency and location of sessions; any charge imposed for missed or cancelled appointments; and the therapist's billing practices. It appears that practitioners of family or couples therapy sometimes use the process of obtaining consent to define or limit the goals of treatment. Thus, a recalcitrant spouse may be willing to enter into family therapy, for example, if he or she is assured that the purpose of the enterprise is to better understand symptoms that have appeared in a child, and not to investigate or reform his or her own character. If consent is being used in such a way, it is important to obtain a fuller or refreshed consent if the therapy later changes course. It is also important to avoid negotiating arrangements with an unstated intention of drawing the reluctant participant into a more free-ranging therapy than he or she initially wishes to accept.

THERAPEUTIC PRIVILEGE

Therapeutic privilege means the voluntary withholding of information, from a competent patient, that he or she ordinarily would be entitled to receive prior to consenting to treatment, on the ground that revealing it would harm the patient. Although virtually every commentator on consent recognizes the existence of the privilege, its contours are indefinite, and it is prudent to seek legal advice before relying on it (*Canterbury v. Spence*, 1972; *Reibl v. Hughes*, 1980; *Pittman Estate v. Bain*, 1994; *Meyers v. Rogers*, 1991; Sharpe, 1987). The doctrine has been variously formulated. At one extreme it extends broadly to include the provision of information so upsetting that it is likely to deprive the patient of the ability to make a 'rational' decision; at the other extreme it is restricted to situations where the provision of the information may expose the patient (or a third party) to tangible harm (e.g., suicide). There is a consensus in the literature that the fact that the provision of information will cause the patient to reject treatment is no ground for exercising therapeutic privilege (Lidz et al, 1988; Appelbaum & Gutheil, 1991; Sharpe, 1987). Therapists should consider whether an intended exercise of therapeutic privilege is not more appropriately dealt with as a case of treatment incompetency. The literature suggests that, where the privilege is exercised, a substitute consent to treatment should be obtained (on which see the material on competency, below). We add that, if the privilege is to be exercised, the patient's chart should include a careful summary of the evidence on which the therapist has relied and his or her reasons for exercising the privilege. It may also be advisable to ask an experienced colleague for advice, albeit perhaps without revealing the patient's identity.

VOLUNTARINESS

The Ontario consent statute stipulates both that a consent must be voluntary and that it must have been obtained without misrepresentation or fraud. In theory the two categories overlap, for a consent obtained by misrepresentation or fraud is not really a voluntary one. Still, there is some utility in distinguishing the two categories, for doing so highlights the subtler forms of coercion to which patients may be exposed. A voluntary consent is one given by a patient who makes his or her own choice to enter into therapy. In practice, voluntariness is most often a problem with institutionalized patients or with those (like many children and adolescents) who enter into therapy at the demand of a parent or guardian. Unlike many of the other elements of consent, voluntariness resists a formulaic treatment because it is hard to draw the line between a realistic response to distressing life circumstances and undue coercion (Appelbaum & Grisso, 1995).

By the term 'competency' we mean the mental ability to provide an informed consent to therapy. In general, therapists should presume that a voluntary adult patient is capable of consenting to treatment unless presented with information or faced with behaviour that would cause a reasonable person to think otherwise. This does not mean that every doubt should translate into a presumption of incapacity, but, rather, that once competency becomes an issue, it must be faced and resolved directly (Madigan, Checkland, & Silberteld, 1994). If the patient is incapable of consenting to treatment, then a substitute consent should be obtained from a close relative before treatment, is initiated. One of the advantages of living in a jurisdiction that has consent legislation is that it will often direct the therapist to an appropriate substitute decider (HCCA, s. 20). In the absence of such an authoritative direction, a therapist should consult someone familiar with local laws, and professional regulations and practices.

Different laws (and different judges) have set different standards of capacity. It is, however, increasingly (and we believe correctly) recognized that the capacity to consent to treatment is *domain-*, *decision-*, and time-specific – domain-specific because capacity is not like a light bulb that is either on or off. Rather, a person may be incapable of making decisions in one domain (e.g., finances), while being perfectly capable of making them in another (e.g., psychotherapy); decision-specific because a person may be incapable of consenting to one medical treatment (e.g., brain surgery) but perfectly capable of consenting to another (e.g., suturing a wound); and time-specific because a patient may be unable to consent to a treatment today (e.g., because he or she is extremely depressed), but may later become able to do so (e.g., after he or she has received a course of antidepressant medication). The general idea is that capacity to consent must be assessed in relation to a particular treatment or treatments that are presently being offered to the patient and not in some general, abstract sense (Weisstub, 1990; President's Commission for the Study of Ethical Problems in Medicine and Biomedical and Behavioral Research, 1982).

Decision specificity entails one extremely important consequence that is increasingly recognized in law. A diagnosis, even a very grave one that often deprives people of the ability to consent to treatment, is not alone sufficient to justify a finding of incapacity. So, for example, a person may be psychotic yet able to consent to treatment if his or her delusions and hallucinations do not impinge on his or her understanding and assessment of the treatment. The same is true of people with developmental handicaps or cognitive impairment. This is not to say that a therapist should not take account of his or her general knowledge of, and past experiences with, a patient. Indeed, the more that the therapist knows about his or her patient, the more accurate his or her assessment of the patient's capacity is likely to be. A valid assessment of capacity does not require the assessor to ignore relevant information, but, rather, to amass as much of it as possible (Freedman, Stuss, & Gordon, 1991). So our objection to relying only on diagnosis or general impressions in making an assessment is that doing so invites cavalier or throw-away judgments formed without considering the patient as an individual (Silberfeld, 1994; Silberfeld & Fish, 1994; Appelbaum, 1994).

If it appears that a patient may be incapable, a therapist should not jump to the conclusion that the patient is, in fact, incapable, or that a formal assessment of capacity (perhaps leading to the patient losing the right to make his or her own treatment decision) is necessary. It may be, for example, that a patient who seems incapable may be only extremely fatigued or anxious. So, before concluding that a patient is or may be incapable, the therapist should conduct an informal assessment of capacity. In large part this consists of nothing more than an exploratory interview with the patient, and perhaps consultation with others who know him or her. An informal assessment serves two purposes. First, it expeditiously determines whether the therapist's doubts about the patient's capacity are justified. Second, it may reveal informal solutions that may overcome the patient's deficits without requiring a formal declaration of incompetence. For example, a patient may be incapable of consenting to one therapy (say, long-term psychotherapy), while being capable of consenting to another (say, brief supportive counselling). The general principle that justifies carrying out an informal assessment of capacity is often formulated as the obligation to employ the means of caring for an incapable person that is least restrictive of his or her liberty (hereinafter, 'the least restrictive alternative'). It may also be formulated as the principle that an intervention into an incapable person's life should be proportional to the extent of the person's incapacity (Madigan & Siberfeld, 1993). More simply, a formal capacity assessment may be hurtful or humiliating, and may lead to a substantial deprivation of liberty and so should not be done unless necessary.

A formal assessment of capacity is required when there are reasonable grounds to think that the patient is incapable of consenting to psychotherapy. In general a therapist ought not to provide treatment without the patient's (or a lawful substitute's) consent, but may not seek a substitute's consent without first finding the patient incapable. In concrete terms, if an informal assessment of capacity suggests that a patient may be incapable there is usually no alternative to performing a formal assessment (Madigan & Siberfeld, 1993). Before starting a formal assessment of capacity (which may involve gathering information from the patient's friends, relatives, and professional caregivers; a medical assessment; psychological testing; and other investigations), the therapist must determine what standard of competency and procedures he or she is required to apply (Silberfeld & Fish, 1994). Under Ontario's consent-to-treatment legislation, the applicable standard is whether the patient 'is able to understand the information that is relevant to making a decision about the treatment ... and able to appreciate the reasonably foreseeable consequences of a decision or lack of decision' (HCCA, s.3). In practice a gloss is placed on this general formula, and the capable patient is one who can:

a. understand the condition for which treatment is proposed;
b. understand the nature of the treatment (including its risks and benefits and the alternatives to it);
c. apply this abstract information to him- or herself (e.g., acknowledge that the condition may affect him or her, and assess how the proposed treatment – or an alternative, including having no treatment – could affect him or her) (Harding, Bursztajn, Gutheil, & Brodsky, 1991; Glass, 1992).

A recent, and extremely careful, review of legal cases has discerned at least four distinct standards of capacity that are applied by American judges, and so this definition is included here primarily as an illustration (Appelbaum & Grisso, 1995): In general the therapist bears the onus of proving that the patient is incapable, that is, if the therapist is unable to prove that the patient is incapable, then he or she should be treated as capable.

When a patient has been found incapable, local laws determine who has the right to make treatment decisions on his or her behalf. Many laws also impose directions or restrictions on how substitute decisions should be made. But, in most places, a substitute consent may be obtained only if the patient is content with the finding of incapacity or has exhausted his or her right to challenge it. The courts are the ultimate arbiters of mental capacity. In some instances the family or friends of a patient may initiate legal proceedings (often called 'guardianship' proceedings) to have the patient authoritatively declared incapable of making his or her own treatment decisions. In other cases, a patient may disagree with a therapist's finding of incapacity and may challenge it either through administrative proceedings (e.g., by applying to an internal board maintained by a facility or to a government review board) or by applying to a judge.

Conclusion

Although we have argued that consent should be viewed as an ongoing dialogue between patient and therapist, the law places more emphasis on the initial disclosure of information – that is, on what is said at a point when the patient's diagnosis, prognosis, and needs may be unclear. With psychotherapy it may well be justifiable to construct a hybrid of the current legalized view of consent and the older view that consent is inferred from the patient's ongoing willingness to participate in therapy (Childress, 1989; Wertheimer, 1993). But these are desiderata, and there is much that can be done within the current doctrine to reduce the potential for conflict between therapist and patient in connection with consent. Indeed, the extent of the practical problem has probably been exaggerated by lawyers and therapists who, in their writing, dwell on the duty to relay information about alternatives and risks to patients while ignoring the corollary duty to disclose the proven and positive benefits of psychotherapy. Indeed, the reader of the consent literature might be forgiven for concluding that every therapy is fraught with risk, and none of them works. The goal of consent to treatment is to allow patients to make their own decisions, aware of *both* the benefits and the risks of treatment.

References

Appelbaum, P.S., (1994). *Almost a revolution.* New York: Oxford University Press.
Appelbaum, P., & Grisso, T. (1995). The Macarthur treatment competence study: I. *Law and Human Behavior, 19,* 105–125.

Appelbaum, P.S., & Gutheil, T.G., (1991). *Clinical handbook of psychiatry and the law.* Baltimore: Williams & Wilkins.

Appelbaum, P.S., Lidz, C.E., Meisel, A. (1987). *Informed consent: Legal theory and clinical practice.* New York: Oxford University Press.

Bloom, H., & Bay, M. (Eds.) (1996). *A practical guide to mental health, capacity and consent law of Ontario.* Toronto: Carswell Thomson Professional.

Bray, J., Shephard, J.N., & Hays, J.R. (1985). *Legal and ethical issues in informed consent to psychotherapy. American Journal of Family Therapy, 13,* 50–58.

Buchanan, A.E., & Brock, D.W. (1989). *Deciding for others: The ethics of surrogate decision-making.* New York: Cambridge University Press.

Canterbury v. Spence, 464 F. 2d 772.

Childress, J. (1989). Autonomy. In: R.M. Veatch (Ed.), *Cross-cultural perspectives in medical ethics: Readings.* Boston: Jones & Bartlet.

Cruzan v. Director, Missouri Health Department (1990) 111 L. Ed. 2d 224.

Fleming v. Reid and Gallagher, (1991) 4 O.R. 3d 74 (C.A.).

Freedman, M., Stuss, D.T., & Gordon, M. (1991). Assessment of competency: The role of neurobehavioral deficits. *Annals of Internal Medicine, 115,* 203–208.

Glass, K.C. (1992). *Elderly persons and decision-making in a medical context: Challenging Canadian law.* Doctoral dissertation, McGill University Faculty of Law.

Grossman, L. (1994). On coming to an agreement about the nature of treatment. *Canadian Journal of Psychoanalysis, 2,* 203–221.

Grunberg, F. (1990). La doctrine du consentement libre et eclaire: Ses fondements ethiques, juridiques et ses applications dans la recherche et la pratique de la psychiatrie. [The doctrine of free and informed consent: its ethical, juridical foundations and its application in psychiatric research and practice]. *Canadian Journal of Psychiatry, 35,* 443–450.

Harding, H.P. Jr, Bursztajn, H.J., Gutheil, T.G., & Brodsky, A.B. (1991). Beyond cognition: The role of disordered affective states in impairing competence to consent to treatment. *Bulletin of the American Psychiatry and Law, 19,* 383–388.

Health Care Consent Act [HCCA] 2 Statues of Ontario, 1996.

Hopp v. Lepp, [1980] 2 S.C.R. 192.

Horowitz, S. (1984). The doctrine of informed consent applied to psychotherapy. *Georgetown Law Journal, 72,* 1637–1664.

Ingelfinger F.J. (1980). Arrogance. *New England Journal of Medicine, 303,* 1507–1511.

Jensen, P., Josephson, A.M., & Frey, J. (1989). Informed consent as a framework for treatment. *American Journal of Psychotherapy, 43,* 378–386.

Katz, J. (1984). *The silent world of doctor and patient.* New York: Free Press.

Klerman, G.L., (1990) The psychiatric patient's right to effective treatment. *American Journal of Psychiatry, 147,* 409–418.

Lidz, C.W., Applebaum, P.S., & Meisel, A. (1988). *Two models for implementing informed consent. Archives of Internal Medicine, 148,* 1385–1389.

Madigan, K.V., & Silberfeld, M. (1993). Clinical application of the least restrictive alternative in competency. *Assessments, Estates and Trusts Journal, 12,* 282–292.

Madigan, K.V., Checkland, D., & Silberfeld, M. (1994).Presumptions respecting mental competence. *Canadian Journal of Psychiatry, 39,*147–152.

Malette v. Shulman, (1990) 72 O.R. 2d 74 (C.A.).

Marta, J., & Lowy, F.H. (1993). Le consentement eclaire: Un atout pour la psychotherpaie? [Informed consent: An asset to psychotherapy?] *Canadian Journal of Psychiatry, 38,* 547–551.

Melton, G.B., Petrila, J., Poythress, N., & Slobogin, C. (1987). *Psychological evaluations for the courts.* New York: Guilford.

Meyer v. Rogers, (1991) 78 D.L.R. (4th) 307.

Nancy B. v. Hôtel-Dieu de Québec, (1992) 86 D.L.R. (4th) 385.

Pittman Estate v. Bain, (1994) 112 D.L.R. (4th) 257.

President's Commission for the Study of Ethical Problems in Medicine and Biomedical and Behavioral Research. (1982). Washington, DC: U.S. Government Printing Office.

Reibl v. Hughes, [1980] 2 S.C.R. 880.

Rodriguez v. British Columbia, [1993] 3 S.C.R. 519.

Rozovsky, L.E. (1995). *The Canadian law of consent to treatment* (2d ed.). Toronto: Butterworths.

Sharpe, G.S. (1987). *The law and medicine in Canada.* Toronto: Butterworths.

Silberfeld, M. (1994). Evaluating decisions in mental capacity assessments. *International Journal of Geriatric Psychiatry, 9,* 365–371.

Silberfeld, M., & Fish, A. (1994). *When the mind fails: A guide to dealing with incompetency.* Toronto: University of Toronto Press.

Stone A.A. (1984). The new paradox of psychiatric malpractice. *New England Journal of Medicine, 311,* 1384–1387.

Tarasoff v. Regents of the University of California, (1976) 529 P. 2d 553 (Cal. 774).

Veatch, R.M. (1987). *The Patient as partner.* Bloomington, Indiana University Press.

Veatch, R.M. (1991). *The physician–patient relation: The patient as partner.* Bloomington: Indiana University Press.

Wenden v. Trikha, (1991) 116 A.R. 81 (C.A.).

Wenning, K. (1993). Long-term psychotherapy and informed consent. *Hospital and Community Psychiatry, 44,* 364–367.

Weisstub, D.N. (Chair). (1990). *Enquiry on Mental Competency: Final report.* Toronto: Queen's Printer for Ontario.

Wertheimer A.A (1993). Philosophical examination of coercion for mental health issues. *Behavioral Sciences and the Law, 11,* 239–258,

Winick, B. (1993). The right to refuse mental health treatment: A therapeutic jurisprudence analysis. *International Journal of Law and Psychiatry, 17,* 99–117.

Zinermon v. Burch, 494 U.S. 113 (1990).

19. Standards and Guidelines for Psychotherapy Record Keeping

Hazen Gandy, Judith Hamilton, Paul Cameron, and Simon Davidson

This chapter reviews important issues of record keeping in psychiatry and psychotherapy. The basic requirements of medical-psychotherapy record keeping are outlined, and some of the more difficult aspects are illustrated.

Record keeping in psychotherapy is recognized as a valuable and important clinical task (Reynolds, Mair, & Fischer, 1992). Psychiatrists are expected to keep track of their patients' progress solely through their records. The reasons therapists cite for producing and maintaining records range from purely medico-legal obligation to the desire to accurately record patient and therapist experiences and interactions. Although surveys suggest there is a direct correlation between the quality of mental health records produced and the quality of patient care delivered, this has never been systematically analysed (Reynolds et al, 1992). Furthermore, psychotherapy records play an increasing role in the systematic evaluation of patient care, therapist accountability, and intervention validity. 'In essence, the patient chart has gone from a simple collection of physician observations, reflections, comments and recollections to a complex hospital medicolegal documentation system' (Soreff, Gulkin, & Pike, 1990, p. 127).

Despite the pivotal role record keeping plays in psychiatric care, it has received remarkably little systematic analysis in the literature. Few mental health organizations in this country have specific guidelines on how to document psychotherapy assessments and progress. Little attention is paid to the teaching of record keeping in psychiatry in residency training programs.

A review of the literature by Reynolds et al (1992) identified three themes: first, there has been relatively little systematic study of mental health records, given the critical role they play in patient care and management; second, mental health practitioners receive surprisingly little training in how to write and read a record, given the amount of time they spend doing both; and, third, communication between professionals in the mental health community is especially complicated as a result of the unusually wide variety of writer/reader backgrounds, care-delivery settings, and documentation standards.

Furthermore, a national survey in the United States conducted in 1981 by Siegel and Fischer revealed a number of interesting observations about patterns of mental health documentation in a variety of settings. The survey consisted of both a nationwide questionnaire and a focused field study. Analysis of the questionnaire indicates that clinical parts of the records were most frequently written and read. Psychiatrists were the highest enterers/writers of information, psychologists the lowest. Nurses and psychiatrists emerged as heavy record users. The survey found that 55.5 per cent of the respondents kept their own personal records (i.e., they kept records other than those required by the care-delivery system) and that respondents in private practice gave 'future use' as their second most common reason for keeping records; those working in state hospitals gave 'communication.' Sixty per cent believed there was at least some relationship between good records and good care, and an additional 26 per cent claimed that this was a strong relationship. The two biggest problems identified were illegible handwriting and too much information.

Results of the field study were often contradictory to the results of the questionnaire. Analysis of the field study revealed that treatment plans were missing from sampled records about one-third of the time. Most records were in a structured format; progress notes were generally unstructured. Mean recording/writing time was 13.2 minutes; mean consulting/reading time was 9.2 minutes per record contact. Records were consulted for specific information rather than a general overview. Information most frequently consulted included the psychiatric findings, psychiatric assessments, and medication planning. The records had varying relevance for different disciplines. Psychiatrists, psychologists, and social workers consulted the records 'to help make decisions.' Other staff consulted the records to 'get instructions.' Respondents to the questionnaires said they both entered and consulted treatment plans frequently; the observational field study did not find that to be true.

'Treatment plans would appear more often if the clinicians regarded them as useful and important, merely beyond fulfilling documentation of care requirements' (Siegel & Fischer, 1981, p. 131). Respondents to the questionnaire said that they most often entered data for clinical reasons, and least often because it was required. Participants in the field-study interviews said they most often entered data because it was required.

Despite the importance of record keeping, some researchers have found that clinician's attitudes pose a significant barrier to the production and development of useful records (Siegel & Fischer, 1981). The belief that writing notes and reports is time-consuming and onerous is prevalent even among senior staff in institutions, teaching centres, and private clinics. This contributes to inadequate training in written communication, which represents the most important barrier to improved record keeping.

Potential Uses of a Psychiatric Record

Psychotherapy records, whether produced in an institutional setting or in a private office, may be used in a variety of ways. Many of these uses may have an impact on the confidentiality of the records. Potentially, information can be exposed to observation, bias, and misinterpretation by individuals for whom it was not intended. This is illustrated by the case of John Tower, who was denied the chance to be George Bush's secretary of state because of records of his alcoholism. Similarly, Thomas Eagleton was denied the chance to be George McGovern's running mate because of records of his shock therapy.

From a clinical perspective, records are used to assist therapists in their treatment through progress review or the reassessment of specific information, or as a guide for future treatment planning. The record can serve as a narrative of content or process, and can help to focus themes and issues in therapy which may have been identified in the initial assessment.

Psychotherapy records can be used for research purposes. In this situation, information may be perused and gathered by individuals other than the primary therapist, and therefore may well be taken out of context for the purposes of data collection. When the record is viewed by a number of others without the knowledge of the patient or the therapist, confidentiality must be maintained.

Not infrequently patients themselves demand to see the records compiled by their therapists. Here the records are perused by individuals who may misinterpret the language and/or technical terms of the record. Or a selective search may distort the information by ignoring the context or perspective from which the record was constructed.

Records are frequently used by licensing bodies in peer reviews to assess the competence of the professionals providing care. In this case several others will examine the records for the indicators of quality of care reflected in the documentation of that care.

Other organizations, such as provincial or private medical insurance companies, or Revenue Canada, may have access to patient records with consent to prove that services were or were not provided, or to determine the validity of claims. Again, several individuals, from various backgrounds and perspectives, may peruse private or sensitive personal information.

Medico-legal purposes such as college investigations, custody suits, compensation cases, and criminal cases are common reasons for others to have access to patient files. This potentially represents the loss of confidentiality as psychotherapy notes become public documents in court proceedings.

Owing to the various potential uses of psychotherapy records, what information is documented and how it is documented is critical to the well-being of both patient and therapist. Certainly psychotherapy records may not be as confidential as therapists might think: there are many potentially authorized examiners of these records. Thus, clinicians must consider who may potentially read the record and the impact such access will have on the patient or the therapist.

Standards for Psychotherapy Records

Psychotherapy records must conform to the legal requirements for all medical records. In Ontario, these are set out in Ontario Regulation 241/94 made under the Medicine Act, 1991 (see appendix). Essentially, these regulations require that physicians must have minimal documentation of each patient visit.

The American Psychological Association's (1993) record-keeping guidelines address five areas: the content of records; construction and control of records; retention of records; outdated records; and disclosure of record-keeping procedures. There are no specific guidelines with respect to psychotherapy documentation.

In 1991, the Ontario Medical Association Section on Psychiatry produced a document outlining standards for psychiatric psychotherapy records. This was revised in 1995 (Joint Task Force on Standards for Medical [Psychiatric] Psychotherapy, 1995) as follows:

I Psychiatric Psychotherapy Records must conform to the standards governing the records of all medical acts as set out in part V, sections 18–21 of Regulation 241/94 of the Medicine Act.

II Psychiatrist's records for patients requiring and receiving psychotherapy should also contain the following:

1. An initial consultation note, which should refer to:
   – the patient's presenting problem
   – the history related to the problem
   – the family and personal history related to the problem

   The note should contain:
   – the patient's mental status, when necessary, and a description of further investigations planned

   There should be:
   – a diagnosis
   – a formulation
   – the prognosis
   – a treatment plan

   This note might follow on one or more than one session with the patient, and is expected to follow the pattern taught in psychiatric training institutions.

2. Progress notes. A progress note should be written for each session. It should be assumed that this note will be of variable length and detail ranging from several words to several paragraphs, depending on the complexity of the treatment. In general, the progress notes for any one patient, taken as a whole over the time of the treatment, should include sufficient material to allow the therapist to reconstruct the themes of the treatment.

   Specifically, Psychiatric Psychotherapy Progress Notes should contain references, when relevant, to the following:

- the state of the relationship
- the state of the transference
- current dynamic issues
- important interventions
- progress made

It is expected that these notes, taken as a whole over the time of the treatment, will demonstrate a recognizable relation to the diagnosis, formulation and treatment plans of the initial note, or revisions thereof, e.g. forms and effects of 'support' delivered and received in 'supportive psychotherapy.'

3. A termination note, which should include:
   - an evaluation of the progress made
   - any final recommendations.

III Finally, in making records, clinicians should be mindful of the possible injurious consequences to the patient of including highly sensitive information or other material. (p. 134)

This document provides specific guidelines based on the principles of medical psychotherapy. Although it makes specific references to psychodynamic psychotherapy, it does not address the specific procedures and processes of other forms of therapy frequently employed by psychiatrists. Nevertheless, it presents a useful guide to structuring the documentation of a psychotherapy process.

Some of the complex issues related to psychotherapy record keeping are illustrated in the following vignettes.

DIAGNOSTIC ISSUES

The following examples from actual records illustrate the importance of documenting diagnoses.

A Consultation Note (abbreviated):
... Impression: ... active fantasy life, ... bizarre dreams, ... hallucinatory experiences – diagnosis: ?psychotic depression, ?schizophreniform illness, ?temporal lobe epilepsy.

The patient was subsequently treated with antidepressant medications resulting in a full resolution of her symptoms. The chart contains no further references to clarify or revise the diagnosis as the treatment proceeded and eventually ended. The patient was subsequently involved in a custody dispute with her husband. After obtaining her psychiatric records by subpoena her husband's lawyer argues that she has schizophrenia and is therefore less fit to care for her children. The husband was successful in obtaining custody of the children on these grounds.

The failure to revise the records to accurately reflect the status of the patient and her current diagnosis led to the appearance of an erroneous diagnosis. In this case, the physicians failed to clearly indicate that she did not have schizophrenia, a diagnosis that favoured the position of her adversary in the eyes of the court. This act of omission had serious consequences, despite the patient's correct diagnosis and treatment.

The following case highlights the potential impact of making a diagnosis without an appropriate initial assessment.

A custody dispute involved a toddler girl placed in the care of a maternal aunt who applied for full custody. When the father sued for custody, the aunt and her husband were assessed by the Family Court Clinic and found to be good parents. However the clinic was obliged to refer in its final report to a psychiatric consultation report written fifteen years earlier. The husband had sought help from a psychiatrist for marital problems related to 'looking at younger women.' According to the husband, the psychiatrist saw him once, gave no feedback and made no follow-up recommendations. Although the record showed no evidence of symptoms or behaviour to support it, the diagnosis on the consultation report was paedophilia.

This case illustrates the potential harm in assigning and documenting a diagnosis based on inadequate information. A history of 'paedophilia' in a man applying for custody of a young child is obviously damaging. The mere use of the word, despite the lack of corroborating evidence, is enough to influence authorities rendering decisions in such a case. The weight placed on final diagnoses in mental health records is substantial. When the impact of recording such diagnoses is not considered, patients can be unintentionally harmed.

DANGEROUSNESS

Psychiatrists receive a great deal of training in assessing risk of harm to self and others, but essentially little or no training in how to appropriately document it. The following example illustrates this point.

14 Feb 1994
Patient feeling angry today after receiving a court order demanding increased support payments form his ex wife. Stated he felt like killing her as he felt that would make his life 'a whole lot easier.' Continues to feel depressed with intermittent thoughts of suicide. Having increasing difficulty concentrating at work as his boss is pressuring him to take on new assignments. Touched on his fear of losing his job and consequently his house that he built himself. Continues to take his Prozac without side effects. See one week.

This note documents that the risks have been identified but does not refer to assessment of the significance of these risks or interventions directed towards these risks. One might presume that the therapist did not believe that the risks of homicide or suicide were significant enough to warrant specific intervention. Alternatively, the therapist might have considered that the risks were significant and undertaken interventions that allowed the patient to safely leave the session. Or the therapist may have not appreciated the risks involved and allowed a highly dangerous patient to leave his office without taking appropriate interventions. This note is inadequate in documenting the presence of risk factors for dangerousness and the response to the identification of these risk factors. In a peer-review chart audit, the note could suggest gross incompetence of the therapist in failing to show a response to the risk factors identified.

Poor documentation not only impacts on patients' well-being, but places therapists at risk by indicating inappropriate or incompetent treatment. Moreover, poor documentation obscures appropriate management if interventions are not recorded.

The note could be revised as follows:

14 Feb 1994
Patient feeling angry today after receiving a court order demanding increased support payments from his ex wife. Stated he felt like killing her as he felt that would make his life 'a whole lot easier.' Depression continues with intermittent thoughts of suicide. Finding work hard. Denied psychotic symptoms. Looked at and ruled out significant intent or risk in his suicidal and homicidal ideation, acknowledging his thoughts are a way of coping

with his stress. Looked at how to respond to his boss's demands and encouraged him to spend some time with his friends who had invited him on a fishing trip for the weekend, stressing the value of taking time for himself in this difficult process. Touched on his fear of losing his job and consequently his house that he built himself. Continues to take his Prozac without side effects. Reinforced that he could contact me or go to Emergency if he felt he was having increasing difficulty coping. See one week.

This revision explicitly addresses the risk factors identified and describes the therapist's interventions. The note reveals that the level of risk has been assessed and appropriately managed. With a different outcome the note might read:

14 Feb 1994
Patient feeling angry today after receiving a court order demanding increased support payments from his ex wife. Stated he felt like killing her as he felt that would make his life 'a whole lot easier.' Depression continues with intermittent thoughts of suicide. Finding work very difficult. Examined his level of functioning – neurovegetative symptoms had worsened. Barely sleeping – pacing the floor at night preoccupied with his ex wife. Noted a fear of losing control of his anger and admitted he had spent the last two nights parked across the street from his ex's house with a loaded rifle which he alternately pointed at her house and placed under his chin. Felt helpless, impotent, becoming increasingly agitated as the session progressed. We reviewed the situation in which I felt he was at a very high risk of harm to himself and/or his ex. After some negotiation he agreed to voluntary hospital admission. Arranged for an emergency assessment and admission after talking to the on-call staff. Escorted him to emergency where we were met by the resident on call. Through out this time he remained cooperative and in good control ...

The record documents that the risks have been identified and assessed. As well, record of the therapist's interventions reflects a respect for the patient's vulnerability.

RECORD LENGTH AND DETAIL

When progress notes consist of a few words or phrases, valuable information serving the clinical needs of the patient or the therapist may be lost. A few words or phrases cannot adequately record the multiple levels of expression, intervention, and interpretation that emerge in a psychotherapy session and impact on the patient's progress or stability.

Conversely psychiatric records often contain too much information. This may consist of irrelevant information or documentation so detailed that it becomes confusing. Consider the following example:

15 Feb 1994
Patient continued to talk about her affair with the President. Examined in detail their sexual relationship – frequency of contact, places of meetings including the executive washrooms at the office and the basement of his home whereby she would sneak in at night after his wife had gone to bed and they would spend the night having sex on the basement floor ...

Documenting this information does not contribute in any meaningful way to the treatment process. The level of detail does not contribute to the understanding of the patient and may reveal more about the therapist than the patient. Furthermore, this information is highly sensitive and could damage the patient or others if this record was scrutinized by other parties for unrelated matters. (See 'Potential Uses of a Psychiatric Record'). Discretion and sensitivity towards the potential impact of written accounts on patients will reduce the risk of unintentionally exposing sensitive information.

The note could be revised as follows:

15 Feb 1994
Pt. continued to talk about her involvement with a VIP in which we examined a variety of aspects of their relationship focusing on the potential impact of this relationship with her family ...

Details are removed so that identification of individuals remains easy for the patient and therapist but difficult for anyone else who might have access to the information. As well, details of the relationship are minimized while its value to the patient is emphasized.

Some situations require a significant amount of detail. Documenting historical accounts of abuse or assault may require enough detail to substantiate or support a patient's claims in court. The importance of this is underscored by recent rulings by the Supreme Court of Canada regarding the disclosure of medical records of sexual assault victims (Sack & Payne, 1996).

Information must be carefully documented. Moscarello (1995) asks: 'How does a therapist know when to trust a patient's self report of symptoms, memories, recollections etc.? Self report measures are used extensively in psychiatric research. The researcher relies upon the patients' perception and memory and not objective findings' (p. 22). When documenting accounts of abuse or neglect, the therapist should carefully note the patient's perceptions and accounts, and avoid accepting these accounts as objective findings.

The final vignette is an example of a progress note that successfully conveys the important, relevant content of a session in a succinct and efficient manner.

> Mrs C. reports improved mood, more energy and better day to day functioning. Continues Parnate 45 mg. daily with minimal side effects. The focus of the working alliance is supporting purchasing a recreational property. This is one of the first times she can pursue pleasure for herself. Secondly, looked at enlisting support from her husband in dealing with her daughter's acting out. Pt. feels she wants his support but does not always agree with him. Examined the conflict of wanting support but needing him to do it her way. This led to her realizing that, in her family, everyone is expected to do things a certain way.
>
> Also looked at how much her husband thinks of her cooking and mothering; her being judged by her parents as a sinner – and how she experienced me. She felt she was not getting better quick enough and wondered if I would not permit her to return to work. Looked at how hard it was to always expect negative judgment – even from me.

This note presents information in a clear and readable manner. Specifically it refers to the progress of pharmacological treatment by identifying her medications and her response and side-effects. It also identifies the working alliance, and transferential issues of her experience of the therapist, and notes the psychodynamic progress of having achieved, for the first time, the ability to pursue pleasure for herself. This note reflects some of the more subtle aspects of a session in terms of content and interaction. In doing so, it maintains a supportive perspective, respectful of the patient's vulnerability to judgment and criticism. In this respect the note reflects the attitude and therapeutic stance of the therapist and conveys this to others reading the note. The note addresses some sensitive issues with sufficient detail so the therapist can identify the issues without being excessive or intrusive. Anyone who reads the note, including the patient, will be able to understand the therapeutic work and its progress, and recognize a trusting partnership.

Summary

Psychotherapy documentation involves balancing a number of opposing concerns. Confidentiality, accuracy, and respect for the patient must be maintained, while reflecting the therapist's professional competence and integrity. As Soreff, Gulkin, and Pike (1990) suggest, 'the clinician must utilize the evolving chart into his practice in a number of ways. The doctor must familiarize himself with the things he must incorporate into his notes. He must demonstrate he is "captain of his chart" by writing notes that 1) show he has read the reports of others and is aware of laboratory results and is cognizant of the work of the members of the treatment team, 2) reflect his unique medical/psychiatric training, background and expertise, and 3) personalize his notes. The clinican should remember that the fundamental purpose of the record is to assist in the treatment of the patient' (pp. 132–133).

Despite careful attention to these guidelines, psychotherapy records inevitably involve the therapist's biases (Reynolds et al, 1992). These personal biases may reflect cultural and historical influences, or involve scientific or academic biases. Records are influenced by the therapist's discipline, be it psychiatry, psychology, or social work; and by setting, community-based care, general hospitals, provincial psychiatric hospitals, or correctional facilities. These factors influence how patients are seen and written about (Reynolds et al, 1992). How therapists define and identify symptoms and disorders, rate their severity, and appreciate their impact will inevitably influence the record.

APPENDIX: ONTARIO REGULATION 241/94 MADE UNDER THE MEDICINE ACT, 1991

Part V, sections 18–21, read:

18. (1) A member shall make records for each patient containing the following information:

1. The name, address and date of birth of the patient.
2. If the patient has an Ontario health number, the health number.

3. For a consultation, the name and address of the primary care physician and of any health professional who referred the patient.
4. Every written report received respecting the patient from another member or health professional.
5. The date of each professional encounter with the patient.
6. A record of the assessment of the patient, including,
    i. the history obtained by the member,
    ii. the particulars of each medical examination by the member, and
    iii. a note of any investigations ordered by the member and the results of the investigations.
7. A record of the disposition of the patient, including,
    i. an indication of each treatment prescribed or administered by the member,
    ii. a record of professional advice given by the member, and
    iii. particulars of any referral made by the member.
8. A record of all fees charged which were not in respect of insured services under the *Health Insurance Act*, which may be kept separately from the clinical record.
9. Any additional records required by regulation.
    (2) A member shall keep a day book, daily diary or appointment record containing the name of each patient who is encountered professionally or treated or for whom a professional service is rendered by the member.
    (3) The records required by regulation shall be,
        (a) egibly written or typewritten or made and kept in accordance with section 20;
        (b) kept in a systematic manner. O. Reg. 241/94, s. 2, *part.*

19. (1) A member shall retain the records required by regulation for at least ten years after the date of the last entry in the record, or until ten years after the day on which the patient reached or would have reached the age of eighteen years, or until the member ceases to practise medicine, whichever occurs first, subject to subsection (2).

   (2) For records of family medicine and primary care, a member who ceases to practise medicine shall,
       (a) transfer them to a member with the same address and telephone number, or
       (b) notify each patient that the records will be destroyed two years after the notification and that the patient may obtain the records or have the member transfer the records to another physician within the two years.

(3) No person shall destroy records of family medicine or primary care except in accordance with subsection (1) or at least two years after compliance with clause (2)(b). O. Reg. 241/94, s. 2, *part*.

20. The records required by regulation may be made and maintained in an electronic computer system only if it has the following characteristics:

1. The system provides a visual display of the recorded information.
2. The system provides a means of access to the record of each patient by the patient's name and, if the patient has an Ontario health number, by health number.
3. The system is capable of printing the recorded information promptly.
4. The system is capably of visually displaying and printing the recorded information for each patient in chronological order.
5. The system maintains an audit trail that,
     i. records the date and time of each entry of information for each patient,
     ii. indicates any changes in the recorded information,
     iii. preserves the original content of the recorded information when changed or updated, and
     iv. is capable of being printed separately from the recorded information for each patient.
6. The system includes a password or otherwise provides reasonable protection against unauthorized access.
7. The system automatically backs up files and allows the recovery of backed-up files or otherwise provides reasonable protection against loss of, damage to, and inaccessibility of, information. O. Reg. 241/94, s. 2, *part*.

21. A member shall make his or her equipment, books, accounts, reports and records relating to his or her medical practice available at reasonable hours for inspection by a person appointed for the purpose under a statute or regulation. O. Reg. 241/94, s. 2, *part*

References

American Psychological Association (APA). Committee on Professional Practice and Standards. (1993). *Record keeping guidelines*. Washington, D.C.: Author.

Joint Task Force on Standards for Medical (Psychiatric) Psychotherapy. (1995). *A Report to Council of the Ontario Psychiatric Association and to Executive of the*

Section on Psychiatry, Ontario Medical Association, on the definition, guidelines and standards for medical (psychiatric) psychotherapy. Toronto: Author.

Moscarello, R., (1995, April). *Memories of sexual abuse: Practice guidelines for psychotherapy.* Presented to the Education Council, Canadian Psychiatric Association.

Reynolds, J.F., Mair, D.C., & Fischer, P.C. (1992). *Writing and reading mental health records.* Newbury Park, CA: Sage.

Sack, J., & Payne, V. (1996, February). Disclosing medical records of assault victims: When is a physician obliged to do so? *Ontario Medical Review,* 90–96.

Siegel, C., & Fischer, S.K. (1981). *Psychiatric records in mental health care.* New York: Brunner/Mazel

Soreff, S., Gulkin,T., & Pike, J.G. (1990). The evolving clinical chart: How it reflects and influences psychiatric and medical practice and the quality of care. *Psychiatric Clinics of North America, 13,* 127–133.

Index

abstinence, 96–7

abuse: of children, 25, 35–7, 85, 192, 256–7, 264–5, 410; of patients, 11, 14, 18–19, 21–4, 232, 434. *See also* physical abuse, sexual abuse, substance abuse

actional model, 200–1

addictive disorders, 112, 174, 206. *See also* substance abuse

adjustment disorders, 64, 235

adolescents, 34, 272–80; confidentiality, 278; countertransference, 274–5; depression, 191; difficulty of treating, 272–3; drop-out rate, 273; in family therapy, 191, 272; in group therapy, 257, 272, 273; hospitalization, 279; individual therapy, 272, 274; informed consent, 262–3; involvement with parents counselling, 242; paradoxical techniques, 278; subphases, 262–3; termination of treatment, 37, 279–80; therapeutic alliance, 275–7; transference, 277. *See also* child psychotherapy

Adult Attachment Interview, 88

adult trauma, 428

advice (clinical intervention), 51–2, 237–8

affirmation (clinical intervention), 51

agoraphobia, 148, 149–50, 189, 298

alcoholism and alcohol abuse. *See* substance abuse

American Association of Directors of Psychiatric Residency Training (AADPRT), 71, 350–1, 374

American Group Psychotherapy Association (AGPA), 199–200, 219–20, 222, 223, 366

American Psychiatric Association (APA), 17, 27–9, 55, 378; *Manual of Psychiatric Peer Review*, 55, 56–7, 58–9, 85; *Treatments of Psychiatric Disorders*, 86

American Psychoanalytic Association, 55

analysibility, 56–7, 115

analytic process, 114–15

anonymity, 96–7

anorexia nervosa, 148, 191, 251

antisocial personality disorder, 407